Enhancing Medical Education Using AI

The use of artificial intelligence (AI) in medicine can deliver significant improvements in the delivery of healthcare. As clinicians learn more about the technology and grow alongside it, so too will new methods of using and analyzing clinical data emerge. Medical education encompasses many levels: medical school, internship, residency, fellowship, and continuing medical education. At each of these levels, AI does, and will, revolutionize the way that healthcare providers learn, teach, and share information. This book is the first of its kind to explore the potential ways in which AI may specifically transform medical education across the globe.

Key Features:

- Discusses a timely, relevant, hot topic in medical schools and beyond
- Focuses on AI in medical education that is relevant to trainees and practicing clinicians across all specialties
- Proves useful for physicians working on continuing medical education activities

AI in Clinical Practice

The Impact of Artificial Intelligence in Radiology
Adam Eltorai, Ian Pan and Henry H Guo

AI and Precision Medicine in Infectious Disease Management
Jen-Tsung Chen

Mastering the Art of Facial Soft Tissue Fillers with Artificial Intelligence: The scientific way to avoid a leap in the dark with hyaluronic acid and AI predictions
Luigi Cursio, Ciro Cursio and Giuila Cursio

Enhancing Medical Education Using AI
Jason E. Liebowitz, Marcy B. Bolster and Philip Seo

For more information about the series, please visit https://www.routledge.com/AI-in-Clinical-Practice/book-series/AICLINICAL

Enhancing Medical Education Using AI

Edited by
Jason E. Liebowitz,
Marcy B. Bolster and Philip Seo

CRC Press
Taylor & Francis Group
Boca Raton London New York

CRC Press is an imprint of the
Taylor & Francis Group, an **informa** business

Designed cover image: Shutterstock image ID: 2458781471

First edition published 2027
by CRC Press
2385 NW Executive Center Drive, Suite 320, Boca Raton FL 33431

and by CRC Press
4 Park Square, Milton Park, Abingdon, Oxon, OX14 4RN

CRC Press is an imprint of Taylor & Francis Group, LLC

ISBN: 978-1-041-01969-5 (hbk)
ISBN: 978-1-041-03304-2 (pbk)
ISBN: 978-1-003-61716-7 (ebk)

DOI: 10.1201/9781003617167

Typeset in Palatino
by Apex CoVantage, LLC

Jason Liebowitz

To my sons Zev and Ori—may you always have a thirst for knowledge, a passion for helping other people, and the inspiration to make the world a better place.

Marcy B. Bolster

I am dedicating this book to my husband, John DiMuzio, who has tremendous vision for the role of technology. John is my partner. He teaches me, and he inspires me. He is always by my side, and for this, I am most grateful.

Philip Seo

I am dedicating this book to my parents, Kyung Hwa Seo, MD, and Hae Ja Yoon, MD. All that I have become, I owe to them.

Contents

Foreword

We're beginning to see the potential for AI to transform the practice of medicine. That includes improved accuracy of interpreting all types of medical scans, like CT, X-ray, ultrasound, and MRI, and images, such as electrocardiogram, pathology slides, and skin. There's increasing use of ambient AI to capture a clinic visit conversation and extrapolate that for the electronic medical record note, along with performing several downstream functions like ordering lab tests, repeat appointments, coding, billing, prescriptions, and insurance prior authorizations. This capability is already reducing the data clerk work of clinicians and giving them the gift of time. Surprisingly, there's mounting evidence that large language models can foster empathy not because they know what empathy is but because they can channel vast sources of human language. Patients are more apt to use chatbots and generative AI to answer their questions, input their lab data, get a second or third opinion, help with making a diagnosis, or prepare for a clinic visit. Given the limitations of access, long wait times, and expense, such an increase in autonomy is welcomed by many. On top of all these encouraging trends, there is the enhanced ability with multimodal AI to predict diseases at the individual level decades ahead, which will propel primary prevention. That's a long-standing dream in medicine that is largely unfulfilled to date.

With all this promise, many concerns detract from an AI-transformation being simple, fast, and free of hazard. There's considerable bias embedded in the inputs to AI models, mirroring those deep-seated in our culture. There are multiple uncertainties of privacy and security of our data, fairness, worsening inequities, hallucinations and errors, appropriate regulatory oversight, and reimbursement. Even after health systems implement AI models, there can be glitches or even adversarial attacks, with potential for harm at scale, warranting continuous surveillance. Added to all of this is lack of transparency of models and medical research results, few compelling studies in the real world of medicine, and, as a result, a lack of trust by the medical community. No less, there is the possibility that clinicians' reliance on AI could promote de-skilling, never-skilling, and reduced clinical reasoning.

The balance of the promise and liabilities is of considerable interest. That's why this new book, *AI in Clinical Practice: Enhancing Medical Education,* edited by Drs. Bolster, Liebowitz, and Seo, fulfills a major unmet need. It systematically addresses many specialties and goes deep into matters pertaining to education, career development, professionalism, and training. The hybridization of human–AI combined efforts to yield optimal performance for diagnosis, management, and communication has yet to be established and may differ for the varied functions and experience of clinicians. Key chapters on clinical reasoning and feedback help to emphasize the obligatory human-in-the-loop concept and, unexpectedly, what may become a norm someday—AI feedback to clinicians to be more empathetic and better communicators.

It is still early in the transition of adopting AI, and there is considerable worry by the public that this will dehumanize medicine, which already has suffered much erosion of the patient–doctor relationship over past decades. Likewise, many clinicians feel threatened by AI, losing control and their valued input, and even, in some cases, their jobs. This trepidation is counterbalanced by the leaders of AI who have all proclaimed healthcare as the singular sweet spot for AI to do good and that the medical community should embrace AI. But we're not there yet. So many pieces need to fall into place. *AI in Clinical Practice* provides a strong foundation for us to build upon in the years ahead.

Eric J. Topol, MD
Professor and EVP, Scripps Research
La Jolla, California

Preface

In October 2025, *The New England Journal of Medicine* published a special article in the "Case Records of the Massachusetts General Hospital" section that was unlike any that had come before it. The "Case Records" section has been in continuous publication since 1923, when it was initially developed under the leadership of Dr. Richard Cabot. A pioneering clinician and educator at the hospital, Cabot believed deeply that trainees needed to recognize clinicopathologic (CPC) correlations in order to develop their skills in diagnostic reasoning. Over the past century, his brainchild has become one of the most enduring and influential CPC series in medical literature.

Against this historic backdrop, the 2025 article stood apart. For the first time, it featured not one but two discussants. The first was Dr. Gurpreet Dhaliwal, Professor of Medicine at the University of California San Francisco School of Medicine and one of the most renowned medical educators in the country. His discussion video and slide deck, made available on the *Journal*'s website, were characteristically masterful, walking viewers through the salient points of the case and arriving at the correct diagnosis with clarity and precision.

The second discussant, however, signaled something entirely new. Dr. CaBot—no relation to Richard Cabot—is an AI system designed to serve as a medical education tool. According to Dr. Arjun Manrai, one of the Harvard Medical School researchers involved in its development, the team wanted to create an AI system that could generate a differential diagnosis and explain its reasoning at the level of an expert diagnostician. The narrated video from Dr. CaBot, also posted online, is a marvel to behold. With a remarkably human-sounding voice, the AI system lays out its step-by-step consideration of the patient's story, generates and refines its differential diagnosis, and elegantly arrives at the correct conclusion—much like Dr. Dhaliwal himself.

Taken together, the two presentations leave viewers contemplating not whether AI will change medical education but rather how it will do so—and how profoundly.

Indeed, over the past several years, the wide availability and user-friendliness of large language models such as ChatGPT, Gemini, Claude, and OpenEvidence have already begun reshaping the educational landscape. Medical students, residents, and subspecialty fellows are rapidly incorporating AI into both their learning and their clinical work. Medical educators similarly strive to keep pace, and many (such as those featured as authors in this book) have done exactly that. While it is true that teachers can, should, and do learn from their students, there must also be a deliberate and coordinated effort within the medical education community to establish thoughtful, evidence-based best practices for AI integration in undergraduate and postgraduate training.

It is precisely this need that inspired the creation of *Enhancing Medical Education Using AI*. We have sought to bring together some of the most thoughtful voices in medicine and medical education to explore the practical and philosophical implications of AI. This book is intended to serve as a landmark reference for understanding the pragmatic applications of AI to medical education, clinical training, and lifelong learning. From the role of AI in educating trainees across specialties, to its impact on teaching empathy, professionalism, ethics, and bedside skills, to the ways in which emerging technologies may reshape curriculum design and recruitment—these topics represent only a portion of the rich and nuanced discussions contained within these pages.

As editors of this volume—and as medical educators ourselves—we have learned a great deal from the expert authors who have contributed to this work. We trust that you, the reader, will likewise gain insight, clarity, and perhaps even inspiration. This book is not intended to be the final word on AI in medical education. Rather, it is a starting point—a foundation upon which future scholarship, innovation, and reflection can build.

Medicine's journey with AI is only beginning. For clinician-educators who have taught for decades before these technologies became widely available, the path forward may at times feel daunting. Yet progress rarely comes all at once. As the ancient Chinese philosopher Lao Tzu reminds us, "A journey of a thousand miles begins with a single step." We hope that this book represents one such step—for educators, trainees, and the profession as a whole.

Editor Biographies

Jason E. Liebowitz, MD, is Assistant Professor of Medicine at Columbia University Vagelos College of Physicians and Surgeons. His research and writings have been published in *The New England Journal of Medicine*, *JAMA*, *JAMA Internal Medicine*, *Arthritis Care and Research*, and *The Journal of Graduate Medical Education.* He is a coeditor of the textbook *Clinical Innovation in Rheumatology: Past, Present, and Future* and a coeditor of the textbook series Interdisciplinary Rheumatology. He has a strong interest in medical education and serves as the codirector of the Rheumatology and Clinical Immunology medical student course at Columbia University.

Marcy B. Bolster, MD, is a rheumatologist and Director of the Rheumatology Fellowship Training Program at the Massachusetts General Hospital, Boston, Massachusetts. She is Professor of Medicine at Harvard Medical School. She has a strong interest in medical education across the spectrum of learners, and she has helped train more than 70 rheumatology fellows. Her commitment to medical education focuses on curriculum design, assessment, mentorship, and professionalism. She is the recipient of the 2019 American College of Rheumatology Distinguished Program Director Award, the 2019 Partners (now Mass General Brigham) Outstanding Program Director Award, and the 2021 Arthritis Foundation Marian Ropes Lifetime Achievement Award.

Philip Seo, MD, MHS, is Associate Professor of Medicine at Johns Hopkins University and the Rheumatology Physician Editor for *UpToDate.* He was Director of the Johns Hopkins Vasculitis Center and Director of the Johns Hopkins Rheumatology Fellowship Training Program for 11 years and recently completed his tenure as Physician Editor for *The Rheumatologist*, a publication of the American College of Rheumatology. In 2021, he received the American College of Rheumatology's Distinguished Clinician Scholar Award, which is bestowed annually to a rheumatologist who makes outstanding contributions in clinical medicine, clinical scholarship, or education.

Contributors

Peter Brodeur, MD, MA
Cardiology Fellow
Harvard Medical School
Beth Israel Deaconess Medical Center
Boston, Massachusetts, USA

Jeffrey R. Curtis, MD, MS, MPH
Professor of Medicine, Epidemiology, and Computer Science
Division of Clinical Immunology & Rheumatology
University of Alabama at Birmingham
Birmingham, Alabama, USA

Michael R. De La Rosa, MD, MSAI
Resident Physician, Department of Neurology
University of Minnesota
Minneapolis, Minnesota, USA

Brian T. Garibaldi, MD, MEHP
Director, Center for Bedside Medicine
Charles Horace Mayo Professor of Medicine
Northwestern University Feinberg School of Medicine
Chicago, Illinois, USA

Steven N. Hart, PhD, ACHIP™
Associate Professor of Biomedical Informatics
Division of Computational Pathology and Informatics
Department of Laboratory Medicine and Pathology
Mayo College of Medicine
Mayo Clinic
Rochester, Minnesota, USA

Wenchao Han, PhD
Assistant Professor of Laboratory Medicine and Pathology
Division of Computational Pathology and Informatics
Department of Laboratory Medicine and Pathology
Mayo College of Medicine
Mayo Clinic
Rochester, Minnesota, USA

Yeji Han, BS
Medical Student
CHA University
Pocheon, Republic of Korea

O. Joe Hines, MD, FACS
Chair, Department of Surgery
David Geffen School of Medicine at UCLA
Los Angeles, California, USA

Poonam Hosamani, MD
Associate Professor, Department of Medicine
Stanford University School of Medicine
Stanford, California, USA

Shalmali Joshi, PhD
Assistant Professor of Biomedical Informatics
Columbia University Vagelos College of Physicians and Surgeons
New York, New York, USA

Ashley Kingon, MS
Associate Director of CUIMC Programs & Service
Columbia University, Center for Teaching & Learning
New York, New York
USA

Nan Liu, PhD
Associate Professor, Centre for Biomedical Data Science
Director, Duke–NUS AI + Medical Sciences Initiative
Duke–NUS Medical School
Singapore, Singapore

Christopher A. Mao, MD, MSAI, MSE
Resident Physician, Department of Internal Medicine
UT Health San Antonio
San Antonio, Texas
USA

Yilin Ning, PhD
Senior Research Fellow, Centre for Biomedical Data Science
Duke–NUS Medical School
Singapore, Singapore

Jasmine Chiat Ling Ong, PharmD
Division of Pharmacy, Singapore General Hospital, Singapore
Duke-NUS Medical School, National University of Singapore, Singapore

John D. Osborne, PhD
Associate Professor
Department of Biomedical Informatics and Data Science
University of Alabama at Birmingham
Birmingham, Alabama, USA

Jordan D. Perchik, MD
Assistant Professor, Department of Diagnostic Radiology
University of Alabama at Birmingham
Birmingham, Alabama, USA

Courtney Reamer, MD
Instructor of Medicine
Center for Bedside Medicine
Northwestern University Feinberg School of Medicine
Chicago, Illinois, USA

Lauren R. Richter, MD
Assistant Professor of Biomedical Informatics & Pediatrics at CUMC
Columbia University Vagelos College of Physicians & Surgeons
New York, New York, USA

Adam Rodman, MD, MPH
Assistant Professor, Harvard Medical School
Director of AI Programs, Carl J Shapiro Institute for Research and Education
Beth Israel Deaconess Medical Center
Boston, Massachusetts, USA

Ronald Rodriguez, MD, PhD
Professor, Medical Education & Urology
UT Health San Antonio
San Antonio, Texas, USA

Arlene Ruiz de Luzuriaga, MD, MPH, MBA
Associate Professor, Section of Dermatology, Department of Medicine
University of Chicago
Chicago, Illinois, USA

Neria Sebastien, MST, EdD
Director of CUIMC Faculty Programs & Service
Center for Teaching & Learning
Columbia University
New York, New York, USA

Bryce Thornton, BS
DMD Student
School of Dentistry
University of Alabama at Birmingham
Birmingham, Alabama, USA

Eric J. Topol, MD
Professor and EVP, Scripps Research
La Jolla, California, USA

Justin P. Wagner, MD, FACS, FAAP
Associate Professor, Department of Surgery
David Geffen School of Medicine at UCLA
Los Angeles, California, USA

Judy J. Wang, MD
Internal Medicine Resident
Department of Medicine
Weill Cornell Medicine
New York, New York, USA

Grace Wei, MD, MPH, MSc
Resident Physician, Section of Dermatology, Department of Medicine
University of Chicago
Chicago, Illinois, USA

Pinar Yilmaz, MD, MSc
Radiology Resident and PhD Candidate
Departments of Radiology & Nuclear Medicine and Epidemiology
Erasmus Medical Center
Rotterdam, the Netherlands

1 What Is Artificial Intelligence?

Shalmali Joshi, Judy J. Wang, Lauren R. Richter

1.1 INTRODUCTION

From molecules to global health, our understanding of medicine, physiology, and disease has changed, though the underlying natural laws of the universe remain constant. Just as the microscope changed the resolution at which we see tissue to reveal cells, organelles, and even matter itself, so too does artificial intelligence (AI) provide the opportunity to further examine and reveal the world around us. Like prior innovations in medicine, AI can change how we perceive and interact with our patients and alter the circumstances in which they present. Unlike prior innovations, AI can analyze, interpret, and even discover– it not only extends human ability but surpasses it. As society enters this new age of AI, we must continue to train physicians on how to turn data into knowledge and knowledge into wisdom, all while staying grounded in critical reasoning and scientific inquiry.

In the context of medical education, we must not only focus on how to educate *about* AI but also *with* AI. AI creates opportunities for learning that previously required tremendous human effort to produce. Now systems are capable of retrieving (and identifying) relevant information, recognizing patterns, generating educational content, simulating clinical scenarios [1–3], and providing meaningful feedback, all at scale. When information gathering and basic interpretation are increasingly automated, how does the physician educator cultivate critical thinking? AI raises a lens to physician training and forces reexamination of which skills are essential to professional competency. How medicine and medical education embrace these new technologies will shape generations of physicians to come.

Integration of artificial intelligence and machine learning (ML) in healthcare has been driven to improve patient outcomes, discover knowledge, and increase efficiency, all with the goal of augmenting clinical practice by increasing the abilities of the human physician. At a broader societal level, AI is integral to the vision of learning health systems,[1] in which data from routine care are continuously analyzed to improve diagnosis, treatment, and prevention. Evolving from the physician's role of information retrieval and sense making, AI/ML has shifted from tools rooted in expert knowledge and logic that is understandable to humans to deep, inexplicable connective networks relying on complex mathematics to predict, categorize, or generate information without explicit instruction on how to do so. Just as physicians may not be able to articulate all of the factors that lead them to particular decisions, so too does AI/ML introduce an opaque, complex decision-making process to medical practice. From a methodological standpoint, the relevance, potential, and impact of AI to healthcare must be understood in terms of fundamental statistical challenges intrinsic to medical data, how AI models consume them to generate insights and how these outputs may be used at point-of-care, that is, human–AI interaction. Without deliberate design and oversight, AI systems risk reinforcing disparities in access, treatment, and outcomes that already hinder healthcare delivery.

Medical educators play a critical role in preparing clinicians to operate effectively in AI-augmented healthcare environments. Traditional medical learning and evidence-based medicine prioritize knowledge acquisition, empirical

DOI: 10.1201/9781003617167-1

reasoning, and context awareness to reduce uncertainty. The fundamental principle of human learning—that, given the same input, a system will produce the same output—is not necessarily true with AI/ML. Machine learning systems are inherently probabilistic without inherent contextual awareness or sensing abilities. The same question may yield different answers despite the underlying information remaining unchanged. Educational curricula must therefore evolve to include foundational concepts in data science and machine learning alongside training in ethical oversight and human–AI collaboration.

The rise of artificial intelligence in healthcare reflects both technological maturation and structural transformation in how health data are generated, interpreted, and used. For clinicians, AI introduces new modes of decision support that require statistical understanding, critical judgment, and ethical responsibility. For medical educators, it demands curricular reform that integrates AI and data literacy with clinical reasoning and patient-centered care. As emphasized throughout this text, realizing the benefits of AI in healthcare depends not only on algorithmic innovation but on deep engagement with data quality, bias, validation, and human–machine collaboration.

1.2 ARTIFICIAL INTELLIGENCE EXPLAINED

AI/ML has benefited from unprecedented progress in the past 20–25 years. Among other factors, massive digitized data availability from the proliferation of the internet and advances in computing infrastructure enabled scaling and innovations in data-driven ML architectures. Subsequent innovations in deep learning led to the now seemingly endless AI potential in the form of large language models (ChatGPT,[2] Gemini [4], Claude[3]). Simultaneously, the digitization and democratization of healthcare data both within and outside the electronic health record (EHR), combined with advances in molecular biology, chemistry, and engineering, have resulted in a paradigm shift in healthcare and the practice of medicine. For physicians and medical educators, the rise of AI necessitates a shift in how clinical knowledge is generated, evaluated, and operationalized in practice. Recent advances have completely changed the paradigms of use, but AI in medicine has existed for decades.

The historical evolution of AI in healthcare contextualizes current developments. Early systems such as MYCIN [5], INTERNIST-I [5, 6], and CASNET[4] relied on rules and expert knowledge to support diagnosis and treatment selection, similar to clinical algorithms and protocols still seen in practice today. These so-called symbolic AI systems, built using predefined logic and discrete data elements (such as diagnosis codes or lab results), achieve narrow success with relatively low cost, but suffer from scalability and maintenance limitations. Subsequent eras introduced probabilistic reasoning, neural networks, and, more recently, deep learning and foundation models. More specifically, newer models rely more heavily on data-driven patterns and much less on expert knowledge, employing large connectionist modeling architectures, popularly known as deep learning, to capture complex representations of the data. While contemporary systems demonstrate improved pattern recognition and adaptability, they also introduce new challenges related to interpretability, generalization, and feedback loops between algorithmic recommendations and clinical behavior.

Though many definitions exist, in its simplest form, AI is a computer-based system that can perform tasks thought to require, or sometimes even exceed, human ability to learn and solve problems. ML describes a subset of AI that uses algorithms to identify patterns within data to improve performance without explicit programming to identify these patterns.

All AI models share common elements: a data source, a task, and a method to achieve the task. Though the details will vary depending on the type of approach used, it is helpful to consider these three elements whenever appraising an AI tool and its fitness for use in a particular scenario. Fundamentally, these models excel at capturing complex associations between such high-dimensional, multimodal inputs to generate insights. Analogous to a physician assessing whether a clinical practice guideline applies to their particular patient at a particular time, one should assess whether an AI tool is appropriate to use and what limitations the model has when generalizing to populations outside of its training.

Health data now includes elements from EHRs—structured and unstructured elements like measurements, diagnosis codes, imaging, laboratory results, genomics, and free-text clinical notes—and, increasingly, data generated outside traditional healthcare systems, such as mobile health applications, wearable sensors, and social media. The digitization of EHRs and the proliferation of consumer health technologies have dramatically expanded the scope and temporal resolution of available data. In the United States, the introduction of the HITECH Act in 2009 and the 21st Century Cures Act in 2016 led to near-ubiquitous use of certified EHRs in both acute and ambulatory settings to maintain health records.[5] As of 2024, 3.6 billion downloads of health and wellness apps were recorded across the world.[6] Modern ML approaches benefit tremendously from the scale of such data. However, having more information does not guarantee knowledge or understanding, particularly in health contexts where data are observational, incomplete, and shaped by complex social and clinical processes. Health datasets are affected by multiple forms of statistical bias, including selection bias, confounding biases, measurement bias, and our current understanding of a particular condition. These statistical issues impact the robustness of AI outputs, their ability to generalize across contexts, and patient subtypes. Therefore, when using AI/ML approaches to address healthcare tasks or using them as a mechanism for education and training, one must adopt such technologies *cautiously/critically*.

There are several ways to categorize modern AI and ML subfields or methods, just as there are many ways to define medical subspecialties. In this chapter, we will discuss the AI/ML subfields of supervised learning, unsupervised learning, reinforcement learning, and generative AI to provide a basic construct around which readers can build their understanding of these systems.

Supervised learning is a foundational paradigm in machine learning in which models are trained using paired inputs and labels to enable an algorithm to learn patterns and accurately classify new, unseen data. An example is a model that correctly identifies pneumonia in a new patient's chest radiograph after learning from a collection of X-rays annotated with potential pulmonary and respiratory conditions [7]. Supervised learning methods can also be used for prediction, outputting a probability or likelihood of an event occurring. Many modern deep neural networks used in medical imaging and clinical risk prediction fall into this category. The Framingham Risk Score, which stratifies patients into low-, medium-, or high-risk groups for cardiovascular disease based on predefined rules, is an example of a curated learned algorithm. In other domains, similar approaches could be applied to predict disease progression, such as identifying asthma subtypes [8] or identifying new disease states to capture variability in multiple sclerosis [9].

In contrast, unsupervised learning—often referred to as clustering or latent variable modeling—aims to uncover structure in data without relying on labeled outcomes. The resulting clusters can then be interpreted by domain experts to infer potential clinical or biological meaning. An example would be flow and mass cytometry analysis methods that do not rely on predefined features or protein markers to differentiate cell types [10]. While unsupervised methods may help identify disease subtypes or novel phenotypes, their findings must be interpreted cautiously as information is transformed into representations that are not necessarily understandable by humans.

Reinforcement learning (RL) represents another major class of machine learning methods, distinguished by its focus on sequential decision-making aimed at optimizing long-term outcomes. In healthcare, an illustrative example is the management of critically ill patients at risk for sepsis in the intensive care unit. Reinforcement learning frameworks could, in principle, learn optimal sequences of interventions—such as the timing and dosing of vasopressors or mechanical ventilation—to maximize the likelihood of survival and successful ICU discharge. Breakthroughs in games such as Go and chess (such as AlphaGo [11] and AlphaZero [11, 12]) highlight the power of these approaches. However, reinforcement learning typically requires large amounts of training data that capture the consequences of diverse actions, often generated through real-world interaction. In healthcare, such experimentation raises significant ethical and safety concerns. As a result, reinforcement learning in clinical settings generally relies on offline learning from observational data, modeling decisions already made by clinicians. Consequently, learned strategies often resemble existing practice patterns, and improvements may be incremental. Nonetheless, RL remains a promising avenue for applications where limited and well-controlled automation is appropriate.

More recent advances in artificial intelligence, including large language models (LLMs) and text-to-image generation systems such as OpenAI's DALL-E[7] and Google's Nano Banana,[8] represent a class of techniques collectively referred to as generative AI. These models are capable of generating new and plausible content by incorporating contrastive learning components to capture complex associations among high-dimensional data. The fundamental paradigm shift is attributable to scalable training using a process known as pretraining—training models on large datasets to solve simple tasks without the need for curated labels (next-word prediction in LLMs or image-generation). These pretrained models are then 'fine-tuned' for task-specific performance enhancement, such as note summarization. The underlying pretrained model is known as a foundation model [13].

LLMs such as OpenAI's GPT are trained on large corpora of web-scale text data to predict the next word or sequence of words, thereby modeling the structure of human language. Similarly, text-to-image systems learn from paired images and textual descriptions to align visual and linguistic concepts, enabling image generation from textual prompts. For example, vision-language models (VLMs) use images and text [14], and techniques known as probabilistic diffusion allow for direct image distribution sampling to create new images [15]. More recently, such generative AI models increasingly consume multiple modalities at a time. Reinforcement learning has been the key ingredient in enhancing the 'reasoning' capabilities of LLMs [16]. In effect, the ability of LLMs to break down a complex question into intermediate reasoning steps emerged as a property of LLMs when trained with 'verifiable' rewards using reinforcement learning. When combined with the ability to act in the world and observe the outcome, LLMs demonstrate the incredible potential of today's coding agents[9] and their ability to solve complex mathematical reasoning problems.[10]

The emergence of generative AI has created new opportunities to enhance clinical workflows. LLMs show promise in applications such as automated transcription of patient–clinician conversations, summarization of clinical documentation, and generating responses to patient messages.[11] For example, when a patient transitions care or is discharged, an LLM could review longitudinal clinical records and generate a concise yet comprehensive summary for the new provider. Likewise, during prolonged and complex hospitalizations, LLMs could synthesize laboratory results, imaging findings, and clinical events into a structured discharge summary, reducing the documentation burden on overextended clinicians. These tools have the potential to save time, improve efficiency, and reduce errors associated with manual information transfer. Analogous advances have taken place in our ability to generate synthetic medical imaging data [17] or train multimodal medical imaging foundation models that enable multimodal capabilities, such as generating radiology reports from radiographic inputs, including incorporating modern reasoning elements of LLMs [18, 19].

For clinicians, AI systems primarily function as components of decision-support pipelines rather than autonomous decision-makers. When used to augment clinical decisions, ML models generate probabilistic risk estimates, predictions of disease progression, or ranked treatment recommendations, all of which require careful interpretation. These applications are still in the minority of the types of AI/ML tools that are currently deployed beyond those leveraging medical imaging. As of November 2025, 950 AI/ML devices were authorized by the FDA, of which 723 were radiology devices (76%).[12] ML supports phenotyping (clustering or categorizing patients along specific aspects), risk prediction, treatment effect estimation, and operational optimization, but its deployment must be governed by principles of equity, transparency, and accountability. When discussing such tools, medical educators must communicate that AI/ML models trained on healthcare data are effectively learning from observational data and continue to emphasize the distinction between correlation and causation. Clinicians must understand the conditions under which the model is trained, evaluated, and when its outputs are valid, as well as the clinical contexts in which algorithmic recommendations may fail. Importantly, responsibility for clinical decisions remains with physicians, making algorithmic literacy a professional necessity rather than an optional technical skill.

Despite AI's promise, significant challenges remain. Supervised learning models often perform best on data resembling their training sets and may fail to generalize to new patient populations, institutions, or time periods. Rare diseases are particularly vulnerable to misclassification due to limited representation in training data. Inter-rater variability among clinicians makes it challenging to incorporate robust supervision that augments capabilities over mimicking such variability. Nonetheless, careful design of tasks can enable AI to be used to improve the standard of care, such as designing a new classification of skin tones over the traditional Fitzpatrick classification [20]. Thoughtful, forward-thinking design incorporating reproducibility, interoperability, and generalizability is essential for continued success.

Overall, such a lack of generalizability can be attributed to the broad notion of 'distribution shifts' [21]. Changes in data acquisition practices, software systems, or patient demographics can lead to distribution shifts in the underlying data that degrade model performance. Moreover, if training data reflect existing biases in healthcare delivery or outcomes, machine learning models may replicate or amplify these biases. Although large generative models are trained on diverse data sources, they face additional concerns, including hallucinated outputs, privacy and copyright risks, and the persistence of subtle biases or spurious correlations. While recent advances have addressed some of these issues, further work is needed to ensure robust real-world performance.

Finally, strong retrospective performance metrics such as area under the receiver operating curve (AUROC), area under the precision-recall curve (AUPRC), or positive predictive value (PPV) do not guarantee clinical benefit. Models must be designed with clinical workflows in mind, and their impact should be evaluated in the populations and settings in which they will be used. This requires prospective validation, including silent trials [22] and randomized controlled studies, to assess how model outputs influence clinician behavior and how those changes affect patient outcomes. Regulatory and publication standards increasingly emphasize such external validation, particularly for systems with greater autonomy [22–27]. Given evolving patient populations, clinical practices, and medical knowledge, continuous monitoring and periodic retraining are essential to maintain model performance and ensure safe, equitable, and effective deployment over time.

1.3 HOW AI WORKS: Basic Concepts and Examples

1.3.1 Examples through Case Vignettes

1.3.1.1 Detecting Lesions on Radiographs

A 52-year-old woman undergoes routine mammogram screening. After completion of her scan, her images go through an AI model, which performs an initial read and highlights a small area of architectural distortion. The radiologist then reviews this flagged region and agrees that it has a high probability of malignancy. The radiologist proceeds to generate a report that recommends additional imaging with biopsy.

Behind the scenes: This AI model, before implementation, already went through a training phase where thousands of mammograms with radiologist-labeled areas of concern were fed into a convolutional neural network (CNN). This model uses all these data points to adjust its internal parameters to recognize imaging patterns associated with these labeled areas and minimize classification errors. Then, when presented with a new image, this model can use its internal parameters to output: (1) a heatmap highlighting regions contributing to the prediction, (2) the probability of a finding (for example, "malignancy probability: 82%").

Clinical significance: These systems support radiologists by flagging suspicious regions, prioritizing studies, or serving as a second reader. This example highlights how AI can learn hierarchical visual features without explicit programming, enabling automated pattern recognition in imaging.

1.3.1.2 Estimating Sepsis Risk from the EHR

A 67-year-old man is admitted with pneumonia. Over several hours, his respiratory rate increases, his blood pressure drifts downward, and his lactate rises. An AI-based early warning system calculates a rising sepsis risk score and triggers an alert to the care team.

Behind the scenes: Time-series variables, such as respiratory rate, mean arterial pressure, and lactate, are each treated as a feature. During training, the model assigns a mathematical weight to each feature based on how frequently it correlates with a "sepsis" diagnosis. For example, a high RR is concerning, but a high RR combined with low BP is much more predictive of septic shock, and weights are assigned accordingly. For a new patient who arrives in the ED and waits several hours with many vital points and lab results, the model can then use temporal trends to output a risk score (for example, "sepsis risk in next 6 hours: 0.67").

Clinical significance: Predicted scores may trigger alerts, prompt earlier clinician review, and support triage decisions. This example highlights how AI can identify multivariable patterns in structured clinical data to estimate risk and support early intervention.

1.3.1.3 Answering Medical Knowledge Questions for Clinicians and Learners

A medical student studying for an exam asks a chatbot, "How do you differentiate Crohn's disease from ulcerative colitis?" The system generates a structured comparison, citing key clinical and pathological differences.

Behind the scenes: Large language models (LLMs) are trained on publicly available biomedical literature, clinical guidelines, and other texts to learn statistical relationships between words and concepts. For example, when a user asks a question—such as "What are the causes of hypercalcemia?"—the model analyzes the entire prompt, identifies the most relevant concepts, and then selects the most likely next word, adds it to the sentence, and repeats this process until the response is complete. The result is coherent, context-aware text that emerges from repeated next-word predictions rather than from the retrieval of prewritten answers.

Clinical significance: Applications include patient education, medical student learning, and drafting clinical documentation automatically. This example highlights how AI can perform language understanding and generation, which enables knowledge retrieval and conversational interfaces.

1.4 AI IN MEDICINE/HEALTHCARE

AI has the potential to make a multitude of positive impacts on the healthcare system, from reducing medical errors to offloading administrative tasks to discovering knowledge. In cancer research, proofs of concept were demonstrated to personalize treatment, improve clinical trial efficiency, and accelerate drug development [28]. Over the last decade, the FDA has been reviewing and authorizing a growing number of AI/ML-Enabled Medical Devices [29]. Much of this attention has been applicable to the fields of radiology and pathology due to the accessibility of imaging data modalities. However, adoption of such technology into the clinical setting has been slow relative to its continued interest and investment. Only a fraction of the approved models have been integrated into the clinical setting, such as using computer-aided diagnostics (CAD) to enhance breast cancer detection and the automating screening of pap smears [30–32]. More recently, there has been an explosion of interest in newer AI methods, such as generative AI and multimodal models. Unlike traditional AI methods that rely on manual feature extraction, models based on deep learning are able to address more complex problems in medical diagnostics because of their strength in image analysis and pattern recognition.

1.4.1 Radiology

Historically relying on trained physicians to visually analyze and assess medical images, radiology has undergone significant progress with the integration of AI-assisted image recognition tasks. Common radiology tasks include abnormality detection, characterization of image findings, and monitoring of imaging changes over time. With the original FDA approval of CAD in mammography in 1998, there have been over 720 FDA-approved AI-assisted devices in radiology as of late 2025, by far the most of any medical specialty. A portion of these devices is used for cancer screening and diagnostics, of which breast, lung, and prostate cancers are the most common. Although AI algorithms have conventionally been used for mammography reading, recent developments are exploring the supplementation of ultrasound and MRI information to improve screening performance [33, 34]. In lung cancer detection, deep learning systems now use 3D CT data that incorporates more diagnostic information, such as surrounding vasculature not part of the main tumor, to perform early detection of malignancy [35, 36]. Such systems are also working on optimizing the detection of tumors 1–3 mm in size that can be easily missed by the human eye (and which are several magnitudes smaller than can be identified by the detection algorithms currently on the market). Developing AI devices is also no longer simply taking the form of detection software. For example, the Virtual Nodule Clinic from Optellum, approved by the FDA in 2021, became the first AI-based decision support system that incorporates a clinically validated lung cancer prediction (LCP) biomarker score for evaluating cancer risk and arranging clinical follow-up [37].

With AI's particular adeptness in imaging analytics, other medical specialties that are seeing increased innovation include ophthalmology and gastroenterology. AI implementation in ophthalmology has been used to augment screening and diagnostics for pathologies including diabetic retinopathy, age-related macular degeneration, and glaucoma, mostly using optical coherence tomography (OCT) and fundus images [38]. More recently, an AI system was developed to identify and classify eyelid tumors with performance comparable to a senior ophthalmologist [39]. In gastroenterology, AI can now identify gastrointestinal bleeds, colorectal polyps, and premalignant lesions in real-time endoscopy with impressive accuracy [40]. Randomized controlled trials comparing the performance of endoscopy with and without AI assistance have shown a significantly higher rate of adenoma detection with the use of AI [41].

1.4.2 Pathology

Where AI applications in radiology have benefited greatly from the native digital nature of radiologic images, pathology has trailed behind. While modern pathology reports are digital, the images themselves are trapped on glass slides that are cumbersome to transport and store. Because of the subcellular resolution of these slides, expensive scanning technology is required for the digitization of pathology images, and only recently has digital pathology moved from a niche product of predominantly academic interest closer to the mainstream, with the FDA authorizing the first system for primary diagnosis via digital pathology in 2017.[13] Adoption rapidly accelerated due to the COVID-19 pandemic and the related relaxation of regulations around the use of digital pathology images for primary diagnosis [42, 43]. Today, large centers boast digital archives of hundreds of thousands to millions of images scanned at or near the resolution available via traditional microscopy.[14] These advances are slowly unlocking pathology image data for use in training and deploying AI models.

An additional bottleneck for AI in pathology is the nature of its image data. The deep learning algorithms that have been so successful in natural image classification are trained on images that are far smaller than scans of pathology slides at full resolution. In fact, fewer than 600 pathology slides contain more pixels than the entirety of ImageNet [44], the most popular natural image computer vision benchmarking dataset. With each slide being one or more gigabytes in size, computational pathology faces unique technical challenges in image processing.

1.4.3 Dermatology

In dermatology, artificial intelligence has been used to advance the classification of skin disease images. While prior works illustrated the use of convolutional neural networks (CNNs) to distinguish between malignant and benign skin lesions [45–47], similar algorithmic applications have extended to improvements in the diagnosis of inflammatory skin diseases and the assessment of diabetic ulcer specifications [48–50]. Both histopathological and clinical images are studied to achieve high sensitivities and diagnostic accuracies. Additional data sources, such as electronic medical records with population-based demographic frequencies and smartphone-based dermoscopic images, are being incorporated in the model training process [51]. In 2019, the American Academy of Dermatology (AAD) published a position commentary on the role of augmented intelligence (AuI) in offering an assistive rather than replacement role for clinicians in dermatology [52]. Recent research has focused on human–computer collaboration to improve image-based diagnostics. Tschandl et al. explored AI-based support in multiple scenarios in order to demonstrate the superior framework of AI-supported clinical decision making compared to either clinician or AI models alone.

In the United States, there are currently isolated FDA-approved AI-based devices in dermatology, such as MelaFind.[15] Several devices and smartphone applications are in the works. MelaFind, a non-invasive tool that uses light to evaluate melanomatous skin lesions up to 2.5 mm beneath the skin surface, was discontinued in 2017 despite achieving high sensitivity and ease of use [53–55]. Moleanalyzer-Pro, a CNN developed in 2018 with dermatologist-level performance on classifying skin lesions, was approved for European markets [56]. 3Derm is the first AI device to receive FDA Breakthrough Device designation in dermatology in 2020.[16] Unique challenges within the dermatology space, including the paucity of diverse skin tone data in publicly available datasets, have rendered fair and inclusive training of AI models and associated clinical translation difficult. Google's 2020 study, which became the backbone for its dermatology app released the following year, saw only 3.5% of its patient data exhibiting Fitzpatrick skin types V and VI, suggesting biased sampling that can impact model performance and clinical diagnostic value when applied across a broad patient population [57].

1.5 OTHER IMPLICATIONS OF AI: Ethical, Legal, Societal

ML systems in healthcare operate within a domain that is already governed by long-standing ethical principles articulated by professional bodies such as the American Medical Association (AMA) and the Canadian Medical Association (CMA). Core principles of beneficence, nonmaleficence, justice, and respect for persons must be operationalized through technical design and evaluation choices. Ethical ML for health, therefore, requires an end-to-end view of the modeling pipeline, recognizing that harms and inequities can be introduced at every stage, from problem formulation to deployment and monitoring [58, 59].

Bias in healthcare ML is rarely confined to a single technical choice; rather, it emerges cumulatively at each decision point across a system's life cycle. Data collection is a major source of distortion. Observational data, typically the main source used for AI training, reflect human decisions, including healthcare access and processes, meaning that administrative and utilization features may be more predictive than underlying physiology, but also more biased. Health insurance claims data introduce additional complexity. While often used as proxies for health outcomes or comorbidity burden, billing codes and costs are shaped more by reimbursement structures than by clinical complexity. Moreover, sensitive demographic attributes such as sexual orientation, gender identity, race, and ethnicity are often missing or inaccurately recorded, further complicating subgroup analysis and fairness assessment.

Modeling decisions compound these issues. Beyond data and labels, technical modeling decisions play a central role in shaping fairness outcomes. Surrogate losses (that is, hinge loss) can disproportionately penalize underrepresented subpopulations when class imbalance is severe. Feature selection practices, including the inclusion or exclusion of protected attributes, can either obscure or legitimize noncausal associations.

Labels in healthcare ML depend on disease prevalence, clinician judgment, access to diagnostic resources, and historical treatment patterns. Consequently, labels may encode systematic biases such as delayed diagnosis, underdiagnosis in marginalized populations, or differential thresholds for intervention. A common failure mode is the use of biased proxy labels. For example, healthcare expenditures have been used as surrogates for disease burden, resulting in inaccurate referrals to proactive care [60]. Similarly, mental health diagnoses may reflect access to care rather than underlying prevalence, and diagnostic delays can produce labels that systematically disadvantage certain populations. Information leakage—where future information inadvertently influences training labels—can further inflate apparent performance without improving clinical validity.

As with other forms of bias, challenges to fairness in machine learning for health arise not from isolated modeling choices but from the interaction of many choices. These decisions span cohort construction, data sources, label definitions, feature engineering, optimization objectives, and deployment context. Importantly, inequities observed in model outputs often reflect preexisting disparities embedded in healthcare systems rather than purely algorithmic failures. Algorithmic fairness has been formalized through multiple statistical criteria. Group fairness frameworks aim to equalize aspects of model performance across protected groups, including selection rates (demographic parity), predictive values (predictive parity), or error rates (equalized odds and equality of opportunity). Each definition encodes a different notion of fairness and entails trade-offs with predictive accuracy and with other fairness criteria.

Individual fairness, by contrast, requires that similar individuals receive similar predictions, though operationalizing similarity in high-dimensional clinical feature spaces remains challenging. Importantly, no single fairness definition is universally appropriate, and some are mutually incompatible.

Causal approaches, such as counterfactual fairness, extend beyond purely statistical parity by asking whether a model's prediction would change under a hypothetical intervention on a protected attribute. For example, would a salary or risk prediction differ if gender were changed while holding all non-descendant variables constant? While conceptually appealing, causal fairness approaches require strong assumptions about the underlying data-generating process and are often difficult to implement in complex clinical settings.

The broader field of algorithmic fairness imposes model-level constraints, or demographic-based corrections [61]. However, fairness constraints applied at the model level cannot fully compensate for biased or misaligned labels. Addressing fairness, therefore, requires scrutiny of what the model is trained to predict, not only how well it predicts. A prominent example is the historical use of demographics-based correction in clinical risk scores, such as vaginal birth after cesarean (VBAC) prediction models. Earlier VBAC algorithms explicitly incorporated race, assigning lower predicted success probabilities to Black and Hispanic women without evidence of a causal biological mechanism. Subsequent analyses demonstrated that systemic differences in care delivery and clinician behavior more plausibly explained these disparities. Newer VBAC models have removed race as an input, illustrating how fairness concerns can motivate substantive changes in model design rather than superficial post hoc adjustments [62]. Hyperparameter tuning and model selection can also introduce group-level overfitting, where performance is optimized for dominant populations at the expense of under-represented groups. These effects are often invisible when evaluation focuses exclusively on aggregate metrics.

Even models that satisfy fairness criteria during development may fail after deployment due to distribution shift. Changes in patient populations, imaging protocols, clinical workflows, or disease prevalence can degrade performance and alter subgroup disparities. Silent trials—where models are evaluated prospectively without influencing clinical decisions—provide a mechanism to detect such failures before deployment [22]. Case studies demonstrate that models with strong retrospective performance can exhibit near-random performance when deployed in new settings, revealing unanticipated correlations or shifts in input distributions. Iterative evaluation, hypothesis generation, and retraining are therefore essential components of safe and fair deployment. Studying human–AI decision-making and providing infrastructure for continual monitoring of AI algorithms is crucial for a successful and positive impact on patient and clinical outcomes.

Regulatory oversight plays an increasingly central role in shaping how ML systems for health are developed and deployed. In the United States, the Food and Drug Administration (FDA) regulates software intended for diagnosis, treatment, mitigation, or prevention of disease. Determining whether an ML system qualifies as a regulated medical device depends on its intended use, level of clinical decision support, and degree of reliance by healthcare professionals.

The FDA's evolving framework for good machine learning practices (GMLP) [63] emphasizes life cycle management rather than static approval. Key requirements include prespecified change management plans, data governance protocols, retraining procedures, performance monitoring, and cybersecurity safeguards. Post-development obligations encompass risk management, traceability from user needs to system requirements, verification and validation, usability testing, and ongoing audit processes [64]. Importantly, regulation increasingly recognizes that ML systems are not fixed artifacts but adaptive tools whose performance and fairness characteristics may change over time [65].

In summary, fairness, safety, and regulation in machine learning for health are inseparable from data quality, evaluation methodology, deployment context, and regulatory oversight. Fragility and unfairness arise from structural features of healthcare systems as well as technical design choices, and they cannot be resolved through algorithmic adjustments alone. Robust fairness assessment requires subgroup-aware evaluation, careful consideration of labels and proxies, and continuous monitoring after deployment. Regulatory frameworks such as FDA good machine learning practices provide essential guardrails, ensuring that performance, safety, and equity are maintained throughout the model life cycle rather than assumed at approval time.

1.5.1 Summary and Key Takeaways

In conclusion, the integration of artificial intelligence and machine learning into healthcare represents a fundamental shift in clinical practice and medical training. While these technologies offer immense potential to improve diagnostic accuracy, clinical efficiency, and patient outcomes, their successful implementation depends on much more than algorithmic innovation. It requires a deep commitment to data quality, algorithmic literacy, and ethical oversight to mitigate risks associated with bias, distribution shifts, and lack of transparency. As AI continues to evolve from static decision-support tools into adaptive, generative systems, medical educators must take a leading role in preparing a new generation of clinicians who can navigate the complexities of human–AI collaboration. Ultimately, the goal is to harness the power of AI to build more equitable and effective learning health systems while ensuring that the final responsibility for clinical decision-making remains firmly rooted in human judgment and patient-centered care.

GLOSSARY

Artificial intelligence (AI): Systems that can perform tasks that typically require a form of intelligence, such as perception, reasoning, learning, and decision-making.

Area under the receiver operating characteristic curve (AUROC): A performance metric for binary classification models that measures a model's ability to trade off false-positive (1-specificity) and true-positive (sensitivity) rates.

Area under the precision-recall curve (AUPRC): A metric for binary classification models that summarizes the trade-off between precision and recall across its score thresholds, especially useful for evaluating models on imbalanced datasets.

Convolutional neural network (CNN): A type of deep learning model designed to process grid-like data, such as images, by using filters to convolve or aggregate across parts of the image to detect spatial patterns.

Electronic health record (EHR): A digital version of a patient's medical history that is maintained within a healthcare system and possibly shared across healthcare systems.

Generative pretrained transformer (GPT): A class of deep learning models that are trained to generate natural language text by learning to predict the next word using long textual context in the training data and the transformer architecture.

Large language model (LLM): A type of AI model, such as a GPT, trained on vast amounts of natural language text data to generate language with high fluency and long contextual awareness.

Machine learning: A type of AI in which algorithms learn statistical patterns from data to make predictions or decisions without being explicitly programmed.

Natural language processing (NLP): A field of AI focused on enabling computers to understand, interpret, and generate human language.

Positive predictive value (PPV): The proportion of positive test results that are true positives, reflecting how likely a positive prediction is to be correct.

Reinforcement learning: A learning paradigm in which an "agent" is trained to act in its environment to optimize a certain utility by receiving rewards or penalties from its interactions with an environment.

Supervised learning: A machine learning approach in which models are trained on labeled data with known inputs and low-dimensional outputs (for example, a diagnosis).

Unsupervised learning: A machine learning approach in which models identify patterns or structure in data without labeled samples.

Vision-language model (VLM): A model that jointly processes, often paired, visual and textual information to perform tasks such as image captioning, visual question answering, or multimodal reasoning.

NOTES

1 https://psnet.ahrq.gov/issue/foundational-science-learning-health-systems
2 https://openai.com/index/chatgpt/
3 https://claude.ai/
4 https://groups.csail.mit.edu/medg/ftp/psz/AIM82/ch2.html#c2_casnet_mode,l
5 https://healthit.gov/data/quickstats/national-trends-hospital-and-physician-adoption-electronic-health-records/
6 https://www.statista.com/topics/9204/health-and-fitness-apps/
7 https://chatgpt.com/g/g-2fkFE8rbu-dall-e

8 https://gemini.google/overview/image-generation/
9 https://code.claude.com/docs/en/overview
10 https://www.wired.com/story/a-new-ai-math-ai-startup-just-cracked-4-previously-unsolved-problems/
11 https://www.epic.com/software/ai-clinicians/
12 https://www.fda.gov/medical-devices/software-medical-device-samd/artificial-intelligence-enabled-medical-devices
13 https://downloads.regulations.gov/FDA-2020-D-1138-0078/attachment_1.pdf
14 https://randolphmn.com/premium/stacker/stories/how-ai-is-speeding-up-cancer-research,148905
15 https://www.accessdata.fda.gov/scripts/cdrh/cfdocs/cfpma/pma.cfm?id=P090012
16 https://www.3derm.com/press/2020-01/breakthrough/

REFERENCES

1. Kokosi T, Harron K. Synthetic data in medical research. *BMJ Med*. 2022 Sep 26;1(1):e000167.
2. Koetzier LR, Wu J, Mastrodicasa D, Lutz A, Chung M, Koszek WA, et al. Generating synthetic data for medical imaging. *Radiology*. 2024 Sep;312(3):e232471.
3. Pang C, Jiang X, Pavinkurve NP, Kalluri KS, Minto EL, Patterson J, et al. CEHR-GPT: Generating electronic health records with chronological patient timelines [Internet]. *arXiv* [cs.LG]. 2024. Available from: http://arxiv.org/abs/2402.04400
4. Saab K, Tu T, Weng WH, Tanno R, Stutz D, Wulczyn E, et al. Capabilities of Gemini models in medicine [Internet]. *arXiv* [cs.AI]. 2024. Available from: http://arxiv.org/abs/2404.18416
5. Shortliffe EH (Ed.). *Computer-based Medical Consultations: MYCIN*. 2012. p. 2. Available from: https://books.google.com/books?hl=en&lr=&id=i9QXugPQw6oC&oi=fnd&pg=PP1&dq=MYCIN&ots=Ib8hZ3cvPF&sig=40pDuUL7IIeHrw9csxCoJNY-Mck
6. Miller RA, Pople HE Jr, Myers JD. INTERNIST-I, an experimental computer-based diagnostic consultant for general internal medicine. In: *Computers and Medicine*. New York, NY: Springer; 1985. p. 139–58.
7. Irvin J, Rajpurkar P, Ko M, Yu Y, Ciurea-Ilcus S, Chute C, et al. CheXpert: A large chest radiograph dataset with uncertainty labels and expert comparison. *AAAI*. 2019 Jul 17;33(01):590–7.
8. Belgrave D, Henderson J, Simpson A, Buchan I, Bishop C, Custovic A. Disaggregating asthma: Big investigation versus big data. *J Allergy Clin Immunol*. 2017 Feb 1;139(2):400–7.
9. Ganjgahi H, Häring DA, Aarden P, Graham G, Sun Y, Gardiner S, et al. AI-driven reclassification of multiple sclerosis progression. *Nat Med*. 2025 Oct;31(10):3414–24.
10. Weber LM, Robinson MD. Comparison of clustering methods for high-dimensional single-cell flow and mass cytometry data. *Cytometry A*. 2016 Dec 1;89(12):1084–96.
11. Silver D, Huang A, Maddison CJ, Guez A, Sifre L, van den Driessche G, et al. Mastering the game of Go with deep neural networks and tree search. *Nature*. 2016 Jan 28;529(7587):484–9.
12. Silver D, Hubert T, Schrittwieser J, Antonoglou I, Lai M, Guez A, et al. Mastering chess and shogi by self-play with a general reinforcement learning algorithm [Internet]. *arXiv* [cs.AI]. 2017 [cited 2026 Feb 8]. Available from: http://arxiv.org/abs/1712.01815

13. Henderson P, Li X, Jurafsky D, Hashimoto T, Lemley MA, Liang P. Foundation models and fair use [Internet]. *arXiv* [cs.CY]. 2023. p. 1–79. Available from: http://arxiv.org/abs/2303.15715
14. Radford A, Kim JW, Hallacy C, Ramesh A, Goh G, Agarwal S, et al. Learning transferable visual models from natural language supervision. Meila M, Zhang T, editors. *ICML*. 2021 Feb 26;139:8748–63.
15. Lai CH, Song Y, Kim D, Mitsufuji Y, Ermon S. The principles of diffusion models [Internet]. *arXiv* [cs.LG]. 2025 [cited 2026 Feb 8]. Available from: http://arxiv.org/abs/2510.21890
16. DeepSeek-AI, Guo D, Yang D, Zhang H, Song J, Wang P, et al. DeepSeek-R1: Incentivizing reasoning capability in LLMs via reinforcement learning [Internet]. *arXiv* [cs.CL]. 2026 [cited 2026 Feb 8]. Available from: http://dx.doi.org/10.48550/arXiv.2501.12948
17. Kazerouni A, Aghdam EK, Heidari M, Azad R, Fayyaz M, Hacihaliloglu I, et al. Diffusion models for medical image analysis: A comprehensive survey [Internet]. *arXiv* [eess.IV]. 2022 [cited 2026 Feb 8]. Available from: http://arxiv.org/abs/2211.07804
18. Acosta JN, Dogra S, Adithan S, Wu K, Moritz M, Kwak S, et al. The impact of AI assistance on radiology reporting: A pilot study using simulated AI draft reports [Internet]. *arXiv* [cs.HC]. 2024. Available from: https://scholar.google.com/citations?view_op=view_citation&hl=en&citation_for_view=QcOG6sgAAAAJ:vbGhcppDl1QC
19. Myronenko A, Yang D, Turkbey B, Aboian M, Azamat S, Akcicek E, et al. Reasoning visual language model for chest X-ray analysis [Internet]. *arXiv* [cs.CV]. 2025. Available from: http://dx.doi.org/10.48550/arXiv.2510.23968
20. Ulrich P, Zink A, Biedermann T, Sitaru S. Beyond Fitzpatrick: Automated artificial intelligence-based skin tone analysis in dermatological patients. *NPJ Digit Med*. 2025 Jun 20;8(1):378.
21. Finlayson SG, Subbaswamy A, Singh K, Bowers J, Kupke A, Zittrain J, et al. The clinician and dataset shift in artificial intelligence. *N Engl J Med*. 2021 Jul 15;385(3):283–6.
22. McCradden MD, London AJ, Gichoya JW, Sendak M, Erdman L, Stedman I, et al. CANAIRI: The collaboration for translational artificial intelligence trials in healthcare. *Nat Med*. 2025 Jan;31(1):9–11.
23. de Kanter E, Kaul T, Heus P, de Groot TM, Kuijten RH, Reitsma JB, et al. Adherence to TRIPOD+AI guideline: An updated reporting assessment tool. *J Clin Epidemiol*. 2025 Dec 23;191:112118.
24. Collins GS, Moons KGM, Dhiman P, Riley RD, Beam AL, Van Calster B, et al. TRIPOD+AI statement: Updated guidance for reporting clinical prediction models that use regression or machine learning methods. *BMJ*. 2024 Apr 16;385:e078378.
25. Vasey B, Novak A, Ather S, Ibrahim M, McCulloch P. DECIDE-AI: A new reporting guideline and its relevance to artificial intelligence studies in radiology. *Clin Radiol*. 2023 Feb;78(2):130–6.
26. Cruz Rivera S, Liu X, Chan AW, Denniston AK, Calvert MJ, SPIRIT-AI and CONSORT-AI Working Group, et al. Guidelines for clinical trial protocols for interventions involving artificial intelligence: The SPIRIT-AI extension. *Nat Med*. 2020 Sep;26(9):1351–63.
27. Liu X, Cruz Rivera S, Moher D, Calvert MJ, Denniston AK, SPIRIT-AI and CONSORT-AI Working Group. Reporting guidelines for clinical trial reports for interventions involving artificial intelligence: The CONSORT-AI extension. *Nat Med*. 2020 Sep;26(9):1364–74.

28. Kourou K, Exarchos KP, Papaloukas C, Sakaloglou P, Exarchos T, Fotiadis DI. Applied machine learning in cancer research: A systematic review for patient diagnosis, classification and prognosis. *Comput Struct Biotechnol J*. 2021 Oct 6;19:5546–55.
29. Singh R, Bapna M, Diab AR, Ruiz ES, Lotter W. How AI is used in FDA-authorized medical devices: A taxonomy across 1,016 authorizations. *NPJ Digit Med*. 2025 Jul 1;8(1):388.
30. Lehman CD, Wellman RD, Buist DSM, Kerlikowske K, Tosteson ANA, Miglioretti DL, et al. Diagnostic accuracy of digital screening mammography with and without computer-aided detection. *JAMA Intern Med*. 2015 Nov;175(11):1828–37.
31. Doi K. Computer-aided diagnosis in medical imaging: Historical review, current status and future potential. *Comput Med Imaging Graph*. 2007 Jun;31(4-5):198–211.
32. Wilbur DC, Prey MU, Miller WM, Pawlick GF, Colgan TJ. The AutoPap system for primary screening in cervical cytology. Comparing the results of a prospective, intended-use study with routine manual practice. *Acta Cytol*. 1998 Jan;42(1):214–20.
33. Bakker MF, de Lange SV, Pijnappel RM, Mann RM, Peeters PHM, Monninkhof EM, et al. Supplemental MRI screening for women with extremely dense breast tissue. *N Engl J Med*. 2019 Nov 28;381(22): 2091–102.
34. Shen Y, Shamout FE, Oliver JR, Witowski J, Kannan K, Park J, et al. Artificial intelligence system reduces false-positive findings in the interpretation of breast ultrasound exams. *Nat Commun*. 2021 Sep 24;12(1):5645.
35. Svoboda E. Artificial intelligence is improving the detection of lung cancer. *Nature*. 2020 Nov;587(7834):S20–2.
36. Ardila D, Kiraly AP, Bharadwaj S, Choi B, Reicher JJ, Peng L, et al. End-to-end lung cancer screening with three-dimensional deep learning on low-dose chest computed tomography. *Nat Med*. 2019 Jun;25(6): 954–61.
37. Kim RY, Oke JL, Pickup LC, Munden RF, Dotson TL, Bellinger CR, et al. Artificial intelligence tool for assessment of indeterminate pulmonary nodules detected with CT. *Radiology*. 2022 Sep;304(3):683–91.
38. Gunasekeran DV, Wong TY. Artificial intelligence in ophthalmology in 2020: A technology on the cusp for translation and implementation: A technology on the cusp for translation and implementation. *Asia Pac J Ophthalmol (Phila)*. 2020 Mar;9(2):61–6.
39. Li Z, Qiang W, Chen H, Pei M, Yu X, Wang L, et al. Artificial intelligence to detect malignant eyelid tumors from photographic images. *NPJ Digit Med*. 2022 Mar 2;5(1):23.
40. Le Berre C, Sandborn WJ, Aridhi S, Devignes MD, Fournier L, Smaïl-Tabbone M, et al. Application of artificial intelligence to gastroenterology and hepatology. *Gastroenterology*. 2020 Jan;158(1):76–94.e2.
41. Wang P, Berzin TM, Glissen Brown JR, Bharadwaj S, Becq A, Xiao X, et al. Real-time automatic detection system increases colonoscopic polyp and adenoma detection rates: A prospective randomised controlled study. *Gut*. 2019 Oct;68(10):1813–9.
42. Lujan GM, Savage J, Shana'ah A, Yearsley M, Thomas D, Allenby P, et al. Digital pathology initiatives and experience of a large academic institution during the Coronavirus disease 2019 (COVID-19) pandemic. *Arch Pathol Lab Med*. 2021 Sep 1;145(9):1051–61.

43. Ardon O, Reuter VE, Hameed M, Corsale L, Manzo A, Sirintrapun SJ, et al. Digital pathology operations at an NYC tertiary cancer center during the first 4 months of COVID-19 pandemic response. *Acad Pathol.* 2021 Jan 28;8(23742895211010276):23742895211010276.
44. Deng J, Dong W, Socher R, Li LJ, Li K, Fei-Fei L. ImageNet: A large-scale hierarchical image database. In: *2009 IEEE Conference on Computer Vision and Pattern Recognition* [Internet]. IEEE; 2009. Available from: http://dx.doi.org/10.1109/cvpr.2009.5206848
45. Das K, Cockerell CJ, Patil A, Pietkiewicz P, Giulini M, Grabbe S, et al. Machine learning and its application in skin cancer. *Int J Environ Res Public Health.* 2021 Dec 20;18(24):13409.
46. Tschandl P, Rosendahl C, Akay BN, Argenziano G, Blum A, Braun RP, et al. Expert-level diagnosis of nonpigmented skin cancer by combined convolutional neural networks. *JAMA Dermatol.* 2019 Jan 1;155(1):58–65.
47. Esteva A, Kuprel B, Novoa RA, Ko J, Swetter SM, Blau HM, et al. Dermatologist-level classification of skin cancer with deep neural networks. *Nature.* 2017 Feb 2;542(7639):115–8.
48. Schäfer Z, Mathisen A, Svendsen K, Engberg S, Rolighed Thomsen T, Kirketerp-Møller K. Toward machine-learning-based decision support in diabetes care: A risk stratification study on diabetic foot ulcer and amputation. *Front Med (Lausanne).* 2020;7:601602.
49. Showalter K, Spiera R, Magro C, Agius P, Martyanov V, Franks JM, et al. Machine learning integration of scleroderma histology and gene expression identifies fibroblast polarisation as a hallmark of clinical severity and improvement. *Ann Rheum Dis.* 2021 Feb;80(2):228–37.
50. Wu H, Yin H, Chen H, Sun M, Liu X, Yu Y, et al. A deep learning, image based approach for automated diagnosis for inflammatory skin diseases. *Ann Transl Med.* 2020 May;8(9):581.
51. Matin RN, Dinnes J. AI-based smartphone apps for risk assessment of skin cancer need more evaluation and better regulation. *Br J Cancer.* 2021 May;124(11):1749–50.
52. Kovarik C, Lee I, Ko J, Ad Hoc Task Force on Augmented Intelligence. Commentary: Position statement on augmented intelligence (AuI). *J Am Acad Dermatol.* 2019 Oct;81(4):998–1000.
53. Fink C, Jaeger C, Jaeger K, Haenssle HA. Diagnostic performance of the MelaFind device in a real-life clinical setting: MelaFind device in a real-life clinical setting. *J Dtsch Dermatol Ges.* 2017 Apr;15(4):414–9.
54. Kupetsky EA, Ferris LK. The diagnostic evaluation of MelaFind multi-spectral objective computer vision system. *Expert Opin Med Diagn.* 2013 Jul;7(4):405–11.
55. Monheit G, Cognetta AB, Ferris L, Rabinovitz H, Gross K, Martini M, et al. The performance of MelaFind: A prospective multicenter study: A prospective multicenter study. *Arch Dermatol.* 2011 Feb;147(2):188–94.
56. Sies K, Winkler JK, Fink C, Bardehle F, Toberer F, Buhl T, et al. Past and present of computer-assisted dermoscopic diagnosis: Performance of a conventional image analyser versus a convolutional neural network in a prospective data set of 1,981 skin lesions. *Eur J Cancer.* 2020 Aug;135:39–46.
57. Liu Y, Jain A, Eng C, Way DH, Lee K, Bui P, et al. A deep learning system for differential diagnosis of skin diseases. *Nat Med.* 2020 Jun;26(6):900–8.
58. Chen IY, Pierson E, Rose S, Joshi S, Ferryman K, Ghassemi M. Ethical machine learning in healthcare. *Annu Rev Biomed Data Sci.* 2021 Jul;4:123–44.
59. Perets O, Stagno E, Yehuda EB, McNichol M, Anthony Celi L, Rappoport N, et al. Inherent bias in electronic health records: A scoping review of sources of bias. *medRxiv* [Internet]. 2024 Apr 12. Available from: https://pmc.ncbi.nlm.nih.gov/articles/PMC11046491/

60. Obermeyer Z, Powers B, Vogeli C, Mullainathan S. Dissecting racial bias in an algorithm used to manage the health of populations. *Science.* 2019 Oct 25;366(6464):447–53.
61. Barocas S, Hardt M, Narayanan A. *Fairness and Machine Learning: Limitations and Opportunities.* MIT Press; 2023.
62. Kimani RW. Reexamining the use of race in medical algorithms: The maternal health calculator debate. *Front Public Health.* 2024 Jun 13;12:1417429.
63. The US Food and Drug Administration, Washington, DC, USA. *Good Machine Learning Practice for Medical Device Development: Guiding Principles* [Internet]. U.S. Food and Drug Administration, FDA; 2023 [cited 2024 Aug 16]. Available from: https://www.fda.gov/medical-devices/software-medical-device-samd/good-machine-learning-practice-medical-device-development-guiding-principles
64. Joshi S, Urteaga I, van Amsterdam WAC, Hripcsak G, Elias P, Amor BRC, et al. AI as an intervention: Improving clinical outcomes relies on a causal approach to AI development and validation. *Journal of the American Medical Informatics Association: JAMIA.* 2025 Jan 7;32:589–94.
65. Center for Devices, Radiological Health. *Marketing Submission Recommendations for a Predetermined Change Control Plan for Artificial Intelligence-Enabled Device Software Functions* [Internet]. U.S. Food and Drug Administration, FDA; 2025 [cited 2026 Feb 8]. Available from: https://www.fda.gov/regulatory-information/search-fda-guidance-documents/marketing-submission-recommendations-predetermined-change-control-plan-artificial-intelligence

2 Generative AI in Medical Education

Michael R. De La Rosa, Christopher A. Mao, Ronald Rodriguez

2.1 INTRODUCTION

With the release of ChatGPT to the public, a spotlight has been shone on generative AI and its applications across nearly every field. The ease of accessibility of ChatGPT, as well as the fact that these models output human language rather than abstract numbers or code, changed the public perception of AI; in the minds of the public, AI was catapulted from an abstract concept to be used far in the future to a tool that can be accessed by anyone with access to a computer or even just a smartphone.

Naturally, this advancement led to a surge of effort in incorporating generative AI into medical education. This chapter will provide a brief overview of the technology, its applications, pitfalls, and future directions as they pertain to medical education.

2.2 GENERATIVE AI

2.2.1 What Is Generative AI?

Generative AI refers to models that can create new content, most commonly in the form of text, images, audio, or video [1]. Unlike traditional AI systems that classify information or predict outcomes, generative AI is designed to "generate" something new. For example, while a predictive system might suggest the next word in an email, a generative model such as ChatGPT can create an entirely original response to a user's prompt.

These models achieve this by learning patterns and relationships within massive amounts of training data. After being exposed to hundreds of millions or even billions of examples, these models can generate outputs resembling the data they were trained on without producing direct copies.

The concept of interactive AI itself is not new. It dates to the 1960s with rule-based systems that generated text using simple if-then rules [2]. One of the best-known examples was ELIZA, a program created to mimic the conversation between a therapist and a patient. ELIZA identified keywords in user input and responded according to preprogrammed rules, allowing a back-and-forth dialogue that resembled a real conversation [3]. The interaction was sufficiently compelling that many people actually felt they were conversing with a real therapist, a phenomenon later called the ELIZA effect.

These early rule-based systems were first developed in the 1950s and formed the basis of what later became the field of natural language processing (NLP). For decades, NLP methods relied on increasingly complex rule sets and statistical techniques, enabling computers to perform tasks such as part-of-speech tagging, machine translation, and information retrieval. While these approaches were important milestones, they were still limited in flexibility and struggled with the nuances of human language.

In the nearly 60 years since ELIZA, generative AI has advanced greatly. The introduction of neural networks—eventually the more advanced form of neural networks called transformer-based architectures—revolutionized NLP, giving rise to LLMs capable of generating coherent, contextually appropriate text across a wide range of topics. This ability to allow models to focus on context across an entire sentence or group of sentences is called attention, and its adoption is one of the most important advancements in the development of generative AI. Along

DOI: 10.1201/9781003617167-2

with advances in computing power, these models have become the foundation for modern generative AI. Today, the field is built around foundation models: large models trained on broad datasets that can be adapted for a variety of applications.

This chapter will cover the main categories of foundational generative AI models, LLMs, text-to-image, text-to-video, text-to-audio, and multimodal systems, with a particular focus on LLMs, as they represent the most significant and widely adopted application in medical education today. The remaining categories will be discussed more briefly, highlighting their emerging potential for future use in the field.

2.2.2 Types of Generative AI

2.2.2.1 LLMs

LLMs are foundational models designed to process and generate natural language. Trained on massive corpora of text, they use statistical patterns to predict the next word in a sequence, enabling them to perform tasks such as answering questions, summarizing material, drafting text, and engaging in dialogue. Their broad generalizability makes them adaptable to specialized domains such as medicine, where they can provide explanations of complex topics, generate practice questions, or simulate patient interactions.

Most generative AI models discussed at the time of this writing are pretrained general LLMs. Popular examples are OpenAI's ChatGPT, Anthropic's Claude, Google's Gemini, X's Grok, and Meta's Llama. Of particular interest is OpenEvidence, a relatively new interactive ChatBot developed for use in the medical field. This model is pretrained on open-source medical research papers and thus is intended to provide more relevant and accurate results in the medical domain. OpenEvidence is being increasingly used by clinicians. Recently, OpenEvidence has even signed content agreements with the *Journal of American Medical Association* and the *New England Journal of Medicine*, allowing their model to use papers from each journal [4, 5]. OpenEvidence has also become HIPAA compliant, allowing users, after signing the necessary paperwork, to enter Protected Health Information (PHI) into the model [6].

2.2.2.2 Text-to-Image

Text-to-image foundational models generate pictures based on written descriptions. These models are trained on large datasets that pair text with images, learning to map words and phrases to corresponding visual features. Popular examples include DALL-E, Stable Diffusion, Adobe Firefly, and Midjourney, which are widely used to create illustrations, concept art, and design prototypes. The process of creating images from text has at its basis a process known as diffusion. As shown in Figure 2.1, diffusion models take real images and introduce random noise incrementally until the image appears to be pure static, and they then reverse the process, removing the noise to "recover" an image guided by the prompt. After training, novel data can be generated by running the denoising process starting from entirely random noise.

Unfortunately, the utility of text-to-image models in medicine is very limited. AI-generated images from most commercial text-to-image systems have serious difficulty reproducing true anatomic detail and frequently incorporate nonsensical features, such as extra fingers or anatomically impossible combinations. As shown in Figure 2.2, images of the cardiovascular system, for instance, may look plausible to a layperson, but, to a medical professional, the details are often clearly inaccurate. This is an area of intense research, and it is expected that, with time, anatomically correct AI image generation will emerge once training is focused on large datasets of real, anatomically correct depictions.

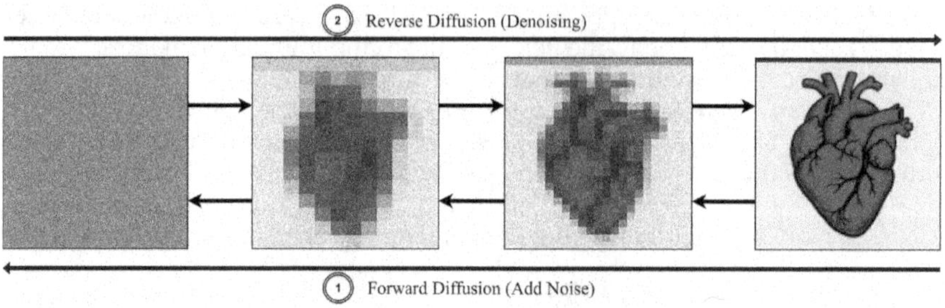

Figure 2.1 Forward and reverse diffusion processes used in text-to-image generative models. This diagram illustrates how diffusion models learn to generate images by progressively adding noise to real images during training in forward diffusion (right to left) and then learning to remove that noise step-by-step in reverse diffusion (left to right). (Figure courtesy of Isaac Alvarez.)

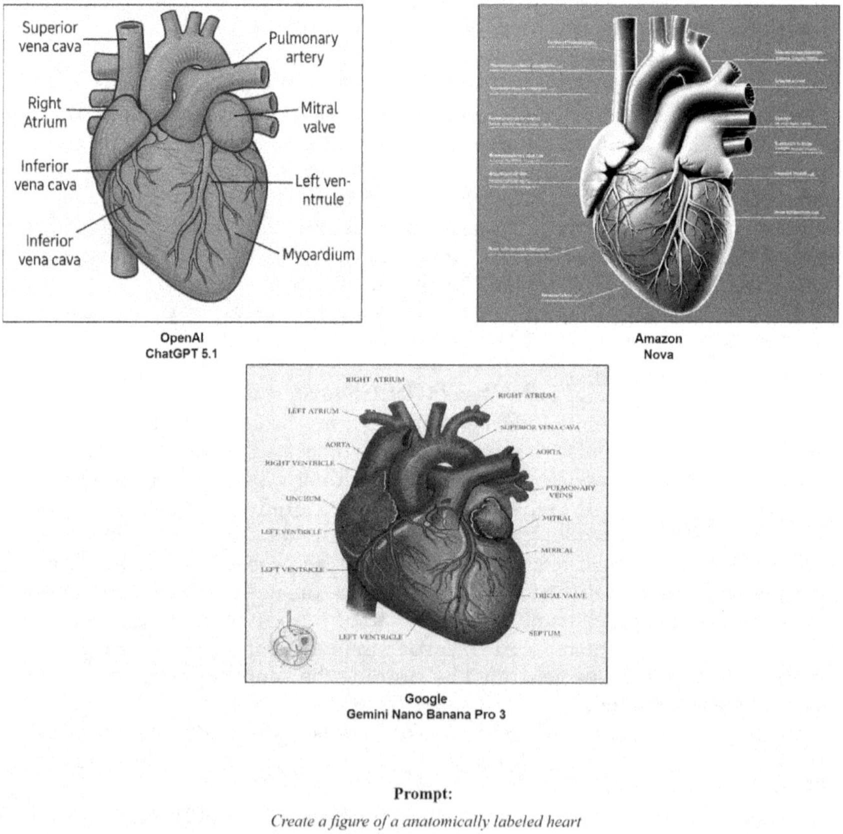

Figure 2.2 Examples of AI-generated illustrations of the human heart created by commercial text-to-image models. These images may appear visually realistic but contain multiple anatomic inaccuracies, including repeated or incorrect labels, fabricated terminology, and illegible text. (Figure courtesy of Isaac Alvarez.)

2.2.2.3 *Text-to-Video*

Text-to-video foundational models extend the capabilities of text-to-image models to generate video sequences directly from text. By training on text–video pairs, these models learn to synthesize not just static visuals but also motion and continuity over time. Examples include Runway Gen-2, Pika Labs, and Sora, which are being developed for creative industries, advertising, and entertainment. Use in medical education is currently more limited, as anatomically correct animations suffer from the same inaccuracy issues as text-to-image models. However, text-to-video technology is well suited for patient encounter simulations, difficult patient interactions, cultural sensitivity training, and other educational scenarios that illustrate key aspects of provider–patient communication and interpersonal skills.

2.2.2.4 *Text-to-Audio*

Text-to-audio foundational models convert written text into sound, including both human speech and nonspeech sounds. They are trained on paired datasets of text and audio recordings, enabling them to mimic voices, accents, and environmental noises. Well-known systems include Google's WaveNet, OpenAI's VALL-E, and ElevenLabs Voice AI, which are widely used for audiobooks, podcasts, dubbing, and sound design. Adaptive medical education tutorials are increasingly being developed to convert existing text-based materials on specific medical concepts into more accessible formats, such as audiobooks and podcasts. As medical students and other medical learners are increasingly accustomed to ingesting new educational materials in audio formats, this area of use is expected to have a dramatic increase in the next few years.

2.2.2.5 *Multimodal*

Multimodal foundational models integrate two or more types of data, such as text, images, audio, or video, into a single system. Unlike unimodal models, they can distinguish relationships across formats and generate outputs that combine them. For example, a multimodal model might take the prompt "describe this picture" while analyzing an image of a dog playing fetch, then produce the response "a golden retriever is catching a ball in the park." Another case might involve uploading a diagram and asking the model to generate a written explanation of it. Examples include GPT-4 with vision, Gemini, and CLIP, which are advancing applications in accessibility, search, and interactive AI systems.

2.3 GENERATIVE AI IN MEDICAL EDUCATION

2.3.1 Learner-Focused Applications of Generative AI

With the widespread adoption of generative AI in society, learners across the full spectrum of education have increasingly integrated these tools into their personal learning and study practices, even without formal instruction. This is also true for medicine, as physicians, advanced practice providers, residents, medical students, and other medical learners continue to find innovative ways to incorporate generative AI into their daily lives [7].

2.3.1.1 *Content Simplification and Explanations*

One of the most common educational uses of generative AI is explaining complex topics. Medicine in general suffers from high linguistic complexity, with excessive use of jargon, abbreviations, and context-specific specialized meanings that often differ from the conventional use of language (e.g., "unremarkable" or "gross"). Students frequently rely on systems such as ChatGPT to clarify concepts, summarize material, and provide simplified explanations when traditional resources fall short. Survey data confirm that "explaining concepts" is the most frequent way medical students apply generative AI in their studies [8].

In mathematics education, for example, AI-generated explanations have produced learning gains comparable to those achieved with human tutor support, indicating that generative AI can function as a scalable and personalizable instructional aid [9].

2.3.1.2 Summarization

One of the greatest strengths of LLMs is the ability to organize and summarize large amounts of information, even when the content is itself poorly organized. Large PDF files of highly technical information, for instance, can be "queried" directly with many AI-enhanced PDF readers. For students working through complicated and dense material, AI can extract key points and condense long documents into more manageable summaries, supporting review, comprehension, and more effective time management. LLMs can effectively summarize peer-reviewed medical abstracts, with physician reviewers rating the outputs as both accurate and high quality [10].

These findings suggest that generative AI holds promise as a tool to help students digest and navigate large volumes of academic reading. However, LLM-derived summaries should be approached with caution due to the possibility of omissions, hallucinations, or misunderstanding of the core concepts. At best, they can serve as a valuable way of reviewing large amounts of material once the content has been vetted.

2.3.1.3 Memory Aids

Generative AI can also enhance learning by creating personalized memory aids designed to improve information retention. By adapting study materials to individual learning preferences, these tools can reinforce key concepts and support long-term recall through repeated and structured engagement.

A particularly promising application lies in the generation of mnemonics. Generative AI can produce high-quality textual mnemonics and pair them with corresponding visual representations to strengthen memory formation. Involving students in the creation of these mnemonic devices further enhances engagement and effectiveness, as learners actively construct memory links that align with their personal cognitive styles [11].

Recent peer-reviewed articles have outlined methods for designing personalized mnemonics, and the topic has also gained attention in online spaces, with instructional videos and forum discussions exploring practical approaches [12]. In parallel, commercial platforms have begun monetizing this process by offering personalized mnemonic-generation tools for medical students [13].

Another widely used category of memory aids involves spaced-repetition systems such as Anki, which strengthen long-term retention through repeated review of digital flashcards at optimized intervals [14]. Thousands of preexisting decks are publicly shared across subjects, allowing students to draw upon extensive community resources. Generative AI has been used to enhance this process by helping learners identify and prioritize flashcards most relevant to their goals, with tools such as AnkiTagger automatically tagging cards aligned with a school's curriculum [15]. Students are also using generative AI to create flashcards directly from lecture notes or study materials, integrating automated content creation with the evidence-based principles of spaced repetition.

2.3.1.4 Simulation and Role Play

Medical simulation and patient–provider role-play are well-established techniques for enhancing performance in clinical communication. In one study, researchers developed a GPT-4–based chatbot that simulated patient interviews for health professions students [16]. The system allowed learners to conduct complete clinical interviews, adapting responses to the student's questioning style. Most participants rated the conversations as realistic and valuable for practicing communication skills, and many prefer the virtual simulations over traditional peer role-play. Unlike human partners, AI-driven simulations do not suffer from social pressures, time pressures, personal judgment, human misinterpretation, or the tendency to place responses into unintended emotional contexts. This can alleviate learners' anxiety about appearing unintelligent, feeling embarrassed about making mistakes, or needing to answer quickly before they are ready.

Similar findings were reported in another study that examined the use of AI-simulated patients to strengthen medical interview skills [17]. Their results showed that generative AI can effectively support the development of communication and clinical reasoning, particularly in scenarios requiring empathy and adaptability. These studies suggest that AI-based simulations can complement traditional role-play by providing flexible, repeatable opportunities for students to rehearse patient interactions in a controlled, nonjudgmental feedback-rich environment.

2.3.1.5 *Generating and Clarifying Practice Questions*

Medical students often rely on practice problems to prepare for exams, yet these resources sometimes lack clear explanations or even correct answers. Generative AI has begun filling this gap, not only by clarifying reasoning but also by creating new, high-quality practice questions tailored to a learner's level. However, because AI-generated content can still contain errors or misleading rationales, human oversight, such as faculty review or alignment with validated question banks, remains essential to ensure accuracy and educational safety.

A turning point came in 2023, when ChatGPT-3.5 passed the USMLE without fine-tuning [18]. Although widely recognized for its precision, the most important finding for education was that its explanations demonstrated concordance, or logical internal consistency, enabling students to follow the reasoning process step by step. In about 90% of cases, its responses also surfaced at least one novel or nonobvious insight, effectively role-modeling the process of clinical reasoning for learners. This made it useful not only as a question-answering system but also as a tutor that explained how and why the answer was correct.

GPT-4 next achieved a significantly improved performance on the USMLE Step 1, with 86% of questions answered correctly [19]. More importantly, it could flexibly adapt explanations to different educational levels: breaking down complex physiology for a first-year student or offering high-level differential reasoning for a senior learner. Students quickly discovered that they could prompt the model to generate entirely new board-style questions, adjust the difficulty, or request analogies that clarified tricky mechanisms. In this way, AI became a study partner that both tested knowledge and expanded understanding.

The educational use cases now extend beyond question-answering. Learners use GenAI to request step-by-step explanations, compare correct and incorrect answer choices, and explore "why not" reasoning. They also create new questions in the style of National Board of Medical Examiners (NBME), tailored to specific organ systems, difficulty levels, or even common errors the student personally struggles with.

2.3.1.6 *Writing and Research*

Medical learners are increasingly turning to generative AI tools for support in their academic work. In research contexts, LLMs are being used to summarize PubMed abstracts into concise notes, to generate outlines for literature reviews, and even to help brainstorm hypotheses and potential statistical approaches [20]. These applications highlight the role of generative AI in streamlining the early stages of research writing and idea development. Beyond research, learners also use generative AI for general writing tasks, including drafting, revising, editing, and summarizing texts [7]. This extends to academic assignments as well as practical communication such as emails or personal statements.

However, because AI can introduce subtle errors, biased interpretations, or fabricated references, ethical use requires active human oversight to verify accuracy, maintain academic integrity, and ensure that final scholarly work reflects the learner's own understanding.

While these uses are highly relevant to learners, they are not unique to medical education and reflect broader trends in how generative AI is being adopted across many fields.

2.3.2 Educator-Focused Applications of Generative AI

While learners have quickly integrated generative AI into their study practices, teachers and faculty are also finding value in these tools to support instruction, curriculum design, and assessment. Unlike learners, who primarily use AI to accelerate self-study, teachers often use it to improve efficiency, clarity, and personalization in educational delivery.

2.3.2.1 Teaching

Generative AI is increasingly being used to develop teaching materials, including lecture slides, diagrams, and case-based learning prompts. Assisted by generative AI, faculty can generate illustrative figures or interactive clinical scenarios in minutes, saving preparation time while expanding the variety of learning experiences. Chatbots serving as "teaching assistants" have also emerged, capable of answering students' questions about course logistics and core content [21]. This approach was first popularized by Georgia Tech and is now being explored conceptually for potential use in health professions education.

2.3.2.2 Knowledge-Based Assessment

Creating high-quality exam questions is challenging, requiring extensive faculty training and editorial oversight. The University of Cincinnati College of Medicine piloted an AI-driven tool that generated USMLE-style questions, answers, and explanations from course content. In a hematology module, faculty reviewers determined that 85% of the AI-generated questions met USMLE criteria, and approximately three-quarters were ultimately shared with students as study material [22]. Importantly, faculty feedback on rejected questions was entered back into the system to improve subsequent outputs. This suggests that AI can reduce cost barriers for students who might otherwise rely on expensive third-party test-preparation services, while also lessening faculty workload.

2.3.2.3 Clinical Skills Assessment

Generative AI is also being explored as a supplement or alternative to standardized patients (SPs). Traditionally, SP encounters require trained actors, faculty observers, and extensive logistical resources, all of which introduce variability and cost [23].

In contrast, AI-generated standardized patients can simulate clinical encounters virtually, with built-in scoring frameworks such as the objective structured clinical examination (OSCE).

At the University of Texas Health Sciences Center at San Antonio, for example, faculty trained an AI system on a broad set of simulated cases and instructed it to provide only accurate, concise responses. Analysis of transcripts revealed useful performance markers. For instance, students who successfully diagnosed cases tended to ask iterative questions throughout the encounter, whereas unsuccessful students often reserved questioning until the end and prematurely ordered tests [22].

A recent innovation in this space is MedSimAI, an AI-powered virtual patient platform developed at Cornell University, in collaboration with Weill Cornell Medicine, Yale University, and the University of California, San Francisco [24]. The simulator features both text-based and voice-interactive modes that approximate real telehealth encounters, allowing students to practice communication, empathy, and diagnostic reasoning in a low-stress environment [24]. MedSimAI uses LLMs to generate realistic patient responses and incorporates a second AI system to evaluate student performance using the same rubrics applied in traditional OSCEs. The model provides immediate, rubric-aligned feedback, highlighting empathetic communication, missed opportunities for inquiry, and diagnostic reasoning quality.

Feedback from early curricular integrations has been strongly positive. Faculty at Weill Cornell reported that MedSimAI provided additional opportunities for deliberate practice and self-directed learning, while students noted its natural conversational flow and usefulness in developing bedside manner [25]. The platform's analytic dashboards and customizable case-blueprints enable institutions to align simulations with their own curricular objectives, building cases from tested blueprints, tailoring feedback frameworks (such as history taking or motivational interviewing checklists), and tracking competency development over time.

While AI-based simulations cannot fully replace human–patient encounters, they demonstrate how generative AI can enhance access to high-quality, standardized clinical training. They provide opportunities for students to refine communication and reasoning skills, bridging the gap between classroom learning and clinical practice.

2.3.2.4 *Procedural Skills Assessment*

Beyond patient interactions, AI is being integrated into virtual reality platforms to assess technical skills. An example is the Intelligent Continuous Expertise Monitoring System (ICEMS), a deep learning application developed for surgical training. By analyzing motor sequences at 0.2-second intervals using long short-term memory (LSTM) neural networks, ICEMS differentiates novice from expert performance, provides real-time feedback, and identifies potential errors [26]. This offers a scalable method to continuously monitor skill acquisition, ultimately aiming to improve both surgical education and patient safety.

2.3.2.5 *Curriculum Design and Accreditation*

Generative AI is also being explored as a tool to support curriculum design and accreditation processes, areas that are traditionally both time-intensive and administratively demanding. LLMs can assist faculty in cross-checking course materials against national standards such as the LCME and ACGME requirements, ensuring that essential competencies are adequately addressed. Beyond compliance, AI can help identify gaps in coverage, such as underrepresented domains including health equity, professionalism, and interprofessional collaboration, thereby strengthening curricular breadth and alignment with modern medical education priorities.

In addition, LLMs are being piloted to draft and refine accreditation documents, reducing the burden on faculty and administrators by generating initial templates, aligning course objectives with regulatory language, and formatting reports to meet institutional or national standards. Similarly, AI has been used to map clinical teaching objectives to the AAMC Core Entrustable Professional Activities (EPAs), providing a systematic way to verify that students are progressing toward expected competencies [27].

By automating these labor-intensive processes, generative AI offers the potential to streamline curriculum oversight and free up educators to focus on higher-order tasks, such as innovating in pedagogy, mentoring learners, and adapting teaching to emerging clinical challenges, while maintaining accountability to accrediting bodies.

2.4 PITFALLS OF GENERATIVE AI

Despite the numerous benefits, the use of generative AI in medicine comes with unique risks. These risks may limit the effectiveness of using generative AI and, in the worst case, may actively harm the educational process. Many of these risks have been documented in other sectors but have special implications for the field of medical education. This section will focus on hallucinations, human overreliance, and ethical concerns.

2.4.1 Hallucinations

A significant problem with current generative AI models is their propensity to "hallucinate," generating information that, while appearing factual and confidently presented, is entirely incorrect, oversimplified, or nonsensical [28]. This phenomenon stems from the probabilistic nature of these models, which are designed to produce the most likely word sequences or patterns based on their training data rather than possessing genuine understanding or a concern for truth. These models are trained on data drawn indiscriminately from both reliable and unreliable sources, with unvetted platforms such as Reddit often contributing a significant portion of the training corpus. This can lead to misleading or even blatantly wrong information being provided by the models, which can sometimes even be traced to a single website or Reddit post [29]. This inherent unreliability creates a "trust deficit" for generative AI, which becomes even more problematic in the context of medicine. It is imperative that generative AI be used with constant vigilance.

Hallucinations in language models come from the way they are trained, by predicting the next word in a sentence based only on statistical patterns in the data. The model sees countless examples of fluent language but is never directly told which facts are true or false [30]. As a result, the more often a collection of terms is found together, the more "accepted" the phrase becomes and the more likely it will be used by an LLM, even when they are incorrect.

To address these challenges, some newer systems incorporate retrieval-augmented generation (RAG), a method that improves accuracy by letting the model search reliable sources before generating a response. As illustrated in Figure 2.3, a RAG system retrieves vetted medical information and then conditions its output on the basis of that evidence. Platforms such as OpenEvidence are applying this approach to connect AI outputs directly to trusted medical literature, thereby reducing the likelihood of hallucinations [31]. However, the effectiveness of RAG ultimately depends on the quality and reliability of the underlying content being retrieved.

In parallel, model developers are experimenting with strategies to reduce overconfidence. For example, OpenAI has noted that language models can be designed to abstain or decline to answer when uncertain and that evaluation metrics should reward this kind of calibrated humility rather than overconfident

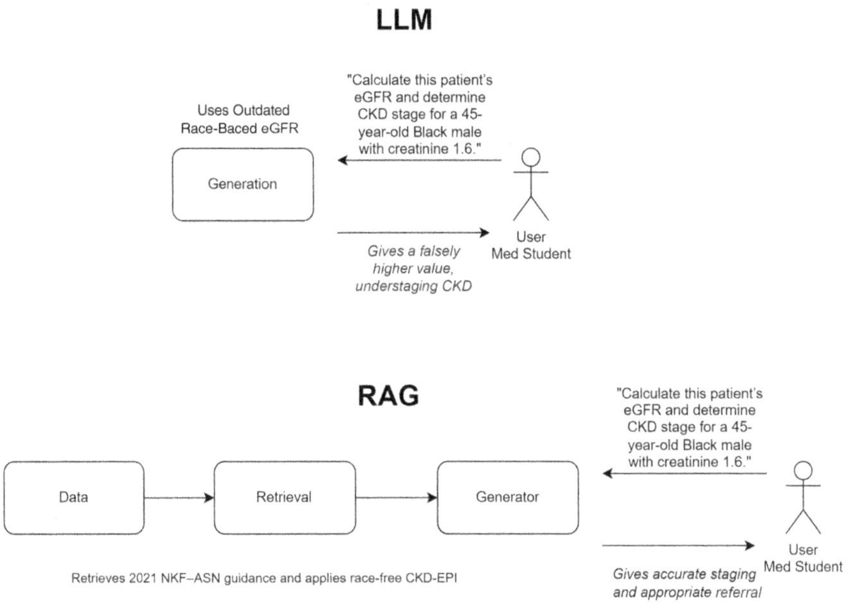

Figure 2.3 Overview of retrieval-augmented generation. A standard language model (top) generates responses using only its internal parameters, which increases the risk of hallucinations and reliance on outdated or incorrect information. In a retrieval-augmented generation system (bottom), the language model first searches vetted medical sources and then conditions its response on the basis of that evidence. (Figure courtesy of Isaac Alvarez.)

guessing [30]. While such approaches do not eliminate hallucinations entirely, they represent early efforts to align AI behavior more closely with the needs of high-stakes domains such as medicine.

2.4.2 Overreliance on AI

A key risk associated with integrating generative AI into medical education is cognitive offloading, the delegation of intellectual work to external systems. While this may streamline certain tasks, persistent reliance may degrade learners' clinical reasoning, diagnostic acumen, and problem-solving resilience. AI can function as an enabler of deep learning or, conversely, as a source of cognitive dependency, depending on how it is integrated into learning contexts [32]; the two are not mutually exclusive.

Recent work in medical education has raised similar concerns, noting that learners may over-rely on generative AI in ways that reduce opportunities for deliberate practice, critical reflection, and knowledge consolidation [33]. These dynamics mirror broader findings in cognitive science, where offloading tasks to AI can diminish active engagement and weaken the very processes necessary for developing independent reasoning.

LLMs can now readily propose differential diagnoses, summarize complex literature, and generate assessment items. If learners accept these outputs unquestioningly, they may circumvent the disciplined processes that underpin rigorous medical reasoning: assembling evidence, weighing competing hypotheses, confronting ambiguity, and refining one's own mental models. Such avoidance of cognitive effort undermines the very practices educators aim to cultivate.

To mitigate this risk, AI must be framed as a support tool rather than a substitute. Curricular design and assessment strategies should preserve and prioritize spaces where learners are compelled to engage in the reasoning work without outsourcing it. Recent empirical work shows that higher AI use is associated with greater cognitive offloading, which in turn is linked to poorer performance on measures of critical thinking, with offloading acting as a partial mediator of that decline [34]. Moreover, reviews of AI dialogue systems warn that unchecked reliance may erode analytical reasoning and decision-making skills [35].

2.4.3 Ethical Concerns

The ethical considerations surrounding generative AI in medical education are numerous, but several are particularly salient for educators and trainees.

2.4.3.1 Bias

LLMs trained on broad, internet-scale datasets often reproduce and even amplify existing racial, gender, and cultural biases. In medical contexts, this can have profound consequences. Recent evaluations of GPT-4 have shown biased outputs across clinically relevant tasks, including the creation of case vignettes for medical education, differential diagnostic reasoning, and treatment planning. These biases exaggerated disease prevalence differences, reinforced stereotypes, and at times generated harmful portrayals of minority groups [36]. In an educational setting, such distortions risk misinforming learners and perpetuating inequities. Mitigation strategies, such as RAG or careful prompt design to ensure appropriate demographic representation, may reduce but not eliminate these risks. For educators, this underscores the need for close oversight and critical appraisal of AI-generated content before it is integrated into teaching [37].

2.4.3.2 Copyright

The training of generative AI models frequently involves the use of copyrighted materials, often without explicit consent from rights holders. While legal frameworks are evolving, they remain unsettled. A recent U.S. legal case illustrates the ongoing uncertainty surrounding copyright and AI training. The court determined that, while the use of copyrighted materials for model training may be permissible, obtaining those materials from unauthorized sources, such as shadow libraries, remains unlawful. In response, Anthropic proposed a multibillion-dollar settlement with affected authors, providing compensation for each copyrighted work used in training [38]. This case underscores the scale of liability at stake and the unsettled nature of intellectual property law in this area. For medical education, where reliance on copyrighted textbooks, journal articles, and exam materials is routine, the use of generative AI–trained on such sources raises unresolved questions of intellectual property and fair use.

2.4.3.3 Sensitive Data and Privacy

Most LLMs not designed for healthcare are not HIPAA compliant, and their use with PHI risks regulatory violations, financial penalties, and professional consequences. Standard ChatGPT models retain data for monitoring and training, a practice that conflicts with HIPAA requirements even when users opt out. Safe deployment in clinical settings requires a HIPAA-compliant platform with a Business Associate Agreement (BAA), zero data retention, and strong PHI safeguards. OpenEvidence is one LLM reported to meet these standards [6].

However, some argue that HIPAA compliance is insufficient. The Privacy Rule assumes that de-identification renders data safe, yet in the era of LLMs, re-identification remains possible and even de-identified data can cause harm. Consequently, HIPAA offers limited protection against modern AI-related risks. Even perfect compliance would not ensure privacy or address broader concerns of power and inequality in the use of patient data [39].

2.5 FUTURE OF GENERATIVE AI IN MEDICINE

As generative AI continues to advance, its role in medical education will expand accordingly. New models and emerging techniques are likely to enhance the applications already discussed, while learners and educators alike will identify novel opportunities for integration. The following subsections highlight four key directions for the future.

2.5.1 Personalized and Adaptive Learning

One of the most persistent challenges in medical education is the imbalance between the large number of learners and limited faculty resources. Generative AI has the potential to narrow this gap by offering personalized, adaptive learning support. Future systems could track a learner's strengths and weaknesses, generating tailored quizzes, adaptive study plans, and targeted explanations. Beyond simple question answering, these tools may incorporate gamification features—quizzes, puzzles, and interactive challenges—that increase engagement and promote self-assessment. Performance prediction is another likely extension: by analyzing learner interactions and progress, AI systems could estimate readiness for major assessments such as USMLE exams or OSCEs. While such tools will not replace educators, they may reduce routine workloads across tasks such as content delivery, remediation, and assessment preparation, freeing faculty to devote more time to higher-value activities, including mentoring, curriculum innovation, scholarly work, and other professional responsibilities beyond day-to-day teaching logistics. Early studies suggest that AI-powered adaptive learning platforms can improve engagement and learning outcomes, though careful oversight remains essential [40].

2.5.2 Photographic and Radiographic Images

Generative AI applications involving photographic and radiographic imagery remain challenging to implement reliably in medical education. The inherent complexity of visual medical data, particularly the fine anatomical structures, subtle contrast differences, and wide spectrum of pathologies, makes it difficult for models to generate images that are both realistic and clinically trustworthy [41].

Nonetheless, progress has been made in both domains. In plastic surgery education, AI systems have successfully produced clinically useful photographs that support visual learning while mitigating privacy concerns associated with real patient images [42].

In radiology, research has shown that synthetic radiographs can be generated, modified for difficulty, and integrated into simulators to aid interpretation training. These tools offer learners opportunities for repetitive, independent practice while reducing the burden on faculty [43].

As generative models continue to improve in resolution, anatomical fidelity, and domain specialization, their potential to create high-quality anatomical diagrams, photographic exemplars, and radiographic case libraries will expand. Future systems may generate adaptive image sets tailored to learner progress or curricular needs, ultimately transforming how visual and spatial knowledge is taught in medicine.

2.5.3 Multimodal Models

Although still limited in performance, multimodal models show considerable potential for medical education. Future iterations could generate detailed anatomical models for study, create customized diagrams and illustrations for learning materials, and integrate diverse data streams into realistic case-based simulations. Recent work has demonstrated their use in simulating patient encounters, where learners interact with "synthetic patients" that combine language, voice, and visual representation to practice sensitive conversations [44]. As these systems mature, they may provide scalable, high-fidelity educational experiences that enhance engagement and better prepare trainees for the complexity of real clinical practice.

2.5.4 AI-Enhanced Clinical Training

Generative AI is poised to transform the ways students acquire clinical and procedural competencies. AI-driven virtual standardized patients can simulate a wide range of demographics and conditions, allowing learners to practice history taking, counseling, and diagnostic reasoning at scale. These interactions can be paired with automated assessment frameworks, such as adaptations of the OSCE, to provide structured and immediate feedback.

In procedural education, integrating AI with extended reality (AR/VR, augmented reality/virtual reality) platforms enables high-fidelity surgical and interventional simulations. The emergence of digital twins—virtual representations of individual patients—has further expanded this potential by allowing trainees to explore anatomy, rehearse procedures, and test interventions within controlled environments [45]. Similarly, recent analyses of AR/VR technologies highlight their capacity to provide immersive, multisensory learning experiences that enhance safety, scalability, and skill retention [46].

Collectively, these innovations reduce dependence on human role-players and faculty observers, lower training costs, and create opportunities for deliberate, data-driven practice. As these systems evolve, they may also assist with clinical documentation, identifying omissions or suggesting clearer phrasing, further integrating AI into the continuum of clinical education and practice.

GLOSSARY

Algorithmic bias: Systematic, inequitable errors in AI outputs (such as by race, gender, or culture) that arise from biased data or model design.

Anki: A spaced repetition flashcard application widely used in medical education to promote long-term retention through adaptive review.

Artificial intelligence (AI): Computer systems capable of performing tasks that typically require human intelligence, such as learning, reasoning, and language processing.

Augmented reality (AR): Technology that overlays digital elements onto the physical world to support interactive and immersive learning.

Business associate agreement (BAA): A legal contract requiring an organization to safeguard PHI on behalf of a covered entity under HIPAA.

Calibrated abstention: Model behavior in which an AI system withholds an answer or indicates uncertainty when confidence is low, improving reliability in high-stakes domains.

ChatGPT: A conversational LLM developed by OpenAI that generates human-like text responses and supports educational, clinical, and research applications.

Cognitive offloading/overreliance: The delegation of thinking or reasoning to AI tools in ways that can reduce independent analysis and problem-solving skills.

De-identification/Re-identification: The removal of personal identifiers from data, and the potential relinking of de-identified data to specific individuals.
Digital Twin: A high-fidelity virtual model of a real patient or system used for simulation, rehearsal, and personalized medical training.
Foundation model: A large, broadly trained model that serves as a base for fine-tuning across a wide range of downstream applications.
Generative AI: A class of AI systems that create new content—such as text, images, audio, or video—based on patterns learned from large datasets.
HIPAA (Health Insurance Portability and Accountability Act): U.S. legislation governing the privacy and security of PHI.
Large language model (LLM): A type of foundation model trained on vast text datasets to understand and generate human language for tasks such as explanation, summarization, and dialogue.
Multimodal model: A model capable of processing and generating across multiple data types (e.g., text, image, audio, and video).
Natural language processing (NLP): The field of AI focused on enabling computers to understand, interpret, and generate human language.
Objective structured clinical examination (OSCE): A standardized assessment method for evaluating clinical, procedural, and communication skills in medical education.
OpenEvidence: An LLM designed specifically for the medical domain.
Protected Health Information (PHI): Individually identifiable health data regulated under HIPAA to ensure patient privacy and data security.
Retrieval-Augmented Generation (RAG): An approach that enhances model accuracy by retrieving trusted source material and conditioning generated responses on it.
Shadow library: An unauthorized online repository that distributes copyrighted academic or literary works without permission from rights holders.
Standardized patient (SP): A trained actor or simulated patient used in medical education to provide realistic clinical encounters for assessment and feedback.
Transformer Architecture: A neural network design introduced in 2017 that enables efficient processing of sequential data and serves as the foundation for most modern LLMs.
USMLE (United States Medical Licensing Examination): A multistep examination sequence required for medical licensure in the United States.
Virtual Reality (VR): Fully immersive digital environments used for clinical simulation, procedural training, and experiential learning.

ABBREVIATIONS

AAMC	Association of American Medical Colleges
ACGME	Accreditation Council for Graduate Medical Education
ACLS	advanced cardiac life support
AI	artificial intelligence
AR	augmented reality
BAA	business associate agreement
EPA	entrustable professional activity
GPT-4	generative pretrained transformer 4
HIPAA	Health Insurance Portability and Accountability Act
ICEMS	Intelligent Continuous Expertise Monitoring System
LCME	Liaison Committee on Medical Education
LLM	large language model
NBME	National Board of Medical Examiners
NLP	natural language processing

OSCE	objective structured clinical examination
PDF	portable document format
PHI	protected health information
RAG	retrieval-augmented generation
SP	standardized patient
USMLE	United States Medical Licensing Examination
VR	virtual reality

REFERENCES

[1] Ronge R, Maier M, Rathgeber B. Towards a definition of generative artificial intelligence. *Philosophy & Technology*. 2025 Mar;38(1):31. Available from: https://link.springer.com/10.1007/s13347-025-00863-y.

[2] He R, Cao J, Tan T. Generative artificial intelligence: A historical perspective. *National Science Review*. 2025 Apr;12(5):nwaf050. Available from: https://academic.oup.com/nsr/article/doi/10.1093/nsr/nwaf050/8029900.

[3] Weizenbaum J. ELIZA—A computer program for the study of natural language communication between man and machine. *Communications of the ACM*. 1966 Jan;9(1):36–45. Association for Computing Machinery, New York, NY, USA. Available from: https://doi.org/10.1145/365153.365168.

[4] OpenEvidence is now HIPAA compliant. *OpenEvidence*; 2025. Available from: https://www.openevidence.com/announcements/openevidence-and-nejm.

[5] OpenEvidence and the JAMA Network sign strategic content agreement. *Journal of American Medical Association*. 2025. Available from: https://media.jamanetwork.com/announcement/openevidence-and-the-jama-network-sign-strategic-content-agreement/.

[6] OpenEvidence and NEJM Group, publisher of the New England Journal of Medicine, sign content agreement. *OpenEvidence*; 2025. Available from: https://www.openevidence.com/announcements/openevidence-and-nejm.

[7] Zhang JS, Yoon C, Williams DKA, Pinkas A. Exploring the usage of ChatGPT among medical students in the United States. *Journal of Medical Education and Curricular Development*. 2024 Jan;11. SAGE Publications. Available from: https://journals.sagepub.com/doi/10.1177/23821205241264695.

[8] Ganjavi C, Eppler M, O'Brien D, Ramacciotti LS, Ghauri MS, Anderson I, et al. ChatGPT and large language models (LLMs) awareness and use. A prospective cross-sectional survey of U.S. medical students. Badawi O, editor. *PLOS Digital Health*. 2024 Sep 5;3(9):e0000596.

[9] Pardos ZA, Bhandari S. ChatGPT-generated help produces learning gains equivalent to human tutor-authored help on mathematics skills. *PLOS ONE*. 2024 May;19(5):e0304013. Available from: https://dx.plos.org/10.1371/journal.pone.0304013.

[10] Hake J, Crowley M, Coy A, Shanks D, Eoff A, Kirmer-Voss K, et al. Quality, accuracy, and bias in ChatGPT-based summarization of medical abstracts. *The Annals of Family Medicine*. 2024 Mar;22(2):113–120. Available from: http://www.annfammed.org/lookup/doi/10.1370/afm.3075.

[11] Pickard-Jones B, Short F. *Mindful mnemonics: Revolutionizing learning with AI-generated mnemonics. Towards AI Literacy: 101+ Creative and Critical Practices, Perspectives and Purposes*. 2024 Jun; p. 154–155. Available from: https://zenodo.org/doi/10.5281/zenodo.11613520.

[12] Elabd N, Rahman ZM, Abu Alinnin SI, Jahan S, Campos LA, Baltatu OC. Designing personalized multimodal mnemonics with AI: A medical student's implementation tutorial. *JMIR Medical Education*. 2025 May;11:e67926–e67926. Available from: https://mededu.jmir.org/2025/1/e67926.

[13] Learvo. Available from: https://www.learvo.com/.
[14] Anki. Available from: https://apps.ankiweb.net/.
[15] Pendergrast T, Chalmers Z. Anki Tagger: A Generative AI tool for aligning third-party resources to preclinical curriculum. *JMIR Medical Education*. 2023 Sep;9:e48780. Available from: https://mededu.jmir.org/2023/1/e48780.
[16] Rädel-Ablass K, Schliz K, Schlick C, Meindl B, Pahr-Hosbach S, Schwendemann H, et al. Teaching opportunities for anamnesis interviews through AI based teaching role plays: a survey with online learning students from health study programs. *BMC Medical Education*. 2025 Feb;25(1):259. Available from: https://bmcmededuc.biomedcentral.com/articles/10.1186/s12909-025-06756-0.
[17] Yamamoto A, Koda M, Ogawa H, Miyoshi T, Maeda Y, Otsuka F, et al. Enhancing medical interview skills through AI-simulated patient interactions: Nonrandomized Controlled Trial. *JMIR Medical Education*. 2024 Sep;10:e58753. Available from: https://mededu.jmir.org/2024/1/e58753.
[18] Kung TH, Cheatham M, Medenilla A, Sillos C, De Leon L, Elepaño C, et al. Performance of ChatGPT on USMLE: Potential for AI-assisted medical education using large language models. *PLOS Digital Health*. 2023 Feb;2(2):e0000198. Available from: https://dx.plos.org/10.1371/journal.pdig.0000198.
[19] Garabet R, Mackey BP, Cross J, Weingarten M. ChatGPT-4 performance on USMLE step 1 style questions and its implications for medical education: A comparative study across systems and disciplines. *Medical Science Educator*. 2023 Dec;34(1):145–152. Available from: https://link.springer.com/10.1007/s40670-023-01956-z.
[20] *AI-Based Literature Review Tools*. Texas A&M University; 2025. Available from: https://tamu.libguides.com/c.php?g=1289555.
[21] Taneja K, Maiti P, Kakar S, Guruprasad P, Rao S, Goel AK. *Jill Watson: A Virtual Teaching Assistant Powered by ChatGPT*. arXiv; 2024. ArXiv:2405.11070 [cs]. Available from: http://arxiv.org/abs/2405.11070.
[22] Boyle P. AI in medical education: 5 ways schools are employing new tools. *AAMCNews*. 2025 Feb. Available from: https://www.aamc.org/news/ai-medical-education-5-ways-schools-are-employing-new-tools.
[23] Peralta Ramirez AA, Trujillo López S, Navarro Armendariz GA, De La Torre Oth´on SA, Sierra Cervantes MR, Medina Aguirre JA. Clinical simulation with ChatGpt: A revolution in medical education? *Journal of CME*. 2025 Dec;14(1):2525615. Available from: https://www.tandfonline.com/doi/full/10.1080/28338073.2025.2525615.
[24] Hicke Y, Geathers J, Rajashekar N, Chan C, Jack AG, Sewell J, et al. *MedSimAI: Simulation and Formative Feedback Generation to Enhance Deliberate Practice in Medical Education*. arXiv; 2025. ArXiv:2503.05793 [cs]. Available from: http://arxiv.org/abs/2503.05793.
[25] Waldron P. Medical students use AI to practice communication skills. *Cornell Chronicle*. 2025 Mar. Available from: https://news.cornell.edu/stories/2025/03/medical-students-use-ai-practice-communication-skills.
[26] Yilmaz R, Winkler-Schwartz A, Mirchi N, Reich A, Christie S, Tran DH, et al. Continuous monitoring of surgical bimanual expertise using deep neural networks in virtual reality simulation. *npj Digital Medicine*. 2022 Apr;5(1):54. Available from: https://www.nature.com/articles/s41746-022-00596-8.
[27] Cooley A, Walji M, Martinez E, Fenton S. *AI Literacy and Education*; 2025. Available from: https://www.utsystem.edu/ai-symposium.

[28] Maleki N, Padmanabhan B, Dutta K. AI hallucinations: A misnomer worth clarifying. In: *2024 IEEE Conference on Artificial Intelligence (CAI)*. Singapore, Singapore: IEEE; 2024. p. 133–138. Available from: https://ieeexplore.ieee.org/document/10605268/.

[29] Jones N. AI hallucinations can't be stopped—But these techniques can limit their damage. *Nature*. 2025 Jan;637(8047):778–780. Available from: https://www.nature.com/articles/d41586-025-00068-5.

[30] Kalai AT, Nachum O, Vempala SS, Zhang E. *Why Language Models Hallucinate*. arXiv; 2025. Version Number: 1. Available from: https://arxiv.org/abs/2509.04664.

[31] Low YS, Jackson ML, Hyde RJ, Brown RE, Sanghavi NM, Baldwin JD, et al. Answering real-world clinical questions using large language model, retrieval-augmented generation, and agentic systems. *Digital Health*. 2025 May;11:20552076251348850. Available from: https://journals.sagepub.com/doi/10.1177/20552076251348850.

[32] Jose B, Cherian J, Verghis AM, Varghise SM, S M, Joseph S. The cognitive paradox of AI in education: Between enhancement and erosion. *Frontiers in Psychology*. 2025 Apr;16:1550621. Available from: https://www.frontiersin.org/articles/10.3389/fpsyg.2025.1550621/full.

[33] Macnamara BN, Berber I, Çavuşoğlu MC, Krupinski EA, Nallapareddy N, Nelson NE, et al. Does using artificial intelligence assistance accelerate skill decay and hinder skill development without performers' awareness? *Cognitive Research: Principles and Implications*. 2024 Jul;9(1):46. Available from: https://cognitiveresearchjournal.springeropen.com/articles/10.1186/s41235-024-00572-8.

[34] Gerlich M. AI tools in society: Impacts on cognitive offloading and the future of critical thinking. *Societies*. 2025 Jan;15(1):6. Available from: https://www.mdpi.com/2075-4698/15/1/6.

[35] Zhai C, Wibowo S, Li LD. The effects of over-reliance on AI dialogue systems on students' cognitive abilities: A systematic review. *Smart Learning Environments*. 2024 Jun;11(1):28. Available from: https://slejournal.springeropen.com/articles/10.1186/s40561-024-00316-7.

[36] Zack T, Lehman E, Suzgun M, Rodriguez JA, Celi LA, Gichoya J, et al. Assessing the potential of GPT-4 to perpetuate racial and gender biases in health care: A model evaluation study. *The Lancet Digital Health*. 2024 Jan;6(1):e12–e22. Available from: https://linkinghub.elsevier.com/retrieve/pii/S258975002300225X.

[37] Hastings J. Preventing harm from non-conscious bias in medical generative AI. *The Lancet Digital Health*. 2024 Jan;6(1):e2–e3. Available from: https://linkinghub.elsevier.com/retrieve/pii/S2589750023002467.

[38] Brittain B, Scarcella M. Anthropic agrees to pay $1.5 billion to settle author class action. *Reuters*. 2025 Sep. Available from: https://www.reuters.com/sustainability/boards-policy-regulation/anthropic-agrees-pay-15-billion-settle-author-class-action-2025-09-05/.

[39] Marks M, Haupt CE. AI chatbots, health privacy, and challenges to HIPAA compliance. *JAMA*. 2023 Jul;330(4):309. Available from: https://jamanetwork.com/journals/jama/fullarticle/2807170.

[40] Alawneh YJJ, Sleema H, Salman FN, Alshammat MF, Oteer RS, ALrashidi NKN. Adaptive learning systems: Revolutionizing higher education through AI-driven curricula. In: *2024 International Conference on Knowledge Engineering and Communication Systems (ICKECS)*. Chikkaballapur, India: IEEE; 2024. p. 1–5. Available from: https://ieeexplore.ieee.org/document/10616675/.

[41] Cagas W, Ko C, Hsiao B, Grandhi S, Bhattacharya R, Zhu K, et al. *Medical Imaging Complexity and Its Effects on GAN Performance*. arXiv; 2024. ArXiv:2410.17959 [eess]. Available from: http://arxiv.org/abs/2410.17959.

[42] Koljonen V. What could we make of AI in plastic surgery education. *Journal of Plastic, Reconstructive & Aesthetic Surgery*. 2023 Jun;81:94–96. Available from: https://linkinghub.elsevier.com/retrieve/pii/S174868152300205X.

[43] Hofmeijer E. *This Is Not a Real Image: Generative Artificial Intelligence to Enhance Radiology Education* [PhD Thesis—Research UT, graduation UT]. University of Twente. Netherlands; 2024.

[44] Chu SN, Goodell AJ. *Synthetic Patients: Simulating Difficult Conversations with Multimodal Generative AI for Medical Education*. arXiv; 2024. ArXiv:2405.19941 [cs]. Available from: http://arxiv.org/abs/2405.19941.

[45] Kyeremeh J, Asciak L, Blackmur JP, Luo X, Picard F, Shu W, et al. Digital twins assisted surgery: A conceptual framework for transforming surgical training and navigation. *The Surgeon*. 2025 Sep; p. S1479666X2500143X. Available from: https://linkinghub.elsevier.com/retrieve/pii/S1479666X2500143X.

[46] Ambrose A. *AR/VR's Potential in Health Care*. Information Technology & Innovation Foundation; 2025. Available from: https://itif.org/publications/2025/06/02/arvrs-potential-in-health-care/.

3 Teaching Empathy in the Era of AI

"Someday We'll Find It, The Human Connection. The Patient, the Computer, and Me"

Poonam Hosamani

A first-year medical student, fresh from having learned the framework of the medical interview, was practicing taking a history with a "real" patient in the simulated setting of a patient exam room. The student had been well-versed on how to conduct the history while building rapport and had been particularly coached on the appropriate responses in the family history, especially in how to respond when a patient disclosed the death of a close relative. When the student asked about the patient's mother, the patient sadly but with notable pride relayed that her mother had recently passed away at a very advanced age. The student, almost as a reflex from their recent feedback said, "I'm sorry to hear that." The patient seemed perplexed in that moment, stopping to consider what reaction she had been hoping for and what had been given. She kindly told the student that she was happy that her mother had lived such a long and full life and that there was no reason to be sorry. The student sheepishly apologized, again, this time for hearing the patient but not listening.

A senior resident, during an introductory session about AI and the novel applications that were already being implemented in the electronic medical record (EMR) raised their hand in excitement. "I was noticing that when I was responding to a patient message the other day, the response that was auto-generated seemed so much nicer than I would have written." There was a chuckle among the rest of the crowd, perhaps a recognition and appreciation that when our own abilities to be empathic are at their lowest, AI can help pull the extra weight to ensure the therapeutic alliance is maintained. Perhaps the response was one of agreement, that AI may be better in some ways in displaying empathy than humans.

In another encounter, a senior physician, upon trialing a similar auto-generated patient inbox message system, stated their annoyance that the responses sounded so unlike their normal tone and that their patients would immediately know that the response had not been generated by the physician who had been caring for them for many years and might make them wary of the advice provided.

The process of cultivating and maintaining empathy has long been a focus of the educational mission of physicians and healthcare professionals. It is a priority of medical schools to recruit those who display natural empathic tendencies. The mission of preclinical medical educators is to promote the application of empathy and compassion in clinical encounters. Clerkship directors and those who work with trainees in the graduate medical education (GME) space are tasked with not only fostering the demonstration of empathy but also preventing the degradation of empathy due to stress and burnout. It is in these same domains where AI may be able to augment these processes. There is an economic and quality benefit to empathy and compassion that should also be considered, especially as it relates to the development and implementation of expensive technological tools. The critical mission of educators will be to keep AI advances from encroaching upon the sanctity of the physician–patient relationship and to define the bounds through which AI can advance the training of practicing and future physicians.

DOI: 10.1201/9781003617167-3

3.1 DEFINITIONS OF EMPATHY AND COMPASSION IN CLINICAL PRACTICE

The assertion that empathy and compassion are foundational to medical practice is incontrovertible. The exact definitions and components of these characteristics are necessary to not only further understand how to nurture them but also understand the ways in which different teaching modalities, technology-based or otherwise, may contribute to their instruction. Empathy can be defined through many different lenses. One that lends itself to technological assistance is the description that Larson and Yao[1] developed based on a term coined by Hochschild:[2] "emotional labor." Larson and Yao describe how providers can provide empathic responses to patients by engaging in both a cognitive processing of the interaction and an affective component to express empathy to patients. They go further to describe the affective process in terms of types of acting, outlining surface acting and deep acting as sequential types of response building. *Surface acting* refers to external facial, verbal, and nonverbal cues that may be selectively chosen to respond in the situation. *Deep acting* refers to a change in attitude that may presumably lead to a more nuanced response. The idea of acting as being central to the display of empathy could lead to the assertion that this response is inauthentic. An additional perspective on the definition of empathy may be considered based on the work of Zaki and Ochsner,[3] which defines the act of experience sharing as the initial partnering in an encounter, mentalizing as the affective component in understanding the others' perspective. Their work includes an additional component of prosocial concern, or the desire to act on the empathy in order to provide aid. It is likely that this reflects many of the qualities medical schools try to identify in their admissions processes.

One model of compassion as it applies to medicine is based on the work of Sinclair et al., saying that compassion could be defined as "a virtuous response that seeks to address the suffering and needs of a person through relational understanding and action."[4] This can be further expanded based on a survey to measure patient perceptions of physician compassion, which found that the display of compassion seemed distinct from even strong communication skills, implying that there may be some intangible component to how patients perceive empathy.[5] It is fascinating to consider expanding further on this indefinable component and how we may further try to bring clarity to this dimension and how it could be defined not only in physician components but also in the ways patients may receive these interactions. It is almost impossible to separate the two, as they are so reliant on each other in a sophisticated dance of physician and patient interactions.

3.2 CURRENT STATE OF CLINICAL EMPATHY TRAINING

The current state of empathy training in medical schools relies on the notion that natural empathic tendencies can be further honed and refined for clinical practice. This is typically done through a variety of evidence-based teaching modalities. The most common methods used for empathy training are role-play and simulation with standardized patients, small group reflection and discussion, guided reflection, and didactics.[6] The influx of the humanities into empathy training has certainly led to a greater appreciation of how a deep understanding of the human condition can enhance the practice of medicine. Dr. Rita Charon eloquently describes the critical role of narratives in the development of the physician–patient relationship.[7] She explains that the entire foundation of the medical interview is based on eliciting a story, building in the elements of differential diagnosis and clinical reasoning, then developing a therapeutic plan or alliance with the patient. All the subsequent actions draw from the initial story that is obtained.

The anecdote at the beginning of this chapter comes to mind as we apply these frameworks of empathy and compassion to early medical training. Most medical schools participate in clinical skills training that emphasizes the role of communication, both verbal and nonverbal, as well as rapport building. As an example, when eliciting the family history, students are introduced to the types of information that would have clinical relevance and are introduced to the types of questions that are asked to procure this information. When we consider the questions that are asked and what the responses may be, this goes beyond what most students will have experienced in their daily lives. Even if they have had significant clinical exposure prior to matriculation into medical school, they were unlikely to have been in a position where they were directly asking questions of patients. Inquiry into some of the most painful moments of a person's life, such as the illness or death of close family members, should be recognized as a high-level skill, though most in medical education would consider it a bare minimum. It should be recognized that strong rapport and eventual trust can be built in the most routine conversations, upon which the rest of the encounter and patient–physician relationship are built.

The different frameworks of empathy lend themselves to being dissected into their components followed by developing strategies for teaching, cultivation, and maintenance. The many modalities to accomplish these goals represent different learning styles and varying uses of technology. One of the earliest and arguably most effective ways of cultivating empathy in early learners is through simulation of patient encounters with standardized patients. Often, these encounters are introduced with scripted responses to give students examples of how rapport can be built, and empathy can be expressed during the more sensitive topics of the patient interview such as the family or social history. Eliciting this information from another individual is often a novel skill for many early learners, and the ability to remember the frameworks of questions while also connecting with a prospective patient to build trust and rapport can be challenging. Scripted responses can often relieve the mental load of generating authentic responses as students internalize patient history frameworks. In addition, multisource feedback is often an integral part of these encounters. The ability to receive structured, high-quality, constructive feedback on communication skills is a cornerstone of this modality of teaching.[8] This type of clinical skills training can be essential. A systematic review of empathy training curricula was able to identify five key behaviors as being most effective: (1) being seated during the interview; (2) detecting nonverbal cues; (3) identifying and responding to opportunities for compassion; (4) nonverbal communication of compassion; and (5) verbal statements of support and validation.

Complementary methodologies of teaching include incorporating the humanities into medicine. Guided reflection has been known to be an effective strategy for promotion of empathy. It can be particularly effective for early learners to help them digest early exposures to patients, empathize with the situations of patients, and think about how they can participate but also about how teams work together to deliver patient care.[9]

Technology has created a fascinating dichotomy that may both enhance as well as limit the ability of educators, administrators, and clinicians to promote empathy and compassion in clinical practice. Even prior to the advent of AI, there were many studies demonstrating the efficacy of technology in training learners in healthcare fields on essential communication skills. These studies emphasized the ability to provide opportunities to do simulation and role-play to practice communication skills and to identify opportunities for improvement and participate in exercises to promote more fulfilling patient interactions in the clinical space.[10] The use of virtual reality to immerse students in different clinical conditions has been shown to lead to a noticeable increase in empathy levels.[11, 12] This is an interesting modification of the empathy paradigm that is rooted in the fact that, despite not experiencing the same symptoms, the physician can still cognitively relate to how the patient might be feeling. The ability to then actually experience, even if temporarily, what a patient may be experiencing, allows for that cognitive process to be even more grounded. At the same time, technological advances, such as the electronic health record, among many others, have been at the forefront of discussions about creating distance in the provider–patient interaction.

The power of the human connection in the physician–patient encounter is still retained, even as technology continues to advance and at times push us in opposite directions.[13] As we embark upon this next major revolution in medical training, we must consider how to utilize these tools to enhance and augment the processes known to cultivate and maintain empathy rather than having these tools replace the critical human connection.

3.3 BARRIERS TO EMPATHIC CARE

The pressures placed on physicians in modern-day practice are numerous. Some that seem to cause the highest levels of burnout are the increasing workload, high documentation and clerical burden, and lack of efficient processes.[14] The move toward increasing demands on providers' time is at the root of the issue and often leads to the shift of the care that is provided from one that is built on a relationship to one that becomes transactional. Instead of the focus of an encounter being the development of rapport and trust, it instead turns into a litany of checkboxes, alerts, and lengthy notes that need to be completed prior to closing an encounter and moving to the next patient. The pursuit of metrics in the name of quality is often the same causes of burnout of the provider and dissatisfaction from the patient, which then lead to worse care and increased dissatisfaction from patients.[15] When these come to a head, it is often when communication breakdowns occur, and the empathy of physicians is tested. The moral injury of attempting to provide care under less-than-ideal circumstances is often what leads to more negative interactions between providers and patients.

One widely observed and well-studied trend is that of the empathy decline that occurs for physicians over time. Some of the steepest declines happen over the course of medical school education, particularly upon entry into clerkships.[16] This decline is unfortunately continually observed over residency training as well with many potential hypotheses.[17] Many of the cited reasons for struggles with empathy include generalized distress from long work hours and high clinical workload, limited social support, mistreatment by superiors, and challenging learning environments, among many others. Interestingly, discontinuity of care has also been brought up at times as a cause of burnout, though one of the reasons for this has been the desire to limit work hours and create more reasonable work hour strategies. The strategies of how to overcome this decline and restore empathy are widely present in the literature. These strategies emphasize the role of simulation or role-play activities, reinforcement on narrative medicine and the humanities, and encouragement of mindfulness and gratitude practices.

It is conceivable that in the face of these challenges, one could postulate that replacement of more of the arduous physician responsibilities with AI could lead to improvements in morale and empathy scores. However, when asked about their preferences, a study performed in German-speaking nations showed that patients generally preferred a human doctor over a human doctor using AI or AI alone.[18] In another study on perspectives of a multinational group of hospitalized patients, while the general perception of AI was positive, this differed significantly based on gender, health status, and familiarity with technology, showing that there is not a generalizable perspective on the use of AI. This study did show that decision-making led by physicians was preferred by most. Given the current data, we can hypothesize that the excessive and increasing workload placed on physicians causes strains on empathy and the physician–patient relationship but that, when presented with an alternative, the human aspect of care is still preferred by patients. It is therefore incumbent on us to define the bounds of AI capabilities to not encroach on the areas of practice that patients and physicians value the most, while guiding AI efforts to tasks that have less importance to the physician–patient relationship.

3.4 AI AS A TOOL TO IMPROVE EMPATHY IN CLINICAL PRACTICE

The emergence of AI as a tool has reframed how technology can impact clinical practice. The applications are numerous, and the potential for implementation is being discussed at every level of the clinical care process. The implications for the role it could play in empathy are strongest in areas where the tasks, as described previously, that cause burnout can be outsourced to AI tools to reduce the clerical or documentation burden. In the outpatient setting, early studies showed that despite no difference in time spent, there were reports of reduction in burnout and exhaustion after the implementation of AI tools to draft responses to patient inbox messages.[19] One of the more intriguing aspects of this particular intervention is that, in addition to potentially reducing burdensome tasks for physicians, AI-generated responses to patient messages were perceived as being more empathic[20]—an interesting observation validated by the resident in the anecdote at the beginning of the chapter. Could AI create an "empathy safety net" of sorts that allows for the maintenance of strong relationships, even when physicians are under stress?

As it relates to the documentation burden within the EMR, the results at this point remain mixed, but this is a rapidly evolving area. The hope for AI tools is that auto-generating more of the perceived time-consuming aspects of documentation will reduce clinician time spent on EMR, enhance time spent with patients during the encounter, and reduce overall feelings of burnout. The results of studies so far are inconclusive but reveal rapidly changing outcomes as the technology improves. One such innovation includes ambient AI tools that can listen to conversations between physicians and patients and generate summaries as well as many components of the written note. Some early studies with ambient AI technologies showed overall reduction in the mental demand, rushed pace, and effort to write notes, although the reduction in mean time spent writing notes was less than 1 minute.[21] Interestingly, in this same study, there were significant differences in the impact between female and male physicians, where the implementation of ambient AI technology led to a larger decrease in time spent per note for female physicians, though they seemed to start with an average time per note spent that was higher than their male counterparts. Similarly, primary care physicians experienced more satisfaction with this tool than medical subspecialty or surgical colleagues, with some suggestions that the ability to adapt to more nuanced specialty-specific details and formats would be appreciated from the AI tools. A separate study of the use of AI scribes showed a similar minor reduction of per encounter documentation time. However, when compounded, AI led to a notable decrease in median daily time in the EMR and, even more importantly, a significant reduction in after-hours EMR use.[22] Many of these early studies show incredible promise but need more widespread adoption to determine their full impact.

As the capabilities of AI continue to evolve, the role of value being added for physicians in healthcare delivery will need to be carefully defined. Indeed, this will need to be clearly elucidated by both physicians and other healthcare providers in the delivery of healthcare, as well as by patients as the recipients. Though the abilities of AI show that it can express adequate and at time superior forms of empathy, it is just that—artificial. Anat Perry describes this as the artificial empathy paradox and that, because the nature of empathy makes it a limited resource, subject to fatigue, burnout, and bias, it has more value.[23] In order to continue to retain its inherent value, educators must make it their mission to emphasize its importance as the basis of the successful delivery of medical care and teach it as such in the medical curriculum.

3.5 AI IN MEDICAL EDUCATION

Acknowledging the central role for the teaching of empathy, it is essential to consider ways we can leverage technology to complement the strategies we know to be evidence-based in this mission. The most apparent use is to create opportunities for learners to practice their communication skills with AI-based simulations. Human-based simulations (standardized and simulated patient actors) comprise a limited resource, require an extensive training process, and are costly. AI-based simulations may provide additional opportunities for learners to practice encounters and for educators to create variations on different aspects of the scenarios to expose students to increased levels of complexity. This gives learners many additional opportunities to test their own skill development and potentially even personally challenge themselves with simulated encounters prior to entering clerkships or clinical practice. It would also allow for a greater degree of personalization of encounters to address the learner's particular improvement areas in a manner that would otherwise be incredibly time and resource intensive to do in a human-simulated setting. AI-based simulation may be equally beneficial for experienced providers as a part of a remediation or clinical improvement process, particularly for those experiencing burnout. The current studies note that the AI technology to simulate realistic and hallucination-free simulations are limited, but this is evolving rapidly.[24]

In addition to actual participation in these simulated activities, AI provides tremendous opportunity to provide formative feedback based on previously validated rubrics and frameworks for compassionate communication techniques. Feedback is critical to the learning process for both students and trainees at all levels, but the process is often challenging on both sides in terms of time needed, specificity, and personalization.[25] When comparing AI to human feedback for a written assignment, students generally preferred the human feedback over AI for its relevance and clarity, among other features, but also reported that the two types of feedback were complementary.[26] AI tools have the ability to perform audio and video analysis to give actionable feedback on communication skills and nonverbal cues. This capability may allow for better implementation of this effective teaching modality to more resource-limited settings and reduce the burden of educators, who may then have greater bandwidth to provide more personalized coaching when needed.

This type of coaching can certainly extend to clerkship students, residents, fellows, and even practicing physicians as well, with AI systems being able to provide individualized guidance on how to approach more challenging conversations or encounters. There are clinical training opportunities where these conversations can be anticipated and can benefit from advanced preparation.[27] The most apparent example would be in a goals of care discussion or in the sharing of difficult news. One could imagine a system in which any student or physician could include the details of the case and use it to gain different communication frameworks and strategies to address the challenges.

Though we have described frameworks of empathy as an emotionally laborious process, it is still at its core the heart of medical care. We understand that even with potential replacements, patients prefer human empathy.[28] We also know that physicians gain greater satisfaction, meaning, and purpose from establishing deep connections with patients, what Suchman and Matthews define as the "connexional" dimension of care, long before many of these technological advances infiltrated medicine.[29] This dimension of care is described as a foundation of medical care and allows for the opportunity to transcend more difficult situations, such as terminal illnesses or when there is more diagnostic uncertainty. These abilities should be centered and celebrated, and the use of technology should be to preserve and enhance the sanctity of this connection, not detract from it.

As with all considerations of ways in which AI will impact medical education and clinical practice, providing and establishing an equitable approach through these systems will be paramount. There are data to show that certain groups may perceive less empathy during clinical encounters than others.[30] We know that these differences in empathy not only impact the patient emotionally but also lead to worse outcomes such as under- or misdiagnosis, undertreatment, and poor quality of care. It is in this space where AI should be leveraged to improve ways in which care is provided to vulnerable groups. Advances such as incorporation of diagnostic algorithms into telemedicine visits can vastly reduce the time to diagnosis for patients in remote communities.[31] Machine learning algorithms can also be fine-tuned to incorporate social determinants of health that may impact marginalized groups, allowing for more personalized treatment plans and better outcomes.[32] Though there is potential for improving equity and access, the danger of perpetuating bias through these systems is not to be ignored and should be studied extensively.[33] It is in these dangerous situations where empathy can serve as a check on the potential harms from algorithmic-based care. It is a fascinating double-edged sword that strict algorithmic-based decision-making can both prevent and perpetuate inequity and that, with proper training, empathy can be the protective shield.

It is in this capacity that medical educators should be imploring technology companies to create products and tools that meet *their* needs and not simply try to be the recipients of products looking for a problem to solve. It is incumbent on educators to define the bounds of what role AI has in an education curriculum and to continually reinforce to students and trainees that it is their presence that brings empathy alive in the encounter. With the promises of efficiency and accessibility that many of these AI tools advertise, it is critical to take advantage of a tremendous opportunity to reclaim the connection with patients, to enhance the ways we communicate and to elevate the human element of patient care.

3.6 CONCLUSION

As we embark on this next phase of medical training in an even more digitally connected and dependent society, it is imperative not only that educators continue to define the tenets of clinical education and skills development but that we role-model that these can be done together with advancing technologies. The rejection of these technologies and the attachment to "the days of the giants" or "the golden age of medicine" might alienate early learners who see the seamless integration of emerging technologies into clinical care as non-negotiable. It will be the physicians and educators who leverage technology to improve the quality of care we deliver to our patients and who effectively role-model how this can be done while retaining the essence of the patient–physician relationship.

GLOSSARY

Connexional dimension of care: Defined by Drs. Suchman and Matthews as the dimension of deep personal connection that is critical to the physician–patient experience.

Family history: A component of the standard medical interview that includes questions regarding a patient's family health history.

Standardized patients: Highly trained individuals who work with different groups of healthcare professionals to simulate patient and medical encounters for the purposes of education and training.

ABBREVIATIONS

AI Artificial intelligence
EMR Electronic medical record
GME Graduate medical education

REFERENCES

1 Larson EB, Yao X. Clinical empathy as emotional labor in the patient–physician relationship. *JAMA.* 2005;293(9):1100–6. https://doi.org/10.1001/jama.293.9.1100

2 Hochschild AR. *The managed heart: Commercialization of human feeling.* Berkeley: University of California Press; 1983.

3 Zaki J, Ochsner K. The neuroscience of empathy: Progress, pitfalls and promise. *Nat Neurosci.* 2012;15:675–80. https://doi.org/10.1038/nn.3085

4 Sinclair S, Beamer K, Hack TF, McClement S, Raffin Bouchal S, Chochinov HM, et al. Compassion in health care: An empirical model. *J Pain Symptom Manage.* 2016;51(2):193–203. https://doi.org/10.1016/j.jpainsymman.2015.10.009

5 Roberts BW, Roberts MB, Yao J, Bosire J, Mazzarelli A, Trzeciak S. Development and validation of a tool to measure patient assessment of clinical compassion. *JAMA Netw Open.* 2019;2(5):e193976. https://doi.org/10.1001/jamanetworkopen.2019.3976

6 Patel S, Pelletier-Bui A, Smith S, Roberts MB, Kilgannon H, Trzeciak S, et al. Curricula for empathy and compassion training in medical education: A systematic review. *PLoS One.* 2019;14(8):e0221412. https://doi.org/10.1371/journal.pone.0221412

7 Charon R. The patient–physician relationship. Narrative medicine: A model for empathy, reflection, profession, and trust. *JAMA.* 2001;286(15):1897–902. https://doi.org/10.1001/jama.286.15.1897

8 Byrne M, Campos C, Daly S, Lok B, Miles A. The current state of empathy, compassion and person-centered communication training in healthcare: An umbrella review. *Patient Educ Couns.* 2024;119:108063. https://doi.org/10.1016/j.pec.2023.108063

9 Savitha, D, Anto T, Tv S. Introducing reflective narrative for first-year medical students to promote empathy as an integral part of physiology curriculum. *Adv Physiol Educ.* 2021;45(2):207–16. https://doi.org/10.1152/advan.00206.2020

10 Chua JYX, Ang E, Lau STL, Shorey S. Effectiveness of simulation-based interventions at improving empathy among healthcare students: A systematic review and meta-analysis. *Nurse Educ Today.* 2021;104:105000. https://doi.org/10.1016/j.nedt.2021.105000

11 Dyer E, Swartzlander BJ, Gugliucci MR. Using virtual reality in medical education to teach empathy. *J Med Libr Assoc.* 2018;106(4):498–500. https://doi.org/10.5195/jmla.2018.518

12 Lin HL, Wang YC, Huang ML, Yu NW, Tang I, Hsu YC, et al. Can virtual reality technology be used for empathy education in medical students: A randomized case-control study. *BMC Med Educ*. 2024;24(1):1254. https://doi.org/10.1186/s12909-024-06009-6

13 Busch F, Hoffmann L, Xu L, Zhang LJ, Hu B, García-Juárez I, et al. Multinational attitudes toward AI in health care and diagnostics among hospital patients. *JAMA Netw Open*. 2025;8(6):e2514452. https://doi.org/10.1001/jamanetworkopen.2025.14452

14 West CP, Dyrbye LN, Shanafelt TD. Physician burnout: Contributors, consequences and solutions. *J Intern Med*. 2018;283(6):516–29. https://doi.org/10.1111/joim.12752

15 Hodkinson A, Zhou A, Johnson J, Geraghty K, Riley R, Panagopoulou E, et al. Associations of physician burnout with career engagement and quality of patient care: Systematic review and meta-analysis. *BMJ*. 2022;378:e070442. https://doi.org/10.1136/bmj-2022-070442

16 Hojat M, Vergare MJ, Maxwell K, Brainard G, Herrine SK, Isenberg GA, et al. The devil is in the third year: A longitudinal study of erosion of empathy in medical school. *Acad Med*. 2009;84(9):1182–91. https://doi.org/10.1097/ACM.0b013e3181b17e55

17 Neumann M, Edelhäuser F, Tauschel D, Fischer MR, Wirtz M, Woopen C, et al. Empathy decline and its reasons: A systematic review of studies with medical students and residents. *Acad Med*. 2011;86(8):996–1009. https://doi.org/10.1097/ACM.0b013e318221e615

18 Riedl R, Hogeterp SA, Reuter M. Do patients prefer a human doctor, artificial intelligence, or a blend, and is this preference dependent on medical discipline? Empirical evidence and implications for medical practice. *Front Psychol*. 2024;15:1422177. https://doi.org/10.3389/fpsyg.2024.1422177

19 Garcia P, Ma SP, Shah S, Smith M, Jeong Y, Devon-Sand A, et al. Artificial intelligence—Generated draft replies to patient inbox messages. *JAMA Netw Open*. 2024;7(3):e243201. https://doi.org/10.1001/jamanetworkopen.2024.3201

20 Small WR, Wiesenfeld B, Brandfield-Harvey B, Jonassen Z, Mandal S, Stevens ER, et al. Large language model–based responses to patients' in-basket messages. *JAMA Netw Open*. 2024;7(7):e2422399. https://doi.org/10.1001/jamanetworkopen.2024.22399

21 Stults CD, Deng S, Martinez MC, Wilcox J, Szwerinski N, Chen KH, et al. Evaluation of an ambient artificial intelligence documentation platform for clinicians. *JAMA Netw Open*. 2025;8(5):e258614. https://doi.org/10.1001/jamanetworkopen.2025.8614

22 Ma SP, Liang AS, Shah SJ, Smith M, Jeong Y, Devon-Sand A, et al. Ambient artificial intelligence scribes: Utilization and impact on documentation time. *J Am Med Inform Assoc*. 2025;32(2):381–5. https://doi.org/10.1093/jamia/ocae304

23 Perry A. AI will never convey the essence of human empathy. *Nat Hum Behav*. 2023;7:1808–9. https://doi.org/10.1038/s41562-023-01675-w

24 Sardesai N, Russo P, Martin J, Sardesai A. Utilizing generative conversational artificial intelligence to create simulated patient encounters: A pilot study for anaesthesia training. *Postgrad Med J*. 2024;100(1182):237–41. https://doi.org/10.1093/postmj/qgad137

25 Schopper H, Rosenbaum M, Axelson R. "I wish someone watched me interview:" Medical student insight into observation and feedback as a method for teaching communication skills during the clinical years. *BMC Med Educ*. 2016;16:286. https://doi.org/10.1186/s12909-016-0813-z

26 Ali M, Harbieh I, Haider KH. Bytes versus brains: A comparative study of AI-generated feedback and human tutor feedback in medical education. *Med Teach.* 2025 Jun 18. https://doi.org/10.1080/0142159X.2025.2519639

27 Chen JH. A physician's surprising encounter with ChatGPT. *Stanford Medicine.* 2023 Nov 10.

28 Rubin M, Li JZ, Zimmerman F, Ong DC, Goldenberg A, Perry A. Comparing the value of perceived human versus AI-generated empathy. *Nat Hum Behav.* 2025 Jun 30. https://doi.org/10.1038/s41562-025-02247-w

29 Suchman AL, Matthews DA. What makes the patient–doctor relationship therapeutic? Exploring the connexional dimension of medical care. *Ann Intern Med.* 1988;108:125–30. https://doi.org/10.7326/0003-4819-108-1-125

30 Roberts BW, Puri NK, Trzeciak CJ, Mazzarelli AJ, Trzeciak S. Socioeconomic, racial and ethnic differences in patient experience of clinician empathy: Results of a systematic review and meta-analysis. *PLoS One.* 2021;16(3):e0247259. https://doi.org/10.1371/journal.pone.0247259

31 Perez K, Wisniewski D, Ari A, Lee K, Lieneck C, Ramamonjiarivelo Z. Investigation into application of AI and telemedicine in rural communities: A systematic literature review. *Healthcare (Basel).* 2025;13(3):324. https://doi.org/10.3390/healthcare13030324

32 Srivastav AK, Singh A, Singh S, Rivers B, Lillard JW Jr, Singh R. Revolutionizing oncology through AI: Addressing cancer disparities by improving screening, treatment, and survival outcomes via integration of social determinants of health. *Cancers (Basel).* 2025;17(17):2866. https://doi.org/10.3390/cancers17172866

33 Seyyed-Kalantari L, Zhang H, McDermott MBA, Chen IY, Ghassemi M. Underdiagnosis bias of artificial intelligence algorithms applied to chest radiographs in under-served patient populations. *Nat Med.* 2021;27(12):2176–82. https://doi.org/10.1038/s41591-021-01595-0

4 Teaching Professionalism and Ethics in the Era of AI

Jasmine Chiat Ling Ong, Yilin Ning, Nan Liu

4.1 PART I: UNDERSTANDING ETHICAL REQUIREMENTS OF AI TOOLS

Ethics is a cornerstone of clinical practice and medical education. The four principles described by Beauchamp and Childress (1), namely beneficence, non-maleficence, autonomy, and justice, continue to guide how clinicians evaluate actions, decisions, and tools used in patient care. Beneficence and non-maleficence focus on promoting good and minimizing harm. Autonomy concerns supporting patients in making informed choices. Justice emphasizes fairness in distributing benefits, risks, and burdens.

As these principles are central to ethical healthcare practice, they are also important for evaluating any tools or technologies used to support care, including artificial intelligence (AI) systems. However, since these principles were originally framed around human actions and decisions, their interpretation in the context of AI is not always straightforward. Health AI introduces new actors into the clinical setting, may alter the traditional relationship between clinician and patient, and creates new ways of interacting with patient information and data that may expose patients to additional risks. For example, AI influences clinical reasoning, reshapes patient–clinician interactions, and relies heavily on sensitive data. These features create ethical challenges that are not fully covered under the traditional biomedical ethics principles. These challenges have expanded with newer technology such as large language models (LLMs) and generative AI, which can support a wide range of clinical and educational tasks but also require additional ethical principles and expectations intended to guide the responsible and trustworthy use of AI in healthcare (2).

The integration of health AI with clinical practice and medical training is inevitable. For clinicians, understanding these ethical considerations and their implications is important for a responsible integration. Ethical literacy allows clinicians to judge whether an AI tool is likely to benefit or harm patients, identify potential inequities or safety risks, and recognize when gaps in transparency or reliability may compromise care. It also prepares clinicians to participate meaningfully in decisions about selecting, implementing, and governing AI tools within their institutions.

In the following subsections, we introduce important ethical requirements for health AI, both familiar principles and newer concerns, organized into practical groups that reflect how these issues arise in clinical practice. Building on established ethical guidance from the World Health Organization (WHO) (3) and European Union (4) and on evidence synthesized from the generative AI literature (2), this section offers a pragmatic structure to help clinicians critically evaluate AI tools and anticipate potential risks.

4.2 BENEFICENCE AND NON-MALEFICENCE IN HEALTH AI

Traditionally, beneficence and non-maleficence describe clinicians' responsibilities to promote patients' well-being and to avoid causing harm. In the context of health AI, these duties extend to how AI systems are designed, how they perform, and how they interact with real clinical workflows. AI tools should not only generate accurate outputs but should also support clinical decisions in ways that genuinely improve patient care.

 DOI: 10.1201/9781003617167-4

Many applications of the health AI focus on disease diagnosis, treatment planning, or risk prediction. In such cases, incorrect predictions or poorly calibrated outputs can lead to suboptimal or harmful clinical actions, whereas accurate and timely predictions can facilitate interventions that improve patient outcomes. In recent years, LLMs have also been adopted for health-related tasks, such as summarizing clinical notes or answering health queries. Although LLMs can provide useful responses across a wide range of topics, their tendency to hallucinate (i.e., producing seemingly plausible yet inaccurate information) introduces risks that may compromise clinical decision-making or patient understanding.

To satisfy the requirements of beneficence and non-maleficence, AI outputs need to meet an acceptable standard of accuracy and reliability. For example, performance metrics such as accuracy, sensitivity, and specificity quantify how well a model predicts the outcome and help determine decision thresholds that balance the consequences of false positives and false negatives. Decision curve analysis offers a complementary approach by emphasizing clinical utility and comparing the net benefits derived from true positives against the harms associated with false positives (5). For LLMs, where outputs are free text and more difficult to evaluate, quality can be assessed through expert review or metrics that compare model outputs with expert-curated references (6).

Yet accurate or high-quality outputs alone are not enough to ensure that these principles are upheld. As highlighted by the GRADE guideline (7), real-world benefits should be evaluated through their impact on patient-important outcomes such as mortality, morbidity, and quality of life. For example, an AI model that reliably detects early-stage disease will not produce meaningful clinical benefit if no effective treatment exists at that stage. Moreover, in settings with limited human and financial resources, cost-effectiveness analysis is useful to determine whether the health gains achieved by an AI tool justify the resources required for its deployment.

Taken together, beneficence and non-maleficence in health AI require more than strong technical performance. They demand evidence that AI tools improve patient care, avoid preventable harms, and integrate safely into clinical practice. Clinicians need to understand these principles because they ultimately decide whether and how AI tools are used. Human oversight is requisite to evaluate AI output quality, anticipate real-world consequences, and judge whether an AI tool is likely to help or harm patients. This oversight is central to ensuring that AI contributes to ethical and responsible care.

4.3 PRIVACY AND SECURITY IN HEALTH AI

Beyond risks from inaccurate outputs, health AI can also expose patients to harm by compromising the privacy and security of their personal data. AI systems typically require large, detailed datasets to learn clinical patterns and generate reliable predictions. This demand increases substantially for deep learning models that analyze medical images or free-text clinical notes, and it is even more pronounced for modern LLMs. As data needs grow, so do the risks associated with collecting, storing, and processing sensitive patient information.

A common safeguard is data de-identification, which involves removing or masking information that could directly or indirectly reveal a patient's identity. Direct identifiers include names, national identification numbers, and hospital registration numbers, while indirect identifiers include time stamps, detailed locations, or rare occupations (e.g., one of the few neurosurgeons in a small region). Importantly, privacy regulations differ across jurisdictions. For example, the Health Insurance Portability and Accountability Act (HIPAA) in the United States and the General Data Protection Regulation (GDPR) in the European Union each set different requirements for what needs to be de-identified before data can be used for AI development. Clinicians therefore need to understand not only which data elements may reveal identity but also how local or regional regulations shape de-identification requirements when working with health AI.

Even when data are de-identified according to regulatory standards, privacy risks remain. Complex models that access rich, multisource datasets may still infer or reconstruct information that points to an individual. These risks are further amplified when AI tools operate on third-party cloud servers (such as proprietary LLMs) because patient data must leave the institution's secure environment for processing. In addition to risks from data handling, AI models (especially complex deep learning models) may inadvertently "memorize" fragments of the training data. In such cases, under certain prompts or conditions, the model might reproduce snippets resembling real patient records. This possibility highlights that protecting privacy should not rely solely on robust IT infrastructure but should also include safeguards within the model development process.

Several technical approaches can help strengthen privacy and security. For example, differential privacy introduces carefully designed noise into the data or model training process so that individual-level information is obscured without meaningfully harming model performance (8). When collaboration across institutions is needed, federated learning allows models to be trained locally within each institution so that only high-level model parameters (instead of raw patient data) are shared (9). Some regulations (e.g., the GDPR) go further by discouraging the reporting of exact statistics for very small patient groups to reduce the risk of re-identification. These practices illustrate the breadth of privacy-preserving strategies needed when working with increasingly granular health data.

Despite these safeguards, protecting patient privacy in health AI remains complex and requires more than technical solutions. Clinicians should not view privacy and security as solely the responsibility of IT departments. They need to recognize which elements of patient data may reveal sensitive information, understand the regulatory requirements in their context, and distinguish whether sufficient privacy-preserving methods are in place during model development and deployment, even if the technical details are handled by experts. This awareness is critical to ensuring that AI tools respect patient confidentiality and uphold long-standing ethical commitments in healthcare.

4.4 EQUITY IN HEALTH AI

Justice is an important ethical principle in medicine, emphasizing fair access to care and the fair distribution of benefits and risks. In health AI, this connects closely to equity, which concerns whether AI tools work reliably for all patient groups and whether they risk widening existing disparities in healthcare.

In practice, defining what seems "fair" in health AI is not straightforward (10). In some situations, fairness means that patients with similar clinical profiles should receive similar predictions regardless of their sex, race, or other sociodemographic characteristics. In other contexts, genuine biological differences may lead to different underlying risks across groups, so the focus shifts from producing similar predicted risk to ensuring that the AI system performs equally well for everyone. Which view is more appropriate depends heavily on the clinical context, making it essential for clinicians to work with AI developers to define equity goals that are both meaningful and feasible (10).

Evaluating equity involves examining whether an AI system makes different types of mistakes or provides different qualities of output for different patient groups (11). For example, a prediction model may tend to overestimate risk in one group and underestimate risk in another, or it may miss certain conditions more often in specific populations. For LLMs, the challenges are even greater (12). Their performance can vary based on demographic characteristics included in the prompt, and language itself becomes a major source of disparity. Many widely used LLMs are developed mainly using English data, which limits their effectiveness for those who are non-English speaking. Patients with limited medical literacy may also be unable to phrase questions in ways these models understand, and this disparity may be perpetuated in the forms of lower-quality health-related responses and suggestions.

Addressing inequities in health AI is often difficult. Some problems can be reduced by ensuring that training data adequately represent all relevant patient groups or by revising the model so it does not consistently favor one group over another (11). When working with LLMs, especially proprietary ones, direct modifications are not possible, and the focus shifts to careful design of prompts, user interfaces, or human–AI interaction modes to reduce the risk of unfair differences in output. Importantly, efforts to improve equity may reduce a model's overall accuracy, so equity goals must be thoughtfully balanced with clinical safety and usefulness.

Given these complexities, clinicians play a crucial role in interpreting equity issues rather than relying solely on technical teams (10). They need to recognize patient groups for whom an AI tool may not perform well, understand how this could affect safety and care quality, and help decide whether an AI system is suitable for a particular patient population. When bias cannot be fully eliminated, it may be appropriate to use the AI tool selectively, develop tailored versions for specific groups, or adjust clinical workflows to ensure equitable care.

4.5 TRANSPARENCY AND INTERPRETABILITY IN HEALTH AI

When making important healthcare decisions, it is essential that both clinicians and patients can understand the basis on which those decisions are made. For this reason, transparency and interpretability are frequently emphasized as key ethical requirements for health AI.

AI is an umbrella term that includes a wide range of models with varying complexity, from simple regression models to deep learning systems and LLMs. These differences in complexity strongly influence how transparent a model can be. Although discussions of AI often focus on complex systems, simpler models, such as logistic regression, decision trees, and clinical risk scores, also fall under this broad category. These models are inherently transparent because the relationship between predictors and the outcome can be expressed explicitly through equations or simple structures, enabling users to fully understand how predictions are made. Despite their simplicity, these transparent models can perform well when data are clean, structured, and contain a manageable number of predictors (13).

As data become more complex, such as when complex interactions and nonlinear relationships are involved, more flexible methods like random forests or XGBoost may be preferred. When the data include images or unstructured clinical text, even more complex deep learning models often outperform simpler approaches. For these "black box" models, it is no longer feasible to infer how any specific predictor contributes to the final prediction simply by inspecting the model. Instead, various explanation techniques are used to approximate model behavior. Among these, LIME and SHAP are commonly applied. LIME builds simple, local approximations to estimate how much each feature influenced a particular prediction (14). SHAP, based on the concept of Shapley values from game theory, partitions a single prediction into contributions from individual predictors (15). While such model-level explanations can be helpful, they provide only a partial view of how the model works and do not replace a thorough evaluation of whether the model is suitable for real clinical use or is in line with clinical understanding.

Because interpretability alone cannot determine whether a model is appropriate, transparency should also include clear reporting about the data, development process, and performance evaluation (16). Clinicians need to understand which patient populations and clinical settings were represented in the training data, how the model was validated, and whether the evaluation reflects the intended application. This process-level transparency is especially crucial for highly complex models such as LLMs, where technical interpretation of the model's internal workings is not feasible or meaningful. Reporting guidelines have therefore been developed to support consistent and comprehensive reporting, including TRIPOD+AI for prediction models (17), CLAIM for image-based AI systems (18), and TRIPOD-LLM for LLM development and evaluation (19).

Beyond transparency about how a model is built, responsible use also requires transparency about a model's capabilities, limitations, and known risks, including how these issues have been mitigated and defining remaining gaps. Every AI model makes assumptions about the data and will have situations in which it performs less reliably. These limitations are not inherently problematic as long as they are recognized, communicated clearly, and considered when deploying the model in practice so that clinicians know when to rely on the model, when to use caution, and when not to use it at all. To help support this broader, governance-level transparency, the TREGAI checklist (2) provides a practical framework for identifying relevant ethical considerations in health AI, documenting mitigation strategies, and highlighting remaining concerns. Ultimately, clinicians need to understand these different layers of transparency and interpretability, at the model level, the development process level, and the governance level in order to support safe, responsible, and trustworthy implementation of health AI.

4.6 AUTONOMY, ACCOUNTABILITY, AND TRUST IN HEALTH AI

The ethical principles discussed earlier largely focus on the properties of health AI, such as their performance, privacy safeguards, equity across groups, and the transparency of their development and behavior. Autonomy extends these considerations by focusing on how humans, particularly clinicians and patients, interact with health AI. These requirements cannot be satisfied through technical design alone but also depend on how AI is integrated into clinical practice and how decisions are ultimately made.

A core aspect of autonomy in healthcare is the patient's right to make informed, independent decisions supported by clear, accurate information that aligns with their values and preferences. Health AI introduces new complexities to this principle. There is currently no consensus on whether the use of AI in care delivery requires explicit patient consent (20), especially when the system is highly complex or opaque, and when explaining its inner workings may overwhelm rather than empower patients. Nevertheless, when consent is sought, well-documented evidence about model performance, safety, and limitations helps clinicians support meaningful communication and shared decision-making.

In most clinical settings, AI tools should not function independently but should operate with clinician oversight. Clinicians remain responsible for interpreting AI outputs, integrating them with other clinical information, and presenting patients with balanced options that reflect both medical evidence and patient values. Supporting autonomy therefore requires not only that clinicians have sufficient understanding of how the AI performs but also that the AI itself provides adequate transparency to enable meaningful clinical interpretation.

Autonomy has another dimension increasingly recognized in the context of health AI: the autonomy of clinicians themselves. As AI becomes more prevalent, clinicians must maintain their professional judgment rather than deferring reflexively to AI recommendations. This expectation aligns with prevailing views on accountability in AI-assisted care. Clinicians remain accountable for the decisions they make, even when AI contributes to those decisions, and must be prepared to challenge or override AI outputs when they appear inaccurate, incorrect, or inappropriate. Accountability also operates at the institutional level, requiring organizations to establish processes for oversight, documentation, and ongoing monitoring throughout the life cycle of AI development, evaluation, deployment, and post-deployment review.

Finally, trust is essential for the responsible use of health AI. Trust reflects confidence that an AI system is ethically developed, technically sound, and used appropriately in practice. Trust must not be assumed but must be earned through transparent processes, careful evaluation, and clear communication about benefits and limitations. For clinicians and patients, trust depends not only on evidence of model performance but also on understanding how the model was built, for which patient groups it is suitable, and the safeguards that are in place to protect privacy and minimize harm. Because AI tools are typically used by clinicians rather than directly by patients, clinicians play a central role in mediating trust. Physicians' confidence, grounded in awareness of the system's strengths, limitations, and governance, strongly influences how patients perceive and accept AI-supported care.

4.7 PART II: TEACHING PROFESSIONALISM WITH AI

4.7.1 Evolving Professional Values in the AI Era

The integration of AI, including generative AI into healthcare practice requires focus and a reexamination of traditional professional values. As AI grows to become the *modus operandi* in various medical practices, debates over diminishing professional identity will likely intensify. Professional values will likely evolve in tandem with this shift in medical practice toward widespread AI adoption. We see this evolution as an adaptation of core ethical commitments described in the previous section rather than a fundamental change in principles.

4.7.1.1 Autonomy: Exercising Judgment without Overreliance

Clinical autonomy has traditionally referred to the physician's capacity to exercise professional judgment in clinical scenarios, to make the best decisions in the interest of the patient. Sometimes referred to as self-determination, the use of AI-augmented decision-making tools will require clinicians to critically appraise algorithmic outputs, recognize different algorithmic failure modes, and exercise independent sound judgment rather than passively accepting them.

The introduction of digital prescribing and clinical decision-support systems (CDSS) have dramatically mitigated patient safety incidents by guiding clinicians toward making the right prescribing decisions. These interfaces have been shown to influence prescribing and diagnostic decisions made by clinicians in real time. Over time, these rules-based systems may reduce vigilance or create "automation bias," described as a tendency for users to overrely on machine recommendations (21). In clinical practice, automation bias may lead clinicians to overlook contradictory evidence or fail to question improbable outputs (22). In particular, generative AI technology such as LLMs are capable of engaging in nuanced, persuasive conversations. However, hallucinations and misinformation remain an unresolved challenge with these models (23). The clinical risks associated with automation bias are heightened when clinicians fail to exercise judgment, skepticism, and contextualization, and accept erroneous AI recommendations.

Professional autonomy in the AI era will require thorough interrogation of all AI outputs, taking into account contextual factors that may not be captured during model training or by clinical data inputs, such as socioeconomic factors, local practice guidelines and drug availability. Clinicians will need to (1) recognize the limitations of the system such as potential model bias when used on unvalidated populations, (2) understand the risks of, or identify, model drift when it happens, and (3) identify and report potential clinical risks associated with use of the model on patients. Clinicians remain the epistemic authority responsible for integrating AI insights into patient-centered medical reasoning.

4.7.1.2 Accountability: Ownership in Human–AI Collaboration

We believe that professional accountability should remain unequivocally in the hands of human stakeholders, including AI model developers, system implementers, end users, and health systems. As AI systems progress toward greater autonomy, questions of liability and responsibility become more complex. However, medical liability frameworks have not evolved to keep up with rapid technological advancements and have transformed clinical practice models. In addition, the black box nature of AI algorithms remains a barrier to establishing causation in the event of patient harm, as some models may adapt themselves over time with new data inputs. This clouds the identification of error source and assessment of foreseeability of harm from model outputs.

At present, even though AI contributes to decision-making, the clinician retains legal and ethical responsibility for patient outcomes. Professional standards across jurisdictions maintain that AI functions as an assistive tool rather than an independent moral agent (24); hence the weight of responsibility lies heavily on clinicians. Accountability in the AI era will require clinicians to (1) clearly document clinical decisions and detail how AI outputs were used (or not used) in crafting diagnosis or treatment plans, (2) override and escalate or report clinically inappropriate AI outputs, and (3) ensure patient consent is sought prior to the use of AI in making significant clinical decisions.

Adopting a framework of shared accountability with other stakeholders may be helpful in partially shifting accountability away from clinicians. In practice, a shared accountability framework for AI in healthcare would function as a clearly defined responsibility matrix across the AI life cycle, where developers are accountable for robust model design, validation, bias mitigation, and transparency; healthcare institutions are responsible for clinical evaluation, safe procurement, integration, staff training, monitoring, and governance oversight; regulators set standards for risk classification, reporting, and post-market surveillance; and clinicians remain accountable for appropriate use, contextual judgment, documentation, and escalation of concerns. When patient harm or adverse events occur, structured audit trails and review processes will allow a systems approach to examining the faults, rather than defaulting to individual clinician blame. Such a model preserves professional responsibility while ensuring that liability and ethical obligations are proportionately distributed according to each stakeholder's level of control and contribution to risk.

4.7.1.3 Excellence: AI Literacy as a Professional Obligation

AI literacy or health AI literacy is the ability to understand, evaluate, and appropriately use AI-enabled health technologies. This can be conceptualized using established health literacy frameworks. Health literacy is commonly described across functional, interactive, and critical domains. Applied to AI, functional literacy refers to understanding AI-generated health information and recommendations. Interactive literacy reflects the ability to engage with AI-enabled systems, such as digital triage tools or decision aids. Critical literacy involves evaluating AI outputs, recognizing limitations, and knowing when to seek human clarification or challenge recommendations. Excellence as a professional value reaches beyond keeping up-to-date with evidence-based medical practice, extending to achieving and maintaining basic AI literacy.

A brief framework for AI literacy encompasses understanding of the following: foundational data science and basic model functioning (such as types and properties of datasets, probabilistic modeling), sources of error and bias, suitable validation methods, appropriate use cases, and limitations of the designed model. Recent frameworks emphasize that clinicians must develop competencies in evaluating and safely implementing AI tools (25). Failure to engage with emerging technologies risks professional obsolescence and may compromise patient safety.

4.7.1.4 Integrity and Transparency: Informed Consent

Across different jurisdictions, there is currently a lack of consensus on the legal and ethical obligations of AI use disclosure during patient care. Professional bodies have yet to develop or endorse any protocol for obtaining informed consent from patients, and research is needed in determining patients' perceived importance of the different AI tool–related information (26). Ethical principles of maintaining transparency and patient autonomy should be upheld during this process, whereby patients are then given the autonomy to decline the use of AI tools in their routine evaluation and management.

While technical explainability of model output may not always be feasible, clinicians should be able to communicate the following prior to the use of AI during consultation: (1) when the AI will be used; (2) an indication of the intended purpose of use; and (3) risks associated with the use of the model, such as when the model gives a wrong prediction or recommendation. In addition to clinical risks, privacy risks related to cybersecurity threats and data leakage should be communicated with patients.

4.7.1.5 Equity: Fairness and Equitable Access

Algorithmic bias, arising from skewed datasets, structural inequities, or flawed proxy variables, can exacerbate disparity in healthcare (27). For clinicians, wearing an equity lens when evaluating and using an AI system will include
(1) distinguishing disparities in model performance across demographic groups,
(2) raising concerns when models consistently produce biased outputs, and
(3) ensuring equitable access to AI tools and technologies across different patient populations, particularly low resourced regions. Frontline clinicians may actively participate in the codesign of AI deployment strategies to best maintain fair and equitable deployment of AI models, ensuring seamless integration into clinical workflows and optimizing benefits to patients.

4.8 PRACTICAL TEACHING STRATEGIES FOR AI-ERA PROFESSIONALISM

Preparing clinicians for an AI-integrated medical practice requires far more than technical training in tool usage. Educational strategies must intentionally cultivate judgment, ethical reasoning, transparency, and accountability within human–AI collaboration. The following approaches embed these professional values into experiential learning environments.

4.8.1 Simulation: Role-Playing AI-Assisted Consultations

Simulation-based education offers a safe, structured environment to explore decisions made in clinical workflows (28). High-fidelity simulation and standardized patient encounters can incorporate AI-generated outputs, such as risk scores, differential diagnoses, triage recommendations, or LLM-generated documentation drafts to create realistic scenarios of human–AI interaction. Professionalism training can be embedded into these simulations to provide exposure to conundrums faced during AI-augmented consultations. For example, learners may encounter:

An AI sepsis alert that conflicts with clinical acumen;

A risk prediction model that appears discordant with patient demographics, suggesting model bias;

An ambient AI scribe-generated clinical summary that contains subtle factual inaccuracies.

The objective is not to test technical fluency with the AI tool but to assess how learners exercise professional judgment. Simulation can explicitly probe automation bias or systematically biased models (29, 30). Learners should be encouraged to question AI outputs, verify data sources, and articulate reasons for accepting or overriding recommendations.

4.8.2 Reflective Practice: Examining AI's Influence on Clinical Reasoning

Reflective practice is central to professional formation and ongoing professional development, and it is particularly important in the context of AI-assisted care. Cognitive offloading, referring to the delegation of mental tasks to technology, may subtly alter clinical reasoning patterns. With the widespread adoption of generative AI tools such as LLM, degradation of clinical reasoning patterns may increasingly become a key concern. Without deliberate reflection, learners may fail to recognize how AI shapes their diagnostic framing, anchoring, or confidence levels.

Intentional, structured, and routine reflection fosters metacognition, enabling learners to identify automation bias and confirmation bias. Evidence suggests that cognitive forcing strategies and structured reflection may mitigate automation bias in clinical settings (31). Writing reflective narratives may also explore various ethical dimensions:

Did the patient understand AI's role in their care?

How would you respond if the AI recommendation conflicted with patient preferences?

Embedding reflection after clinical encounters reinforces that AI use is not purely technical but relational and ethical. Over time, learners develop a disciplined habit of interrogating both their own reasoning and algorithmic outputs. Generative AI–based chatbots may also take on the role of facilitating such reflections.

4.8.3 Using AI as a Feedback Tool: Pedagogical and Ethical Implications

Generative AI systems can themselves be integrated into feedback processes, by generating structured peer feedback on clinical notes, reflective essays, or simulated encounters. Such tools may improve efficiency and standardization of formative assessment. However, these tools will require rigorous evaluation and validation, as well as critical examination of reliability, prior to adoption. Studies evaluating LLM-generated feedback demonstrate variability in quality and potential reinforcement of biases (32). AI-generated feedback may appear authoritative while lacking contextual nuance.

4.9 CONCLUSION

The rise of AI in healthcare does not replace professionalism, but rather it intensifies its importance. Educational strategies must therefore move beyond technical training toward cultivating reflective, ethically grounded, and digitally competent professionals capable of stewarding AI responsibly in patient care.

GLOSSARY

Artificial intelligence (AI): A broad field of computer science focused on developing systems that can perform tasks typically requiring human intelligence, such as pattern recognition, prediction, decision-making, and language understanding. AI encompasses a range of approaches, from relatively simple rule-based or statistical models to more complex machine learning methods. Deep learning is a subtype of AI that uses multilayered neural networks to analyze complex data such as images or text.

Generative AI: AI systems that generate new content, such as text, images, audio, or video, by learning patterns from large volumes of training data.

Health AI: Health AI encompasses machine learning, deep learning, and generative AI systems that analyze structured and unstructured health data such as medical records, imaging, physiological signals, and clinical text to assist with diagnosis, prognosis, treatment decision-making, clinical documentation, and other patient-facing applications.

Large language model (LLM): A type of AI model trained on vast amounts of text data to understand and generate human-like language. LLMs are commonly used for tasks such as text summarization, question answering, and conversational interaction, and represent a major category of generative AI focused on text-based inputs and outputs.

ABBREVIATIONS

AI	Artificial Intelligence
CDSS	Clinical Decision Support System
CLAIM	Checklist for Artificial Intelligence in Medical Imaging
GDPR	General Data Protection Regulation
GRADE	Grading of Recommendations Assessment, Development, and Evaluation
HIPAA	Health Insurance Portability and Accountability Act
IT	Information Technology
LIME	Local interpretable model-agnostic explanations
LLM	Large Language Model
SHAP	SHapley Additive explanations
TREGAI	Transparent Reporting of Ethics for Generative AI
TRIPOD	Transparent Reporting of a multivariable prediction model for Individual Prognosis Or Diagnosis
WHO	World Health Organization
XGBoost	eXtreme Gradient Boosting

REFERENCES

1. Beauchamp TL. *Principles of Biomedical Ethics*. Childress JF, editor. New York: Oxford University Press; 2019.
2. Ning Y, Teixayavong S, Shang Y, Savulescu J, Nagaraj V, Miao D, et al. Generative artificial intelligence and ethical considerations in health care: A scoping review and ethics checklist. *The Lancet Digital Health*. 2024 Nov 1;6(11):e848–56.
3. WHO Guidance. *Ethics and Governance of Artificial Intelligence for Health* [Internet]. [cited 2023 Dec 20]. Available from: https://www.who.int/publications-detail-redirect/9789240029200
4. *Ethics Guidelines for Trustworthy AI | Shaping Europe's Digital Future* [Internet]. 2019 [cited 2024 Apr 30]. Available from: https://digital-strategy.ec.europa.eu/en/library/ethics-guidelines-trustworthy-ai
5. AJ V, EB E. Decision curve analysis: A novel method for evaluating prediction models. *Medical Decision making: An International Journal of the Society for Medical Decision Making*. 2006 Nov;26(6):565–74.
6. Hong C, Chowdhury A, Sorrentino AD, Wang H, Agrawal M, Bedoya A, et al. Application of unified health large language model evaluation framework to In-Basket message replies: Bridging qualitative and quantitative assessments. *J Am Med Inform Assoc*. 2025 Apr 1;32(4):626–37.
7. Schünemann HJ, Mustafa RA, Brozek J, Santesso N, Bossuyt PM, Steingart KR, et al. GRADE guidelines: 22. The GRADE approach for tests and strategies-from test accuracy to patient-important outcomes and recommendations. *J Clin Epidemiol*. 2019 July;111:69–82.
8. Ficek J, Wang W, Chen H, Dagne G, Daley E. Differential privacy in health research: A scoping review. *J Am Med Inform Assoc*. 2021 Oct 1;28(10):2269–76.
9. Li S, Liu P, Nascimento GG, Wang X, Leite FRM, Chakraborty B, et al. Federated and distributed learning applications for electronic health records and structured medical data: A scoping review. *J Am Med Inform Assoc*. 2023 Dec 1;30(12):2041–9.
10. Liu M, Ning Y, Teixayavong S, Mertens M, Xu J, Ting DSW, et al. A translational perspective towards clinical AI fairness. *npj Digital Medicine*. 2023 Sept 14;6(1):172.
11. Liu M, Ning Y, Teixayavong S, Liu X, Mertens M, Shang Y, et al. A scoping review and evidence gap analysis of clinical AI fairness. *npj Digit Med*. 2025 June 14;8(1):360.
12. Omar M, Soffer S, Agbareia R, Bragazzi NL, Apakama DU, Horowitz CR, et al. Sociodemographic biases in medical decision making by large language models. *Nat Med*. 2025 June;31(6):1873–81.
13. Cowling TE, Cromwell DA, Bellot A, Sharples LD, van der Meulen J. Logistic regression and machine learning predicted patient mortality from large sets of diagnosis codes comparably. *Journal of Clinical Epidemiology*. 2021 May;133:43–52.
14. Ribeiro MT, Singh S, Guestrin C. "Why should I trust you?" Explaining the predictions of any classifier. In: *Proceedings of the ACM SIGKDD International Conference on Knowledge Discovery and Data Mining*. Association for Computing Machinery; 2016. p. 1135–44.
15. Lundberg SM, Lee SI. A Unified approach to interpreting model predictions. In: *Proceedings of the 31st International Conference on Neural Information Processing Systems*. Neural Information Processing Systems; 2017. p. 4768–77.
16. Ning Y, Liu M, Liu N. Advancing ethical AI in healthcare through interpretability. *Patterns (N Y)*. 2025 June 13;6(6):101290.

17. Collins GS, Moons KGM, Dhiman P, Riley RD, Beam AL, Calster BV, et al. TRIPOD+AI statement: Updated guidance for reporting clinical prediction models that use regression or machine learning methods. *BMJ*. 2024 Apr 16;385:e078378.
18. Tejani AS, Klontzas ME, Gatti AA, Mongan J, Moy L, Park SH, et al. Updating the checklist for Artificial Intelligence in medical imaging (CLAIM) for reporting AI research. *Nat Mach Intell*. 2023 Sept;5(9):950–1.
19. Gallifant J, Afshar M, Ameen S, Aphinyanaphongs Y, Chen S, Cacciamani G, et al. The TRIPOD-LLM reporting guideline for studies using large language models. *Nat Med*. 2025 Jan;31(1):60–9.
20. Mello MM, Char D, Xu SH. Ethical obligations to inform patients about use of AI tools. *JAMA*. 2025 Sept 2;334(9):767–70.
21. Goddard K, Roudsari A, Wyatt JC. Automation bias—A hidden issue for clinical decision support system use. *Stud Health Technol Inform*. 2011;164:17–22.
22. Hasanzadeh F, Josephson CB, Waters G, Adedinsewo D, Azizi Z, White JA. Bias recognition and mitigation strategies in artificial intelligence healthcare applications. *npj Digit Med*. 2025;8:154.
23. Ong JCL, Ning Y, Yang R, Bitterman DS, Liu X, Tham YC, Collins GS. Large language models in global health. *Nat Health* 2026;1:35–47.
24. World Health Organization. *Ethics and Governance of Artificial Intelligence for Health: WHO Guidance*. WHO; 2021.
25. Topol E. *Deep Medicine: How Artificial Intelligence Can Make Healthcare Human again*. Basic Books; 2019.
26. Park HJ. Patient perspectives on informed consent for medical AI: A web-based experiment. *Digit Health*. 2024 Apr 30;10:20552076241247938.
27. Obermeyer Z, Powers B, Vogeli C, Mullainathan S. Dissecting racial bias in an algorithm used to manage the health of populations. *Science*. 2019;366(6464):447–53.
28. Lateef F. Maximizing learning and creativity: Understanding psychological safety in simulation-based learning. *J Emerg Trauma Shock*. 2020 Jan–Mar;13(1):5–14.
29. Khera R, Simon MA, Ross JS. Automation bias and assistive AI: Risk of harm from AI-driven clinical decision support. *JAMA*. 2023;330(23):2255–7.
30. Jabbour S, Fouhey D, Shepard S, Valley TS, Kazerooni EA, Banovic N, et al. Measuring the impact of AI in the diagnosis of hospitalized patients: A Randomized Clinical Vignette Survey Study. *JAMA*. 2023;330(23):2275–84.
31. Lyell D, Coiera E. Automation bias and verification complexity: A systematic review. *Journal of the American Medical Informatics Association*. 2017 Mar;24(2):423–31.
32. Zhui L, Yhap N, Liping L, Zhengjie W, Zhonghao X, Xiaoshu Y, Hong C, Xuexiu L, Wei R. Impact of large language models on medical education and teaching adaptations. *JMIR Med Inform*. 2024 Jul 25;12:e55933.

5 AI and Surgical Training

Justin P. Wagner, O. Joe Hines

5.1 INTRODUCTION

The *Halstedian* apprenticeship model of surgical training has shifted toward a competency-based paradigm that attempts to redefine surgical decisions and operative performance as measurable steps that are optimizable. This shift was accelerated by the technical and educational demands of minimally invasive and robotic approaches, which require deliberate practice, objective assessments, and structured exposure to achieve safe, reproducible outcomes.[1] As these practices have become common, training programs have identified gaps in technical skills, spatial reasoning, and team-based dynamics that were not reliably addressed by case logs and summative assessments alone. Accordingly, simulation, standardized assessments, and milestone-guided progression have become critical features of current surgical training.[2]

Within this modern paradigm, artificial intelligence (AI) offers a path of customizable learning beyond static drills. Operative simulators allow computer vision and sensor analytics to translate video and motion into coaching, while adaptive virtual environments can render variations in case content and intraoperative findings that approximate real cases.[3, 4] Nonetheless, AI technology in surgical training demands ethical and practical considerations around privacy, transparency, bias, faculty preparation and training, and governance that must be addressed.[5] Given the rapid pace of AI innovation and growing interest across departments and societies, surgical curricula must account for AI literacy and validated AI-enabled assessments, ensuring that the technology enhances—rather than weakens—supervision and autonomy.[6]

Since 2010, there has been tremendous effort to develop systems capable of performing discrete technical tasks autonomously. These systems have rapidly progressed from robots capable of venipuncture[7] to those that can perform *in vivo* laparoscopic bowel anastomosis.[8] In 2025, Kim et al. described a stepwise policy algorithm for an AI-powered surgical transformer to perform *ex vivo* laparoscopic cholecystectomies. This system performed the operation with metrics of economy of motion and smooth action, outperforming expert surgeons, albeit with longer task durations.[9] Surgical educators have long recognized that innovation produces great interest in applying technology to surgical skills acquisition. As early as 1999, Gorman et al. cautioned that simulation and technical skills laboratories comprise distinct technical practices from traditional elements of clinical training.[10] It remains salient that surgical trainees must assimilate AI technology in a way that sustains the evolving craft. This evolution may result in surgeons ceding algorithmic technical tasks in favor of a dynamic approach to decision-making and patient-centered care in collaboration with generative AI systems.

In this chapter, we summarize frameworks for integrating AI in surgical education, applications employed, policy and AI oversight, the fine balance of clinical efficiency with experiential training, and implications for the future of surgical training in the AI era.

5.2 SURGICAL EDUCATION FRAMEWORKS

Building durable AI capacity in surgical education requires data management resources from departments and time from surgical faculty. Training programs

DOI: 10.1201/9781003617167-5

need educators who can interpret algorithmic outputs, translate them into coachable behaviors for surgical trainees, and engage in local policy development. Departments must secure equipment for video acquisition, motion capture, computing, and data management. Surgical and educational societies must develop shared professional standards so AI models may be trained, tested, implemented, and maintained over time.[11]

AI-derived measures of competency should map explicitly to existing assessment frameworks, such as the Accreditation Council for Graduate Medical Education (ACGME) Milestones[12] and the American Board of Surgery (ABS) Entrustable Professional Activities (EPAs).[13] In practice, this entails specifying how specific AI signals correspond to particular competencies, setting validated thresholds, and using concordance checks with expert surgeons before being employed in a high-stakes environment.[14] Table 5.1 illustrates a sample of how select AI-derived metrics may be mapped to ACGME Milestones and ABS EPAs. Using this mapping scaffold, a training program may cite specific applications of the technology in achieving its goals and objectives. For example, a residency program may use generative AI to create adaptive learning materials and provide structured feedback for surgical residents as they demonstrate patient care, medical knowledge, and professionalism while performing an EPA such as an initial trauma survey.

To validate these objective-focused AI practices, surgical faculty must develop literacy with the technology. The progression of faculty literacy begins with baseline exposure to AI interfaces, progresses to intermediate skills, and culminates in advanced stewardship (Figure 5.1). Following initial exposure, the surgical faculty will explore whether and how AI may be applicable to their teaching methods. They will then demonstrate intermediate skills in explicitly adapting AI applications to tailor instruction to their trainees. This intermediate level of faculty literacy has been validated in several studies. For instance, AI signals previously mapped to ACGME Milestones independently reproduce faculty ratings that effectively discriminate experts from novices.[15, 16] Surgeon-educators with advanced literacy may then conduct their own reviews of AI decision support tools, comparing them with faculty-led benchmarks of Milestones and EPA assessments. This allows them to provide oversight and stewardship of the technology in the training environment. Studies using external validation cohorts across varied surgical training centers have shown that faculty at this advanced level of literacy deliver equitable structured feedback, standardized video annotation schemas, and scalable data use protocols.[17–19] This framework provides a means for surgical training programs to provide objectives for faculty development in AI literacy.

Training programs are supported in accelerating faculty literacy in AI through professional development as may occur via institutional graduate medical education programs, industry-led efforts, and surgical societies. Some key offerings from surgical societies include core concepts of AI development and training, projected AI capabilities, and limitations in ethical AI practices among surgeons and trainees.[4, 19, 20] Within local institutions, surgical education programs should also include instruction for both faculty and trainees in recognizing bias, issues of generalizability, and hallucinations. Professional development programs should teach when to question or override a suggested algorithm. They should also ensure that the adopted AI algorithms support the teacher's articulated observations of a trainee's performance without replacing or redirecting their critical assessments.[21]

Table 5.1: Sample Mapping of AI-Derived Metrics[15–19, 22] to ACGME Milestones[12], American Board of Surgery EPAs[13]

		ABS EPAs[9]							
		Appendicitis	Gallbladder	Hernia	Acute Abd/SBO	Consultation	Critically Ill Periop	Flex GI Endoscopy	Trauma Eval/Initial
ACGME Milestones[8]	PC	PSR, KIN	PSR, KIN	PSR, KIN	PR, KIN	ADAPT	PSR, ADAPT	PSR, KIN	PSR, ADAPT
	MK	ADAPT	ADAPT	ADAPT	ADAPT	ADAPT	ADAPT	ADAPT	ADAPT
	PBLI	NLP, ADAPT	NLP, ADAPT	NLP, ADAPT	NLP, ADAPT	NLP, ADAPT	NLP, ADAPT	NLP, ADAPT	NLP, ADAPT
	SBP	CASE	CASE	CASE	CASE	CASE	CASE	CASE	CASE
	PROF	NLP	NLP	NLP	NLP	NLP	NLP	NLP	NLP
	ICS	NLP	NLP	NLP	NLP	NLP	NLP	NLP	NLP

Abd = abdomen; ABS = American Board of Surgery; ACGME = Accreditation Council for Graduate Medical Education; ADAPT = adaptive curriculum; CASE = case-based exposure dashboard; EPA = entrustable professional activity; GI = gastrointestinal; ICS = interpersonal communication skills; KIN = kinematics/errors; MK = medical knowledge; NLP = structured narrative feedback via natural language processing; PBLI = practice-based learning and improvement; PC = patient care; PROF = professionalism; PSR = phase/step recognition; SBO = small bowel obstruction; SBP = systems-based practice

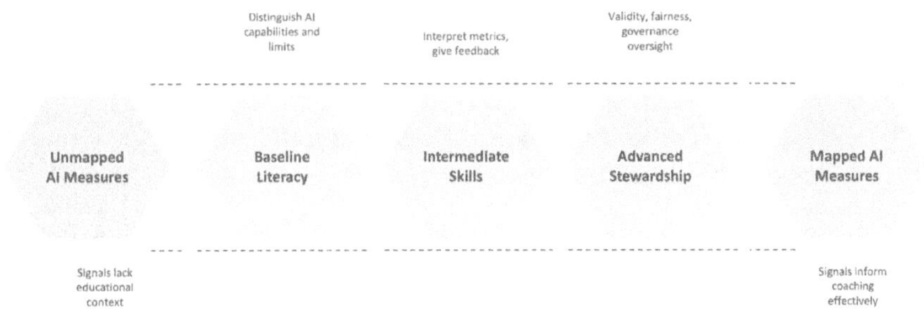

Figure 5.1 Flowchart of AI integration into surgical education curriculum.

5.3 APPLICATIONS OF AI IN SURGICAL EDUCATION

The growth of AI in surgical training is rapid, and the technology has resulted in demonstrable change in teaching practices. In simulation, computer vision and kinematics help surgeons envision potential intraoperative decisions. In the assessment process, automated standardized metrics may be employed to provide timely, targeted feedback to accelerate learning. In adaptive curricula, learner-specific AI models may sequence the next best task to guide and maintain deliberate practice.[23] This section illustrates these applications and clarifies how they add value while preserving faculty judgment and supervised autonomy.

5.3.1 Enhanced Simulation and Skills Acquisition

AI-augmented simulation empowers assessments to discriminate between expert and learner behaviors in low- or high-fidelity environments. Trainees use LLMs to generate low-fidelity, text-based simulations of cases, quizzes, and steps of surgical procedures. In high-fidelity immersive platforms, computer vision and motion capture streams can translate instrument kinematics and error events into metrics that align with those of experts. These data facilitate highly targeted assessment and feedback.[15, 24] AI-mediated simulation can also create unintended actions in practice, such as optimizing efficiency of the non-dominant hand at the expense of economy of motion of the dominant hand.[23] This side effect of AI training may be offset by varying the techniques required in simulated tasks, modifying objectives, and conducting periodic standard simulations without AI to independently assess the trainee's competence.

Simulated task difficulty can also adjust in real time to keep learners in a targeted challenge zone. AI simulators can automatically change the strictness of assessment criteria, alter tissue behavior during a simulation, or add realistic disruptions as performance improves. Generative models can create new case content, include comorbid conditions and develop branching decision points. These systems may be used to produce a library of simulated cases that challenge judgment and psychomotor skills.[25] While these iterative simulations will mimic clinical decision support, there is no current guideline to support best practices in this field. To serve the goals of a surgical training program, it is crucial to create a clear distinction between trainees' learning via simulated cases and demonstrating autonomous surgical practice with the help of a clinical support tool.[26, 27]

Oral examination can also be simulated with AI. A pilot study from 2025 describes an LLM-powered platform that presents standardized vignettes, interrogates reasoning in a conversational format, and scores responses against a rubric before faculty perform their assessment.[28] This AI application addresses the problems of variability in examiners' assessments and the burden of scheduling traditional mock oral exams. Additionally, it provides learners with an opportunity to articulate real-time surgical decisions and receive feedback on demand. This form of deliberate practice—verbalizing clinical decisions—is associated with high first-time pass rates on the high-stakes ABS Certifying Examination.[29]

5.3.2 Assessment and Feedback

AI systems allow a feedback process rooted in data by summarizing clear measures of performance that support faculty judgment. In contrast to traditional means of subjective, instructor-led assessments, AI performance assessments may be uniformly engineered to reflect the specific objectives of the training program, faculty member, or trainee. For instance, within an operative EPA, objectives may include enumerating steps completed in an operation, achieving a target instrument path length, idle time, smooth motions, or error events requiring corrections. For narrative assessments, AI may distill and summarize large amounts of verbal feedback using natural language processing (NLP). With automated AI reviews of these sources of data, feedback may be anchored with consistency. This process allows a program to follow longitudinal trainee performance trends.[25, 26, 30]

In a simulator or video-enabled operation, AI may also automate video analysis. Using a case-specific rubric with distinct phases of the operation, a video-based AI assessment program can detect deviations and show performance alerts in near-real time. This practice supports timely, focused debriefs and intraoperative prompts for the teaching surgeon to reinforce correct technique.[16] When faculty surgeons are provided with prompts preemptively (such as curated clips, a list of operative steps, and video overlays of the trainee's performance metrics), their feedback is less biased and has greater generalizability and reproducibility.[17] These applications of AI empower teaching surgeons to provide more effective coaching and mentorship.

Trainees may receive feedback in multiple AI-generated formats. An AI feedback dashboard may include curated or annotated video clips, data summaries, micro-objectives aligning with stage of training, longitudinal performance data, or a recent error summary. These systems can also provide a trainee with a custom priority list of next tasks to practice, highlight exemplary performances for comparison, isolate particular motions, and generate prompts for face-to-face feedback sessions with faculty surgeons.[17, 31] Figure 5.2 depicts a simplified progression from video and sensor stream input to precise, targeted performance feedback.

5.3.3 Intelligent Curriculum Adaptation

Surgical trainees have already demonstrated initiative in using AI to adapt curricula outside of the operating room to meet their needs. Use cases have been described in which learners have designed custom prompts for educational chatbots. These prompts include patient education resources, coaching in research study design and analysis, and on-demand generation of multiple-choice subject exam items.[32]

In AI-generated operative simulations, adaptive curricula may provide an appropriate level of challenge for the trainee's level of experience. After each case or simulation, instructive models may update with fresh metrics and generate the next best action. Generative systems may create an additional micro-practice on a recurrent error, a targeted video review, or a slightly modified scenario so trainees remain appropriately challenged without stagnating or becoming discouraged. These systems may also track secondary measures (such as tissue handling while working on speed) to ensure trainees acquire skills in a balanced fashion.[33]

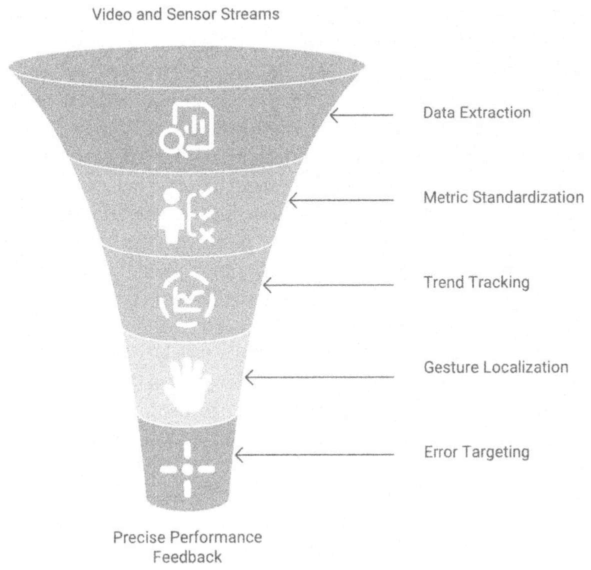

Figure 5.2 Refining performance feedback with AI.

In both technical and nontechnical domains, AI assessment tools can provide specific materials in real time based on a trainee's recent performance. By reviewing a trainee's performance data and cross-referencing clinical guidelines, these systems may provide reinforcement for trainees' specific decisions. One prospective study showed that this type of AI-mediated adaptation supports learning more efficiently than static curricula.[3] As mentioned in the preceding sections, adaptive curricula mapped to competency frameworks like Milestones and EPAs provide high-quality data in tracking a trainee's progression. These assessments may clarify when supervision can be tapered or where focused remediation is indicated. Importantly, surgical faculty retain the discretion to assess a trainee's entrustability while being informed by these data.[26, 34]

5.4 POLICY, GOVERNANCE, AND PROFESSIONAL GUIDELINES

Surgical training programs must adopt a common consensus for data privacy, algorithmic fairness, and regulatory fit, with the following specific practices: (1) secure captured video and data streams with a clear schedule for retention and access controls; (2) document clear attributions of datasets used to train AI models; (3) audit AI model performance across learner subgroups to detect unintended biased behaviors; and (4) clearly distinguish educational analytics from data that can be misconstrued as clinical decision support. Local processes of review must be devised prior to any high-stakes use of AI-based surgical education models. These reviews must include benchmark evaluations of AI model performance relative to standard assessments and protocols for when AI models fail.[18, 27] A practical data policy should include de-identification of any captured audio or video material. Specifically, face and voice distortion and restraints in field of view may be employed to avoid inadvertent capture of protected health information.

As with innovations in healthcare delivery, the quality of AI models in surgical education requires continuous oversight. Training programs should distinguish internal educational or quality improvement projects from research that would require evaluation by an Institutional Review Board. Recording policies must specify language for consent, opting out, and retention of video and data streams for education. External sharing of AI programs and data require separate processes and approvals than those required for initial development. Information security is especially sensitive in the perioperative environment, and data storage regarding a trainee's performance must use encryption, restricted access, and predefined schedules of data retention and archiving. Interinstitutional use of these data should proceed only under uniform data use agreements. Administrators should also plan for the durations of AI vendor and model agreements with clear schedules for performance audits, updates to infrastructure, and rollback plans for underperforming models.

Surgical societies have initiated this important work (Figure 5.3). The Society of American Gastrointestinal and Endoscopic Surgeons (SAGES) released consensus documents establishing common AI annotation schemas for video, defining expectations for data use and sharing, and encouraging multi-institution comparability.[18, 19] These technical standards complement broader professional perspectives that frame surgeons' roles as stewards for their patients, workplace leaders, and educators. The ACS has also published commentaries on the responsibilities of surgeons as AI integrates into surgical practice and education, while guidance from nonsurgical professional societies also inform best practices in surgical education to best prepare for the evolving training paradigm.[18, 19, 35, 36]

A remaining gap is alignment with accreditation structures. ACGME Milestones and ABS EPAs are well suited to integrating validated AI metrics, but neither yet

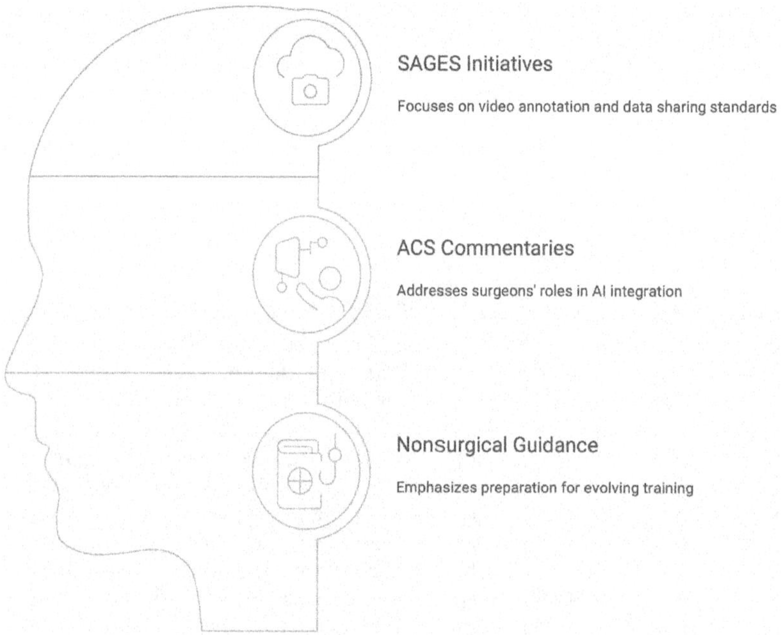

Figure 5.3 Society-based practices in advancing standards for AI in surgical training (ACS: American College of Surgeons; SAGES: Society of American Gastrointestinal and Endoscopic Surgeons).

offers AI-specific requirements. Accordingly, training programs must reconcile their adoption of AI technology with existing expectations for patient safety, informed consent, supervision, and documentation. Programs must make explicit when and how AI-derived evidence informs entrustment, that appeals and arbitration pathways should exist, and how future refinements will achieve greater fairness and reliability.[12]

5.5 BALANCING EFFICIENCY WITH TRAINEE EXPERIENCE

AI offers value in the efficiency of surgical practice. These gains should be reinvested to prioritize direct supervision of surgical trainees. Consensus and society statements consistently suggest AI should augment and not replace clinical acumen, emphasizing that entrustment remains a human decision anchored to performance, context, and risk tolerance. Training programs should establish minimums for hands-on exposure at index steps in each Milestone or EPA, use systematic processes to provide feedback, and explicitly dictate how to allocate time saved to additional direct clinical observation.[3, 14, 37]

At this time, the most ubiquitous AI tools used among surgeons encompass several aspects of clinical practice. As described previously in this chapter, computer vision enables real-time interpretation of anatomical landmarks, the character of tissues, and guidance during minimally invasive procedures.[1, 38, 39] Robotic surgery platforms offer incorporated AI programs for enhanced intraoperative navigation, precision of movement, and real-time feedback.[1, 39] AI-driven models integrate with the electronic health record (EHR) and provide clinical decision support, including prediction of perioperative risk, patient selection, and resource allocation.[22, 40–42] NLP programs increase surgeons' efficiency in generating operative summaries, extracting clinically relevant data, constructing narratives, and communicating with insurers.[38, 43] These examples expose the rapid pace with which AI aspires to become a fixture of surgical practice.

Technological disruptions such as AI are often framed as tools to relieve surgeon-educators of administrative burden and liberate time for teaching. In practice, this framing remains aspirational. Figure 5.4 illustrates the factors that dissuade surgeons from prioritizing teaching when clinical efficiency increases. There is currently no direct evidence to support that increases in efficient clinical practices attributable to AI manifest in increasing surgeons' teaching activities. A 2024 scoping review by Isaacs et al. emphasizes the need to evaluate the real-world effects of AI implementation on surgical faculty workload, teaching time, and educational outcomes.[31] Furthermore, in a 2021 study by Bohnen and colleagues, 2006–2012 data trends from the National Surgical Quality Improvement Program showed differences in operative times for "teaching" and "non-teaching" cases reduced by 36%.[44] Taken together with data from thematic analysis, despite technologies that historically increased clinical efficiency (such as ubiquitous adoption of EHRs, evidence-based protocols for clinical care, enhanced recovery pathways, and refinements in minimally invasive techniques), surgeons remain more likely to prioritize patient safety and efficient workflow over educational activities when time constraints are perceived.[45]

Concerning AI, the principal perceived hazard among surgeon-educators is overreliance, which may erode one's capacity for independent judgment.[14] To counter this, trainees may be assigned to generate a pre-AI plan, compare it with model outputs, and articulate an explanation for the resulting agreement or disagreement. Training programs should require periodic "AI-off" assessments to demonstrate the capabilities of both teachers and learners without decision support. Audits for concordance and appeal processes should be incorporated into

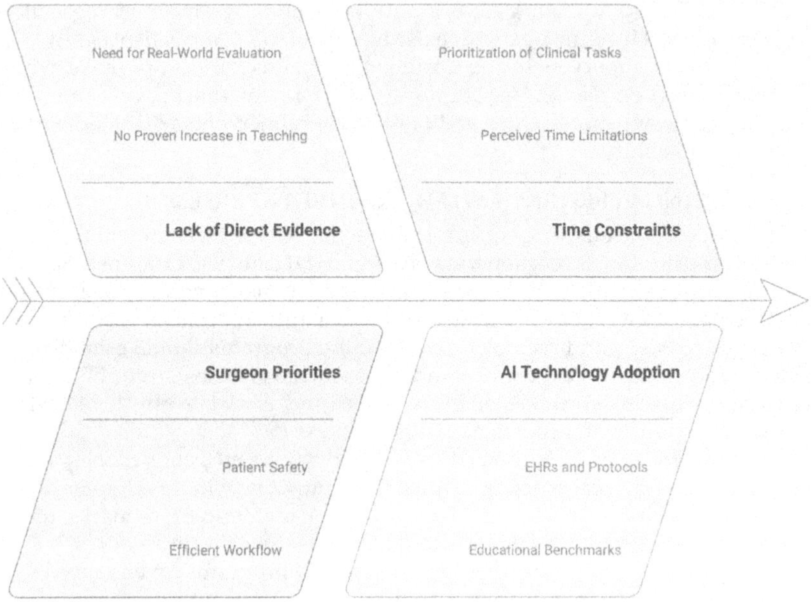
Need for Real-World Evaluation
No Proven Increase in Teaching
Lack of Direct Evidence
Prioritization of Clinical Tasks
Perceived Time Limitations
Time Constraints
Surgeon Priorities
Patient Safety
Efficient Workflow
AI Technology Adoption
EHRs and Protocols
Educational Benchmarks

Figure 5.4 Challenges to prioritizing teaching activities with increased clinical efficiency in surgical practice (EHRs: electronic health records).

EPA reviews of trainee performance.[3, 46] Expert perspectives on educating future surgeons underscore this stewardship model, which explicitly trains surgeons to critically appraise algorithms, manage uncertainty, and prioritize patient safety. The efficiency afforded by AI systems should reinforce the redundancy of clinical interface necessary for surgeons to develop independent clinical reasoning skills.

AI has been criticized for its susceptibility to discrimination on the basis of gender, race, and ethnicity because of biased input data. Several systematic reviews and empirical studies show AI models often reflect and amplify existing biases that lead to disparities in diagnostic accuracy, risk prediction, and treatment recommendations for historically underserved populations, including women, Black, Hispanic, and socioeconomically disadvantaged patients.[47–51] Equity in AI surgical education models will require routine subgroup performance assessments by demographic factors, and corrective actions must be undertaken when disparities arise. Potential solutions may include expansion of datasets used to train AI models, retraining with more balanced samples, adjustment of performance thresholds to reflect equitable assessment methods, and policies to engage human oversight in continuous validation of the models employed.

Surgical trainees maintain an optimistic perspective about AI. While many report concerns about information security, overreliance and clinical skills decline, and ethical practices, the majority of trainees are enthusiastic.[46] A 2024 survey study of general surgery residents by St. John et al. found that most expressed excitement about AI's automation of repetitive tasks and contributions to advancing their own medical knowledge. Additionally, those with greater familiarity with AI reported more positive attitudes about its integration.[52] Surgical trainees' attitudes signify the broad cultural acceptance of AI as an extension of contemporary life. Accordingly, surgery will inexorably evolve with AI, and it is up to our training programs to determine how deliberately they will contribute to this evolution.

5.6 FUTURE DIRECTIONS AND RESEARCH OPPORTUNITIES

Promising research lies in pairing generative AI with multimodal data in surgical education. Some opportunities for this exploration include operative video assessments, surgeons' motion data, telemetry of instruments or devices, verbal articulation of surgical decision-making, and narrative feedback.[46] Generative AI models may process vast amounts of this multimodal data and engineer new instructional methods for surgical trainees.

Scholastic interest regarding AI in surgical training continues to accelerate rapidly, with reports of AI integration in surgery surging over 400% since 2020.[53] The generation of new scholarly works will provide greater evidence to inform best practices in assimilating AI technology in surgical training. Additionally, surgeons trained with AI are empowered to produce and critically appraise these scholarly works.[54] Consequently, surgeons' academic productivity will likely manifest in the extent to which they employ AI effectively.

As of 2025, studies of AI in surgical education must advance beyond single-center convenience samples. Loftus and colleagues identified a deficiency of scientific rigor among studies of AI implementation for surgical decision support.[22] Additional multi-institutional trials with specified end points, standardized data use and annotation schemas, and external validation studies are needed.[24] Study outcomes should extend beyond purely technical metrics. Potential areas of study include faculty decisions of trainee entrustability, trainee skills retention, clinical outcomes, and patient-centered indicators of care quality.

Finally, implementation of AI in surgical education should follow the American Association of Medical Colleges (AAMC) framework that situates the technology across people, processes, and systems.[55] Training programs encourage AI literacy among all stakeholders, develop policies for acceptable use, map AI indicators to goals and objectives (such as Milestones and EPAs), and test whether AI-enabled curricula encourage autonomous practice or inadvertently narrow it. Generative systems and multimodal data can support surgical instruction and accelerate scholarly works, provided outputs are transparently sourced and accepted by faculty prior to use in teaching and assessment. In sum, the AAMC framework positions surgical educators to adopt AI responsibly while protecting the core goal of surgical training: to prepare surgeons to provide informed, safe, and compassionate care to our patients.

5.7 CONCLUSION

Responsible integration of AI in surgical training demands ethical stewardship. There is already demonstrated value of AI tools in standardizing assessment, accelerating formative feedback, and informing competency-based progress. Equally important are the preservation of transparency, safeguards against bias, and protection of learner and patient data. Programs should demonstrate these principles with clear governance: policies for use and retention of data, reviews of fairness, and explicit separation of educational analytics from clinical decision support. Professional consensus and technical standards from SAGES, ACS, AAMC, and ACGME provide practical guidelines for implementation across the surgical education community with uniform shared practices.

Surgical training with AI requires active trainee participation. AI-derived signals should be mapped to ACGME Milestones and ABS EPAs. Future surgeons should be taught to critically appraise AI models, manage clinical uncertainty, and treat AI decision support as an adjunct to (not a replacement for) clinical reasoning and entrustment decisions. Surgical training programs must cultivate their trainees' professional identities as stewards of AI technology. Literacy in data science should be integrated as a part of surgical training curriculum, and trainees should participate actively in AI validation and quality review processes. In short, trainees must forecast how to cooperate with AI to shape practice, advocate for policies that protect patient safety, and execute implementation plans that keep our field humane and relevant as our capabilities evolve.

5.8 ACKNOWLEDGMENTS

The authors acknowledge the contributions of the AAMC, ABS, ACGME, ACS, Association for Surgical Education, SAGES in their progressive work to rapidly assimilate standards of AI in surgical education. We also acknowledge the forthcoming efforts of our current faculty, trainees, and students in defining the future of our field with this exciting technology.

5.9 STATEMENTS ON AI USE

The authors used AI-enabled tools in the preparation of this chapter. Specifically, GPT-5 (OpenAI, San Francisco, CA) was used to assist in literature organization, language polishing, and consistency checks. Literature search assistance was provided by OpenEvidence (Cambridge, MA). Reference management assistance was provided by Zotero (Corporation for Digital Scholarship, Fairfax, VA). Graphics and illustrations were prepared using Napkin (Napkin.io, Los Altos, CA). All conceptual framing, interpretation of evidence, and final prose were conceived, written, and approved by the authors.

GLOSSARY

Adaptive curriculum: An instructional approach that adjusts content and difficulty to a learner's recent performance.

Augmented intelligence: Human-centered use of AI to support (not replace) expert judgment.

Computer vision (CV): Algorithms that analyze surgical videos to recognize phases, steps, gestures, or events.

Concordance check: Comparison of AI outputs with expert ratings to evaluate agreement and fitness for use.

Deliberate practice: Structured, goal-oriented training on tasks just beyond current ability, repeated with focused attention, immediate feedback, and refinement under expert guidance to drive measurable performance improvement.

Entrustable professional activity (EPA): A unit of work that can be entrusted to a trainee once competence is demonstrated.

Generative AI: Models that create new content (text, images, or scenarios) from learned patterns.

Hallucination: In generative AI, the production of plausible-sounding content that is not grounded in the input, training data, or objective data.

Kinematics: Quantitative motion data (such as instrument paths, speed, idle time) used to assess technical performance.

Kinematic streams: Time-ordered sequences of position, velocity, and acceleration data of hands or instruments capturing motion dynamics for analysis and assessment.

Milestones (ACGME): Developmental competencies and subcompetencies and level descriptors used to assess trainee progression.

Natural language processing (NLP): AI methods that structure and summarize narrative feedback or transcripts.

Supervised autonomy: A graded training state in which the trainee performs tasks independently while an attending surgeon maintains the option to intervene, calibrated to the trainee's demonstrated proficiency.

Telemetry: Continuous remote measurement and transmission of device or performance signals to a receiving system for monitoring and analysis.

ABBREVIATIONS

Abd	abdomen
ABS	American Board of Surgery
ACGME	Accreditation Council for Graduate Medical Education
ACS	American College of Surgeons
ADAPT	adaptive curriculum
AI	artificial intelligence
CASE	case-based exposure dashboard
CV	computer vision
EPA	entrustable professional activity
GI	gastrointestinal
ICS	interpersonal and communication skills
KIN	kinematics/errors
LLM	large language model
MK	medical knowledge
NLP	natural language processing
OR	operating room
OSATS	objective structured assessment of technical skill
PBLI	practice-based learning and improvement
PC	patient care
PROF	professionalism
PSR	phase/step recognition
SAGES	Society of American Gastrointestinal and Endoscopic Surgeons
SBO	small bowel obstruction
SBP	systems-based practice

REFERENCES

1. Hashimoto DA, Rosman G, Rus D, Meireles OR. Artificial intelligence in surgery: Promises and perils. *Ann Surg*. 2018;268(1):70–76. https://doi.org/10.1097/SLA.0000000000002693
2. Bilgic E, Gorgy A, Yang A, et al. Exploring the roles of artificial intelligence in surgical education: A scoping review. *Am J Surg*. 2022;224(1):205–216. https://doi.org/10.1016/j.amjsurg.2021.11.023
3. Guerrero DT, Asaad M, Rajesh A, Hassan A, Butler CE. Advancing surgical education: The use of artificial intelligence in surgical training. *Am Surg*. 2023;89(1):49–54. https://doi.org/10.1177/00031348221101503
4. Fried GM, Varas J, Telem DA, et al. Opportunities and applications of educational technologies in surgical education and assessment. *Ann Surg*. 2025;281(1):34–39. https://doi.org/10.1097/SLA.0000000000006367
5. How artificial intelligence is expected to transform surgical training. *ACS*. Accessed September 4, 2025. https://www.facs.org/for-medical-professionals/news-publications/news-and-articles/bulletin/2023/august-2023-volume-108-issue-8/how-artificial-intelligence-is-expected-to-transform-surgical-training/
6. Satapathy P, Hermis AH, Rustagi S, Pradhan KB, Padhi BK, Sah R. Artificial intelligence in surgical education and training: Opportunities, challenges, and ethical considerations—Correspondence. *Int J Surg*. 2023;109(5):1543–1544. https://doi.org/10.1097/JS9.0000000000000387

7. *Profile: Veebot—IEEE Spectrum*. Accessed October 5, 2025. https://spectrum.ieee.org/profile-veebot
8. Saeidi H, Opfermann JD, Kam M, et al. Autonomous robotic laparoscopic surgery for intestinal anastomosis. *Sci Robot*. 2022;7(62):eabj2908. https://doi.org/10.1126/scirobotics.abj2908
9. Kim JW (Brian), Chen JT, Hansen P, et al. SRT-H: A hierarchical framework for autonomous surgery via language-conditioned imitation learning. *Sci Robot*. 2025;10(104):eadt5254. https://doi.org/10.1126/scirobotics.adt5254
10. Gorman PJ, Meier AH, Krummel TM. Simulation and virtual reality in surgical education: Real or unreal? *Arch Surg*. 1999;134(11):1203–1208. https://doi.org/10.1001/archsurg.134.11.1203
11. Silva C, Nascimento D, Dantas GG, et al. Impact of artificial intelligence on the training of general surgeons of the future: a scoping review of the advances and challenges. *Acta Cirúrgica Bras*. 2024;39:e396224. https://doi.org/10.1590/acb396224
12. *ACGME Surgery Milestones*. Accessed September 4, 2025. https://www.acgme.org/specialties/surgery/milestones/
13. EPAs for General Surgery. *American Board of Surgery*. Accessed September 5, 2025. https://www.absurgery.org/get-certified/epas/general-surgery/
14. Vedula SS, Ghazi A, Collins JW, et al. Artificial intelligence methods and artificial intelligence-enabled metrics for surgical education: A multidisciplinary consensus. *J Am Coll Surg*. 2022;234(6):1181–1192. https://doi.org/10.1097/XCS.0000000000000190
15. Winkler-Schwartz A, Bissonnette V, Mirchi N, et al. Artificial intelligence in medical education: Best practices using machine learning to assess surgical expertise in virtual reality simulation. *J Surg Educ*. 2019;76(6):1681–1690. https://doi.org/10.1016/j.jsurg.2019.05.015
16. Pedrett R, Mascagni P, Beldi G, Padoy N, Lavanchy JL. Technical skill assessment in minimally invasive surgery using artificial intelligence: A systematic review. *Surg Endosc*. 2023;37(10):7412–7424. https://doi.org/10.1007/s00464-023-10335-z
17. Kiyasseh D, Laca J, Haque TF, et al. A multi-institutional study using artificial intelligence to provide reliable and fair feedback to surgeons. *Commun Med*. 2023;3(1):42. https://doi.org/10.1038/s43856-023-00263-3
18. Meireles OR, Rosman G, Altieri MS, et al. SAGES consensus recommendations on an annotation framework for surgical video. *Surg Endosc*. 2021;35(9):4918–4929. https://doi.org/10.1007/s00464-021-08578-9
19. Eckhoff JA, Rosman G, Altieri MS, et al. SAGES consensus recommendations on surgical video data use, structure, and exploration (for research in artificial intelligence, clinical quality improvement, and surgical education). *Surg Endosc*. 2023;37(11):8690–8707. https://doi.org/10.1007/s00464-023-10288-3
20. Cobianchi L, Verde JM, Loftus TJ, et al. Artificial intelligence and surgery: Ethical dilemmas and open issues. *J Am Coll Surg*. 2022;235(2):268–275. https://doi.org/10.1097/XCS.0000000000000242
21. Pesapane F, Volonté C, Codari M, Sardanelli F. Artificial intelligence as a medical device in radiology: Ethical and regulatory issues in Europe and the United States. *Insights Imaging*. 2018;9(5):745–753. https://doi.org/10.1007/s13244-018-0645-y
22. Loftus TJ, Altieri MS, Balch JA, et al. Artificial intelligence—Enabled decision support in surgery: State-of-the-art and future directions. *Ann Surg*. 2023;278(1):51–58. https://doi.org/10.1097/SLA.0000000000005853
23. Fazlollahi AM, Yilmaz R, Winkler-Schwartz A, et al. AI in surgical curriculum design and unintended outcomes for technical competencies in simulation training. *JAMA Netw Open*. 2023;6(9):e2334658. https://doi.org/10.1001/jamanetworkopen.2023.34658

24. Rao L, Yang E, Dissanayake S, Cuomo R, Seth I, Rozen WM. The use of generative artificial intelligence in surgical education: A narrative review. *Plast Aesthetic Res*. Published online November 27, 2024. https://doi.org/10.20517/2347-9264.2024.102
25. Hla DA, Hindin DI. Generative AI & machine learning in surgical education. *Curr Probl Surg*. 2025;63:101701. https://doi.org/10.1016/j.cpsurg.2024.101701
26. Booth GJ, Ross B, Cronin WA, et al. Competency-based assessments: Leveraging artificial intelligence to predict subcompetency content. *Acad Med*. 2023;98(4):497–504. https://doi.org/10.1097/ACM.0000000000005115
27. Robinson JR, Stey A, Schneider DF, et al. Generative artificial intelligence in academic surgery: Ethical implications and transformative potential. *J Surg Res*. 2025;307:212–220. https://doi.org/10.1016/j.jss.2024.12.059
28. Rao AS, Prasad S, Lee RS, Farrell S, McKinley S, Succi MD. Development and evaluation of an artificial intelligence—Powered surgical oral examination simulator: A Pilot Study. *Mayo Clin Proc Digit Health*. 2025;3(3):100241. https://doi.org/10.1016/j.mcpdig.2025.100241
29. Pennell C, McCulloch P. The effectiveness of public simulated oral examinations in preparation for the American Board of Surgery certifying examination: A systematic review. *J Surg Educ*. 2015;72(5):1026–1031. https://doi.org/10.1016/j.jsurg.2015.03.018
30. Valente DS, Brasil LJ, Spinelli LDF, Vilela MAP, Rhoden EL. A narrative review of transforming surgical education with artificial intelligence: Opportunities and challenges. *AME Surg J*. 2025;5:1. https://doi.org/10.21037/asj-24-25
31. Isaac S, Phillips MR, Chen KA, Carlson R, Greenberg CC, Khairat S. Usability, acceptability, and implementation of artificial intelligence (AI) and machine learning (ML) techniques in surgical coaching and training: A scoping review. *J Surg Educ*. Published online May 2024:S193172042400165X. https://doi.org/10.1016/j.jsurg.2024.03.018
32. Sathe TS, Roshal J, Naaseh A, L'Huillier JC, Navarro SM, Silvestri C. How I GPT It: Development of custom artificial intelligence (AI) chatbots for surgical education. *J Surg Educ*. 2024;81(6):772–775. https://doi.org/10.1016/j.jsurg.2024.03.004
33. Shaw K, Henning MA, Webster CS. Artificial intelligence in medical education: A scoping review of the evidence for efficacy and future directions. *Med Sci Educ*. 2025;35(3):1803–1816. https://doi.org/10.1007/s40670-025-02373-0
34. Thanawala R. The impact of AI on surgery residency programs: Improving competency, performance, and the future. *Glob Surg Educ—J Assoc Surg Educ*. 2024;3(1):55. https://doi.org/10.1007/s44186-024-00255-4
35. The Topol Review—NHS Health Education England. *The Topol Review—NHS Health Education England*. Accessed September 4, 2025. https://topol.hee.nhs.uk/
36. Olsen GH, Jopling JK. Artificial intelligence in surgery: The American College of Surgeons and the future of the profession. *J Am Coll Surg*. 2022;235(1):146–147. https://doi.org/10.1097/XCS.0000000000000189
37. AI is poised to "Revolutionize" surgery. *ACS*. Accessed September 4, 2025. https://www.facs.org/for-medical-professionals/news-publications/news-and-articles/bulletin/2023/june-2023-volume-108-issue-6/ai-is-poised-to-revolutionize-surgery/
38. Dagli MM, Rajesh A, Asaad M, Butler CE. The use of artificial intelligence and machine learning in surgery: A comprehensive literature review. *Am Surg*. 2023;89(5):1980–1988. https://doi.org/10.1177/00031348211065101

39. Chevalier O, Dubey G, Benkabbou A, Majbar MA, Souadka A. Comprehensive overview of artificial intelligence in surgery: A systematic review and perspectives. *Pflugers Arch*. 2025;477(4):617–626. https://doi.org/10.1007/s00424-025-03076-6
40. Hassan AM, Rajesh A, Asaad M, et al. A surgeon's guide to artificial intelligence – Driven predictive models. *Am Surg*. 2023;89(1):11–19. https://doi.org/10.1177/00031348221103648
41. Kenig N, Monton Echeverria J, Muntaner Vives A. Artificial intelligence in surgery: A systematic review of use and validation. *J Clin Med*. 2024;13(23):7108. https://doi.org/10.3390/jcm13237108
42. Loftus TJ, Tighe PJ, Filiberto AC, et al. Artificial intelligence and surgical decision-making. *JAMA Surg*. 2020;155(2):148–158. https://doi.org/10.1001/jamasurg.2019.4917
43. Douglas MJ, Callcut R, Celi LA, Merchant N. Interpretation and use of applied/operational machine learning and artificial intelligence in surgery. *Surg Clin North Am*. 2023;103(2):317–333. https://doi.org/10.1016/j.suc.2022.11.004
44. Bohnen JD, Chang DC, George BC. Operating room times for teaching and nonteaching cases are converging: Less time for learning? *J Surg Educ*. 2021;78(1):148–159. https://doi.org/10.1016/j.jsurg.2020.06.029
45. Woelfel I, Wang T, Pieper H, Meara M, Chen XP. Distortions in the balance between teaching and efficiency in the operating room. *J Surg Res*. 2023;283:110–117. https://doi.org/10.1016/j.jss.2022.10.032
46. Leon S, Lee S, Perez JE, Hashimoto DA. Artificial intelligence and the education of future surgeons. *Am J Surg*. 2025;246:116257. https://doi.org/10.1016/j.amjsurg.2025.116257
47. Colacci M, Huang YQ, Postill G, et al. Sociodemographic bias in clinical machine learning models: A scoping review of algorithmic bias instances and mechanisms. *J Clin Epidemiol*. 2025;178:111606. https://doi.org/10.1016/j.jclinepi.2024.111606
48. Seyyed-Kalantari L, Zhang H, McDermott MBA, Chen IY, Ghassemi M. Underdiagnosis bias of artificial intelligence algorithms applied to chest radiographs in under-served patient populations. *Nat Med*. 2021;27(12):2176–2182. https://doi.org/10.1038/s41591-021-01595-0
49. Hussain SA, Bresnahan M, Zhuang J. The bias algorithm: How AI in healthcare exacerbates ethnic and racial disparities—A scoping review. *Ethn Health*. 2025;30(2):197–214. https://doi.org/10.1080/13557858.2024.2422848
50. Marko JGO, Neagu CD, Anand PB. Examining inclusivity: The use of AI and diverse populations in health and social care: A systematic review. *BMC Med Inform Decis Mak*. 2025;25(1):57. https://doi.org/10.1186/s12911-025-02884-1
51. Omar M, Sorin V, Agbareia R, et al. Evaluating and addressing demographic disparities in medical large language models: A systematic review. *Int J Equity Health*. 2025;24(1):57. https://doi.org/10.1186/s12939-025-02419-0
52. St John A, Cooper L, Kavic SM. The role of artificial intelligence in surgery: What do general surgery residents think? *Am Surg*. 2024;90(4):541–549. https://doi.org/10.1177/00031348231209524
53. Malik AP, Ahmad W, Iqbal J. The AI surge in surgery: Evolution, challenges, and ethical considerations. *Ann Biomed Eng*. 2025;53(9):1989–1992. https://doi.org/10.1007/s10439-025-03813-z
54. Li B, Kayssi A, McLean LJ. Generative artificial intelligence in surgical publishing. *JAMA Surg*. 2025;160(4):366. https://doi.org/10.1001/jamasurg.2024.6446
55. Principles for the responsible use of artificial intelligence in and for medical education. *AAMC*. Accessed September 4, 2025. https://www.aamc.org/about-us/mission-areas/medical-education/principles-ai-use

6 AI and Pathology Training

Wenchao Han, Steven N. Hart

6.1 INTRODUCTION

Artificial intelligence (AI) is no longer an abstract technological concept confined to computer science laboratories. In pathology, it is becoming a daily reality. Advances in digital pathology, machine learning, and natural language processing have created tools that can, for example, classify tissue, segment tumors, predict biomarkers, and even generate structured pathology reports. (See Figure 6.1.) The emergence of generative AI (1), primarily driven by advancements in transformer architectures, has marked a pivotal time, with transformative impacts across all aspects of society, including medicine (2). For the pathologist in training, this presents both an opportunity and a challenge (3). The opportunity lies in learning to work with systems that can increase diagnostic efficiency and uncover patterns imperceptible to the human eye. The challenge, however, is to do so responsibly, with a clear understanding of both the strengths and limitations of AI.

The pathologist-in-training need not be an AI engineer but must be a discerning and critical user of AI tools. Unlike microscopes or immunohistochemical stains,

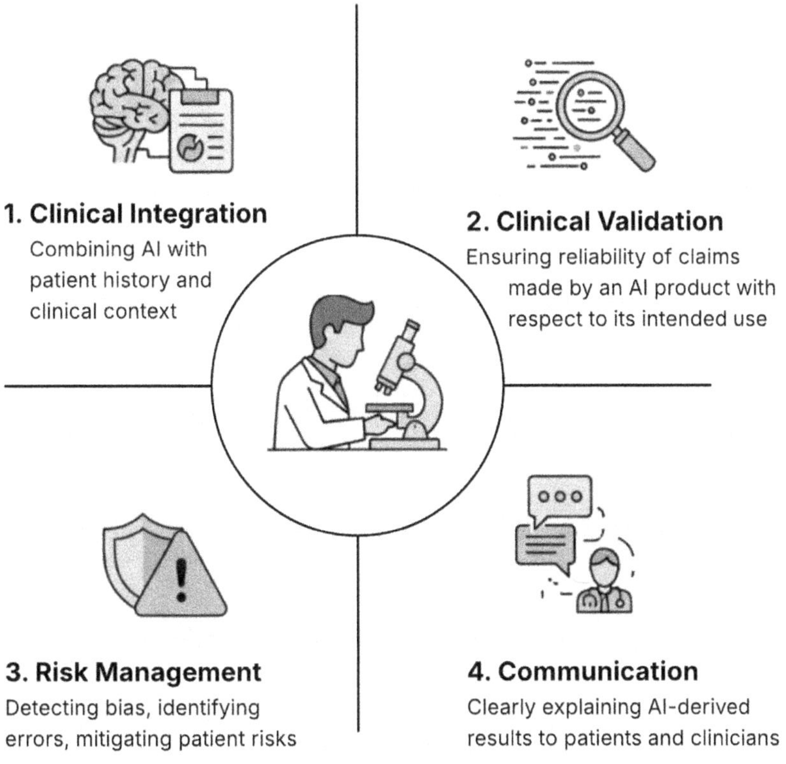
1. Clinical Integration
Combining AI with patient history and clinical context
2. Clinical Validation
Ensuring reliability of claims made by an AI product with respect to its intended use
3. Risk Management
Detecting bias, identifying errors, mitigating patient risks
4. Communication
Clearly explaining AI-derived results to patients and clinicians

Figure 6.1 Pathologist's role in AI stewardship.

DOI: 10.1201/9781003617167-6

AI algorithms are dynamic, probabilistic, and subject to failure modes that are not always obvious. The risk of automation bias—blindly accepting machine output without critical scrutiny—can be particularly dangerous in a clinical environment (4). Just as past generations of pathologists were expected to master molecular diagnostics and quality assurance principles, the new generation must learn to evaluate AI performance, distinguish its vulnerabilities, and integrate it thoughtfully into diagnostic practice.

This chapter is framed by three broad questions: (1) What should the trainee learn? (2) How should the trainee learn to use AI responsibly? And (3) how can AI be practically and ethically embedded into pathology practice?

6.2 WHAT PATHOLOGY TRAINEES NEED TO KNOW

AI already has wide-ranging applications in pathology, with many more on the horizon. Studying current examples provides a practical foundation, while learning machine-learning fundamentals deepens understanding of how models function and where they fail. Equally important is early recognition of risks and limitations so AI can be used safely in clinical practice.

Digital and computational pathology companies are rapidly expanding, offering AI solutions across diagnosis, research, clinical workflows, and education. For trainees, familiarity with these applications—and the principles on which they are built—provides an essential basis for assessing clinical safety and validity, ensuring that patient care is not compromised by the uncritical adoption of vendor claims. A clear example is automated immunohistochemistry (IHC) quantification. Several platforms now provide AI-based scoring of Ki-67 expression in breast cancer, illustrating how machine learning can streamline repetitive, labor-intensive tasks and reduce interobserver variability. Many promising applications are currently translational, enabling discovery and innovation. Emerging models that predict genomic expression profiles directly from hematoxylin and eosin (H&E)–stained tissue sections suggest more cost-effective approaches to advanced diagnostics, although they remain under development and validation. Similarly, multimodal models that integrate histopathology, genomics, and clinical variables may accelerate prognostic algorithms and reveal previously unrecognized biomarkers.

The starting point for any discussion of AI in pathology is data. Unlike human experts, who adapt fluidly to new contexts, AI models are constrained by the characteristics of the datasets on which they were trained. Trainees should recognize that specimen quality, assay variability, reference interval mismatches, and temporal changes in patient populations all exert a profound influence on performance. For example, a system trained on well-fixed, high-resolution slides may falter when confronted with suboptimally processed tissue or a different scanner. Likewise, a model developed on one immunohistochemistry (IHC) platform may yield inconsistent results on another. Even seemingly minor differences in laboratory reference intervals can cause clinical AI tools to misclassify results. AI reliability is therefore not intrinsic to an algorithm; it depends critically on the quality and relevance of the data used in model development, making both data literacy and active human oversight essential for interpretation.

Navigating these principles requires familiarity with fundamental machine-learning concepts. In supervised learning, a model is trained on labeled examples—for instance, distinguishing tumors from non-tumor tissue on histologic slides. In contrast, unsupervised learning identifies patterns without predefined labels, such as clustering patients who share similar molecular profiles. A common pitfall is overfitting, in which a model performs exceptionally well on its training data but fails to replicate those results on external datasets. The ability to maintain accuracy across populations, institutions, and technical platforms—generalizability—is therefore essential for clinical application. Generative AI adds further challenges, including hallucinations, where the system produces outputs that appear plausible but are not grounded in the underlying data or clinical reality.

Pathology trainees must also understand bias in AI (5). Bias extends beyond demographic factors and may arise from technical artifacts, institutional practice patterns, or imbalances in training datasets. A digital pathology model developed on slides from a single academic center may perform poorly in community settings where staining protocols, case distributions, or scanner characteristics differ. Appreciating these sources of bias equips trainees to critically appraise AI outputs and underscores the importance of validating tools across diverse clinical environments.

Another essential competency is the ability to recognize AI "failure zones." Models are often brittle: They perform well under familiar conditions yet may fail abruptly when exposed to novel inputs. Rare or underrepresented entities in training data—such as uncommon tumor subtypes—are frequent blind spots. Artifacts in digital images, including tissue folds, staining variability, or poor digitization, can mislead otherwise accurate systems. A related problem is dataset shift, in which deployment data differs from training data; this can occur, for example, when a laboratory changes an analyte or adopts a new staining protocol, invalidating prior assumptions. Trainees should cultivate the habit of asking, *"Under what circumstances might this output be wrong?"*

Human judgment remains essential. The pathologist-in-the-loop paradigm is the safest approach: AI highlights regions of interest, suggests preliminary interpretations, or drafts report elements, while the pathologist retains responsibility for confirmation, integration, and final diagnosis. Trainees need both technical literacies to understand AI's role and the professional mindset to safeguard patients against its limitations. Unlike a human pathologist, an AI model generally lacks awareness of the broader clinical picture, specifically prior treatment history or discordant radiologic findings. It functions strictly within the mathematical boundaries of its training data. Consequently, the trainee's responsibility extends beyond simply verifying technical accuracy. They must ensure that the narrow output provided by AI is appropriately integrated into the complex and patient-centered reality of medical practice.

6.3 FUNDAMENTALS OF AI IN DIGITAL AND COMPUTATIONAL PATHOLOGY

The growing adoption of digital pathology has created fertile ground for AI to transform the practice of pathology. At its simplest, AI refers to the ability of computers to perform tasks that would otherwise require human intelligence—such as recognizing tumor regions, distinguishing between benign and malignant cells, or predicting patient outcomes based on subtle morphologic patterns. For trainees, the value lies not in learning to build AI models from scratch but in understanding what AI is, how these models are constructed, and what their limitations may be. These foundations enable trainees to leverage AI in pathology practice, contribute to research, and participate meaningfully in evaluation and integration.

In digital and computational pathology, AI models are built by training on large numbers of whole-slide images (WSIs), clinical notes, diagnostic labels, pathology reports, and laboratory results. During training, the model is exposed to examples—such as annotated tumor regions, mitotic figures, or immunohistochemistry stains—and gradually learns to recognize the relevant patterns. Once trained, the model can be assessed on unseen slides to evaluate whether it generalizes well beyond its training data. Poorly designed or narrowly trained models may perform well on familiar slides but fail when applied in a different clinical setting, highlighting the importance of diverse data and external validation.

Different approaches to AI offer different capabilities. Supervised learning, the most common form of machine learning used to train AI models, relies on labeled data provided by pathologists—such as tumor boundaries, grades, or biomarker scores—to guide model training (Table 6.1). This has been successfully applied to tasks such as prostate Gleason grading or automated HER2 and Ki-67 scoring. Unsupervised learning does not require labels but instead finds hidden patterns in the data, such as clustering-based methods, and has been used in research to identify cellular phenotypes. A related paradigm is self-supervised learning, in which the model creates proxy prediction tasks and learns generalizable representations without exhaustive manual annotations. This approach underpins modern foundation models in vision and language (including large language models) and is particularly advantageous in pathology, where detailed annotations are time-consuming and require expert effort.

Real-world use cases illustrate the breadth of AI's applications. Automated mitosis detection can reduce the burden of counting mitotic figures in breast cancer grading. AI-based IHC quantification provides reproducible and standardized scoring for biomarkers such as HER2, PD-L1, and Ki-67, improving consistency across observers. In research, advanced models are now capable of predicting molecular alterations directly from H&E-stained slides—for example, microsatellite instability or gene expression signatures—pointing to a future where image-based AI could complement or even reduce the need for costly molecular assays.

One of the most exciting frontiers in computational pathology is the integration of large language models (LLMs) with image analysis. Traditional

Table 6.1 Common AI Training Approaches in Pathology

Approach	Definition	Data Requirements	Common Pathology Applications
Supervised learning	The model learns to map input images to specific outputs based on explicit examples.	**High:** Requires large datasets labeled by pathologists (for example, tumor boundaries, grades).	Prostate Gleason grading HER2 and Ki-67 scoring Tumor detection
Unsupervised learning	The model identifies hidden structures, patterns, or clusters within the data without predefined categories.	**Low:** Does not require diagnostic labels or annotations.	Discovery of new cellular phenotypes Patient stratification by morphology
Self-supervised learning	A type of unsupervised learning where the model generates its own training signals (proxy tasks) to learn generalizable features.	**Low:** Reduces the need for exhaustive manual annotation, making it scalable for large datasets.	Foundation models (e.g., vision transformers) Feature extraction for downstream tasks

AI in pathology has focused primarily on image-based tasks—detecting tumor regions, quantifying biomarkers, or predicting molecular profiles. However, pathology is not just visual; it is also a highly textual discipline. Reports, synoptic templates, and free-text comments are integral to diagnostic practice, and combining language with image understanding has the potential to transform both efficiency and consistency in reporting. LLMs, such as those that underpin modern generative AI systems, are trained on vast amounts of textual data and can generate coherent, context-sensitive language outputs. In pathology, these models can be adapted to draft structured diagnostic reports, summarize complex findings, or standardize synoptic elements across cases. For example, after an AI system analyzes an H&E slide and identifies invasive carcinoma with positive margins, an LLM could draft a preliminary report that integrates these findings into the correct reporting format. While the pathologist must always review and finalize the report, such systems could significantly reduce administrative burden and improve consistency.

An even more transformative possibility lies in multimodal AI models that combine pathology images with text. These models are trained simultaneously on digitized pathology images and corresponding pathological descriptions, enabling them to learn how histologic patterns relate to diagnostic language. Early research has shown that such models can "explain" their predictions by generating human-readable rationales or even link histologic features to prognostic descriptors automatically. For instance, a multimodal model might highlight a tumor region on a slide while also generating a text explanation such as "poorly differentiated adenocarcinoma with high mitotic activity," providing both visual and narrative reasoning. These approaches open the door to explainable AI in pathology. Unlike conventional image-only models, which output a probability or score without justification, image–language models can provide interpretable narratives that align more closely with the ways pathologists think and communicate. This not only enhances trust in AI output but also facilitates education and training, as trainees can see side by side the features detected by the model and the textual reasoning behind them.

For pathology trainees, literacy in LLMs and multimodal AI is essential to prepare for the next phase of digital transformation. These tools are poised to streamline reporting, standardize communication, and provide novel forms of decision support. Just as importantly, they introduce a new paradigm where AI not only sees but also explains—bridging the gap between quantitative image analysis and the interpretive language of pathology practice.

For pathology trainees, it is important to recognize that AI models are not replacements for clinical judgment but tools designed to augment efficiency, standardization, and discovery. Their strengths include handling large-scale image data, automating repetitive tasks, and revealing novel patterns. Their limitations include dependence on training data quality, vulnerability to bias, and the need for ongoing monitoring once deployed in clinical practice.

As AI continues to advance, trainees will increasingly encounter these tools in both clinical and research settings. By gaining literacy in how AI models are built and applied, pathologists in training can critically evaluate their use, contribute to their responsible adoption, and help shape a future where digital and computational pathology are deeply integrated into precision medicine.

6.4 HOW PATHOLOGY TRAINEES SHOULD APPROACH AI

Pathology trainees should approach AI with the same critical rigor applied to any diagnostic test. Each new system warrants interrogation: *What data were used for training, and how was the model developed? How was performance evaluated and externally validated? How should reported metrics be interpreted for clinical use? How might performance change outside the original development context?* These questions align with evidence-based medicine and should become second nature when evaluating assertions made by AI.

Educational theory provides useful frameworks for structuring this new domain of knowledge. Adult learning theory emphasizes that adults learn most effectively when material is relevant, self-directed, and problem-centered (6). Thus AI literacy should not be taught as abstract computer science but as clinically embedded, case-driven instruction. Bloom's taxonomy provides another scaffold, beginning with basic recognition of concepts, progressing through application in clinical examples, and culminating in evaluation and synthesis. Bloom's earlier work on the "2 sigma problem" highlighted the power of individualized instruction, a principle that resonates with the adaptive potential of AI in medical education (7). Competency-based medical education offers yet another lens: The goal is not exposure time to AI but demonstrable competence, such as the ability to evaluate a validation study, detect potential dataset shifts, or communicate AI limitations in a tumor board (8).

Human oversight remains indispensable. No AI system is infallible, so risk mitigation strategies must become an integral part of education and training. AI outputs should be treated as preliminary opinions rather than as definitive answers, subject always to human arbitration. Audit trails are essential to maintain accountability, allowing institutions to review how AI was used in a diagnostic decision. Interpretability tools, such as attention maps or feature attribution scores, can help pathologists determine whether the AI based its conclusion on relevant features or on spurious artifacts. Clear escalation pathways should be defined for situations in which AI outputs conflict with the trainee's or attending's impressions.

Ethical and professional responsibilities are equally important. Transparency requires that patients and clinical colleagues know when AI contributed to a report. Bias mitigation demands vigilance for inequities introduced by unbalanced training data. Professional communication includes explaining limitations to patients and providers. Regulatory awareness is essential, as AI intersects with FDA, CLIA, CAP, and HIPAA frameworks. Ethical guidance emphasizes transparency, accountability, and governance as cornerstones of responsible integration (9, 10). For trainees, this means recognizing that their professional role extends beyond diagnosis to stewardship of AI's responsible use in medicine.

6.5 HOW AI CAN BE EMBEDDED INTO PATHOLOGY PRACTICE

The practical embedding of AI into pathology should balance innovation with caution. Educational use provides an accessible entry point (1). Generative models can produce practice questions across multiple levels, simulate oral examinations, and support virtual sign-out by comparing draft reports with reference standards. Such exercises foster iterative case review, error recognition, and correction. Large language models can also accelerate journal clubs by summarizing new publications and highlighting methodological issues, helping residents keep pace with rapid literature growth.

Transitioning from education to clinical practice requires additional safeguards. In diagnostic workflows, AI can prescreen or detect regions of interest on whole slide imaging (WSI), quantify cell populations, and flag abnormal laboratory results. Decision support systems may suggest differential diagnoses or ancillary stains for pathologist review. In structured reporting, AI can prepopulate sections, with final synthesis and sign-out by the pathologist. In each of these contexts, the principle of the "pathologist-in-the-loop" must remain paramount: AI aids and supports, but human judgment is the final arbiter.

Successful implementation depends on seamless integration with clinical systems and a clear understanding of end-to-end pathology workflows. Many translational AI systems have not reached clinical deployment because of complicated workflows, failure to deliver meaningful efficiency gains, or marginal diagnostic improvements. Pathology training and clinical experience prepare future pathologists to participate actively in integration. By collaborating as informed end users with AI scientists, engineers, and clinical informaticists, pathologists can guide and accelerate effective deployment.

Interactive platforms that integrate augmented reality with AI overlays may allow trainees to experience sign-out sessions enhanced by live, context-sensitive guidance. These developments, while exciting, underscore the need for trainees to cultivate flexibility and a lifelong learning mindset. The tools available today are evolving rapidly; the essential skill is not mastery of a particular platform but the ability to be nimble and critically adapt to new AI systems as they emerge.

6.6 INSTRUCTIONAL MODULES: Applied Learning

Clinical vignettes are an effective means to anchor abstract principles in the realities of practice. Consider, for example, the case of an AI system that classifies atypical cells in cytology. A trainee may encounter an algorithm that flags numerous cells as suspicious, only to realize upon review that the changes are reactive rather than malignant. The lesson is clear: AI lacks contextual judgment, and, without human arbitration, overtreatment would result.

Another example arises when a laboratory transitions to a new immunohistochemistry platform. A breast cancer biomarker model, which was previously reliable, begins to misclassify cases. The trainee learns to recognize that assay variability and dataset shift can undermine the generalizability of AI systems.

Interpretability tools further illustrate the importance of skepticism. Imagine a lymphoma case in which an AI system confidently predicts malignancy. Attention maps reveal that necrotic areas, rather than viable tumor tissue, drove the model's conclusion. Here, interpretability exposes misattribution, highlighting the necessity of human review.

Communication is the most important competency of all. At an interdisciplinary tumor board, a trainee may present a case where an AI-generated prognosis diverges from traditional staging. The skill lies not only in recognizing the limitations of the AI but in articulating them clearly: "This model was trained on a narrow population and may not generalize to our patient." Such moments underscore the significant role of the pathologist as both diagnostician and communicator, and it is imperative to ensure that AI enhances shared decision-making rather than impeding it.

6.7 CONCLUSION

Artificial intelligence is becoming integral to pathology, and trainees should view AI literacy as a core competency alongside morphologic interpretation, molecular pathology, and laboratory management. The aim is not to become an AI engineer but to cultivate professional habits: (1) proactive learning, (2) data literacy, (3) skepticism about error modes, and (4) a commitment to human oversight. Pathologists must remain the final authority both in rendering diagnoses and in protecting patients from the risks of poorly deployed technology.

Pathology has repeatedly absorbed innovative technologies—from immunohistochemistry to next-generation sequencing—each of which initially raised concern but ultimately proved to be indispensable. AI follows a similar trajectory, at broader scale and faster pace. Unlike static reagents, AI systems are evolving algorithms that require continuous evaluation, monitoring, and risk management. The goal for trainees is to learn how to use AI responsibly today and to adapt to the systems of tomorrow. The future of pathology is not human versus machine but human with machine—pathologists and AI working together to both advance and safeguard diagnostic rigor and patient care.

GLOSSARY

Algorithmic bias: Systematic error in AI models that produces unfair or misleading results, often reflecting imbalances in training data.

Artificial intelligence (AI): The field of computer science focused on creating systems capable of tasks that normally require human intelligence, such as pattern recognition and natural language processing.

Automation bias: The human tendency to over-trust or uncritically accept machine-generated outputs.

Bloom's taxonomy: An educational framework that categorizes levels of learning from basic recall to higher-order evaluation and synthesis.

Competency-based medical education (CBME): A framework that measures trainee progression based on mastery of defined competencies rather than time in training.

Dataset shift: A change in the statistical distribution of data between model training and deployment, leading to reduced accuracy.

Explainability/interpretability: Tools and methods that make AI decision-making processes comprehensible to human users.

Generative AI: A form of AI capable of producing new data or content, such as text, images, or synthetic training slides.

Hallucination (AI): An AI-generated statement or output that is plausible but factually incorrect or fabricated.

Large language models (LLMs): Transformer-based AI systems trained on vast corpora of text, capable of generating human-like language.

Machine learning (ML): A subset of AI that allows systems to learn patterns from data and improve performance without explicit programming.

Multimodal AI: AI models capable of integrating and processing multiple forms of input, such as text, images, and clinical data.

Overfitting: A modeling error in which an algorithm performs well on training data but fails to generalize to new data.

Pathologist-in-the-loop: A model of AI deployment in which the human pathologist reviews, confirms, and remains accountable for all AI outputs.

Reference interval mismatch: A discrepancy between laboratory reference ranges used in training data versus those applied in clinical deployment.

Synthetic data: Artificially generated data that mimic real-world characteristics, often used for training AI models while preserving privacy.

Transformer architecture: A neural network design introduced in 2017 that uses attention mechanisms to process sequential data, forming the foundation of LLMs.

ABBREVIATIONS

ABPath	American Board of Pathology
AI	artificial intelligence
AGI	artificial general intelligence
CAP	College of American Pathologists
CLIA	Clinical Laboratory Improvement Amendments
CME	continuing medical education
FDA	Food and Drug Administration
HIPAA	Health Insurance Portability and Accountability Act

LLM	large language model
ML	machine learning
NETs	neutrophil extracellular traps
USMLE	United States Medical Licensing Examination

REFERENCES

1. Cecchini MJ, Borowitz MJ, Glassy EF, Gullapalli RR, Hart SN, Hassell LA, et al. Harnessing the power of generative artificial intelligence in pathology education: Opportunities, challenges, and future directions. *Arch Pathol Lab Med*. 2025 Feb 1;149(2):142–51.
2. Lee P, Bubeck S, Petro J. Benefits, limits, and risks of GPT-4 as an AI chatbot for medicine. *N Engl J Med*. 2023 Mar 29;388(13):1233–9.
3. Boscardin CK, Gin B, Golde PB, Hauer KE. ChatGPT and generative artificial intelligence for medical education: Potential impact and opportunity. *Acad Med J Assoc Am Med Coll*. 2024 Jan 1;99(1):22–7.
4. Hassell LA, Absar SF, Chauhan C, Dintzis S, Farver CF, Fathima S, et al. Pathology education powered by virtual and digital transformation: Now and the future. *Arch Pathol Lab Med*. 2023 Apr 1;147(4):474–91.
5. Cross JL, Choma MA, Onofrey JA. Bias in medical AI: Implications for clinical decision-making. *PLOS Digit Health*. 2024 Nov;3(11):e0000651.
6. Knowles MS, Holton III EF, Robinson PA, Swanson RA, Robinson PA. *The Adult Learner: The Definitive Classic in Adult Education and Human Resource Development*. 9th ed. London: Routledge; 2020. 406 p.
7. *The 2 Sigma Problem: The Search for Methods of Group Instruction as Effective as One-to-One Tutoring—Bejamin S. Bloom, 1984* [Internet]. [cited 2025 Sep 5]. Available from: https://journals.sagepub.com/doi/10.3102/0013189X013006004
8. Hagemann IS, Elliott R, Kalof A, Keung ES, Patil N, Peterson JEG. Advancing fellowship training in selective pathology. *Arch Pathol Lab Med*. 2022 Apr 1;146(4):501–6.
9. Chauhan C, Gullapalli RR. Ethics of AI in pathology: Current paradigms and emerging issues. *Am J Pathol*. 2021 Oct;191(10):1673–83.
10. Jackson BR, Ye Y, Crawford JM, Becich MJ, Roy S, Botkin JR, et al. The ethics of artificial intelligence in pathology and laboratory medicine: Principles and practice. *Acad Pathol*. 2021 Jan 1;8:2374289521990784.

7 AI in Radiology Training

Jordan D. Perchik, Yeji Han, Pinar Yilmaz

7.1 INTRODUCTION

Radiology and the field of medical imaging more broadly have found themselves at the center of the AI boom in healthcare. Radiology has been the dominant force in the AI marketplace, and the number of FDA-approved AI applications in radiology continues to increase every year. The field is, in many ways, uniquely well suited to AI development and implementation, and AI promises to alleviate many of the problems faced by the specialty today and into the near future [1]. Radiology finds itself poised in an unusual position: The development and implementation of AI has outpaced opportunities for AI training for practicing radiologists. Internationally, the need for AI education in radiology training is being recognized as an emerging issue. Here, we discuss the history of AI in radiology, highlight the ways different health systems have addressed the need for AI education, and highlight the immediate need for improved access to AI education in radiology.

7.2 BRIEF HISTORY OF AI IN RADIOLOGY

7.2.1 A Natural Fit

Radiology is a technology-driven specialty that requires effective coordination among physicians, technologists, IT personnel, and clinic staff to function efficiently. For each radiology exam, there are a number of informatics steps in the electronic health record (EHR) and non-interpretive processes that occur between exam ordering, patient scheduling, and exam acquisition (Figure 7.1). This multistep process is well suited for AI integration to increase efficiency between these multiple systems and steps in the radiology exam life cycle. Additionally, for modalities that involve extensive image processing, such as computed tomography (CT) and magnetic resonance imaging (MRI), these processes can be optimized by AI techniques to improve image quality using less radiation and a lower dose of contrast, and requiring less time to acquire and process images. Even the radiologist's image interpretation parallels how AI applications can detect patterns from images and use these patterns to make diagnoses. In the early 2000s, radiology departments around the United States began to digitize their workflow using a system known as picture archiving and communication systems (PACS) [1–3]. In addition to making medical images more accessible, the use of the Digital Imaging Storage and Communications in Medicine (DICOM) format provided a standardized "language" for image storage and transmission, providing an abundance of available, annotated medical images for algorithm training [4–6].

7.2.2 Meteoric Rise

Between 2010 and 2020, radiology saw an exponential increase in research and publications in AI, and the radiology AI development boom has continued into the 2020s [7, 8]. The 2010s saw a series of advancements in AI and developments in the AI marketplace that precipitated this rapid growth. First, advancements in machine learning techniques and the rise of convolutional neural networks and deep learning allowed computer systems to perform more advanced tasks than ever before, particularly in the area of image processing [9]. Second, access to anonymized, publicly available—and, importantly, labeled—data sets was made available to AI researchers [10–12]. Compiling sufficient numbers of anonymized

DOI: 10.1201/9781003617167-7

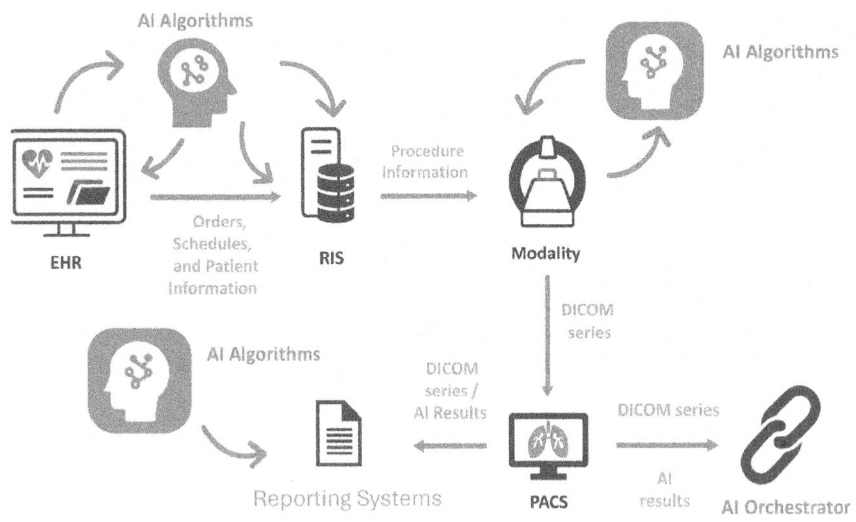

Figure 7.1 Overview of how AI can integrate into the different steps of the radiology exam life cycle.

studies for algorithm training, which can require tens of thousands or hundreds of thousands of cases, serves as a major roadblock. These anonymized data sets drastically lowered the barriers to algorithm development, particularly for cardiothoracic and neuroimaging. Finally, the first deep learning enabled AI application, Arterys, which performs automated segmentation of ventricle volumes on cardiac MRI, gained Food and Drug Administration (FDA) clearance in 2016 and a European Conformity (CE) Mark in 2017 [1]. Arterys was not the first AI-enabled tool to gain clearance for medical use, but its approval served as a precedent for medical AI approval through a Software as a Medical Device (SaMD) pathway. This opened the floodgates for the hundreds of AI applications that have acquired FDA clearance since 2016.

7.2.3 Promise, Panic, and Hype

The prospect of an AI Future has led radiologists and AI developers to imagine what AI could really do once it reached clinical practice. Reports were published demonstrating the effectiveness of AI algorithms in detecting pneumonia and breast cancers, often performing as well as or better than human radiologists [13]. This prompted some in radiology to wonder if the days of the human radiologist were numbered [14–16]. Drastic predictions of AI replacing radiologists by 2021 and totally autonomous AI algorithms have not come to pass, but more modest predictions of AI-supported daily workflow interventions have seen considerable growth [17]. Fears of replacement persist, but as Curtis Langlotz, a radiologist at Stanford University, has said, "AI will not replace radiologists, but radiologists who use AI will replace radiologists who don't" [18].

7.3 AI AND RADIOLOGY EDUCATION

AI is already an established presence in the daily practice of radiology and has been for decades. One of the most widely used examples of clinical radiology AI was first implemented in 1998 and is colloquially referred to as CAD (computer-aided detection); this tool assists radiologists in the detection of suspicious breast lesions for screening mammograms [19]. A survey of radiologists in 2020 by Allen et al. showed that one-third of practicing radiologists used AI in their clinical practice, and it is likely that this number has only increased since that time [20]. Access to clinical AI tools has vastly outpaced access to AI education and training. Fundamental topics in AI education were not widely incorporated in radiology training until the 2020s, and the scope and topics included remain highly variable between programs. A year after the survey by Allen et al. was published, another survey by Li et al. showed that fewer than half of the 62 highest-funded US radiology programs had any AI education in their radiology training curricula [21]. This disconnect between the availability of AI tools and their actual use underscores a pressing need for structured AI education. Without foundational knowledge, radiologists may struggle to interpret AI outputs responsibly or assess the validity and limitations of different AI tools. This disconnect is even more pronounced for radiologists in low- and middle-income countries (LMICs). In low-income health systems, strained resources and high need could reap the most benefits from AI tools that increase efficiency, raise proficiency, and can offload burdensome and low-value tasks [22], but unfortunately it is in these regions where AI education and training has historically been the least accessible.

Medical students, radiology trainees, and practicing radiologists all over the world recognize the integral role that AI will play in the future of radiology practice and the imperative to integrate AI into radiology education [23–27]. Both a challenge and a strength of the current state of AI education in radiology is the diverse and multifaceted approach to how AI should be taught to radiology trainees. Some AI education programs are organized and led through individual institutions, while others are led by professional organizations or aligned with national health service initiatives (Figure 7.2). Programs can vary in duration from weeks or months to an entire year of study. Some programs are in-person with hands-on components, while others are remote in order to increase accessibility for asynchronous learners. Some courses are free, while still others require a fee [27–33]. The variability in program curricula, format, and learning objectives allows us to compare and contrast the different methods of delivering AI education to radiology trainees and how each method reflects the needs and resources of the learners and health systems it serves.

7.3.1 United States

Radiology residency in the United States occurs after completion of four years of medical school and a one-year internship and is typically four years with an option for a one- to two-year fellowship after completion of residency. Radiology is a highly competitive residency, although there was a significant decrease in applications during the height of the AI panic in 2016 and 2017 [34].

Overall, there is significant interest in AI education among radiology trainees and educators, and access to AI education among U.S. radiology trainees is relatively high (with options for in-person and remote courses). Access to hands-on experiences and opportunities for research and scholarship in AI vary between high- and low-resource programs. Larger programs may have AI research labs as well as dedicated AI or informatics pathways or fellowships for their trainees. As an example, the University of Washington offers a six-month Deep Learning Pathway for its radiology residents. Residents learn about the fundamental methods and structure of a deep learning application, how to prepare data to train and test a deep learning application, and how to use deep learning to solve clinical problems with the program culminating in a capstone project at the end of the six-month pathway [35]. Other training programs opt to integrate AI education

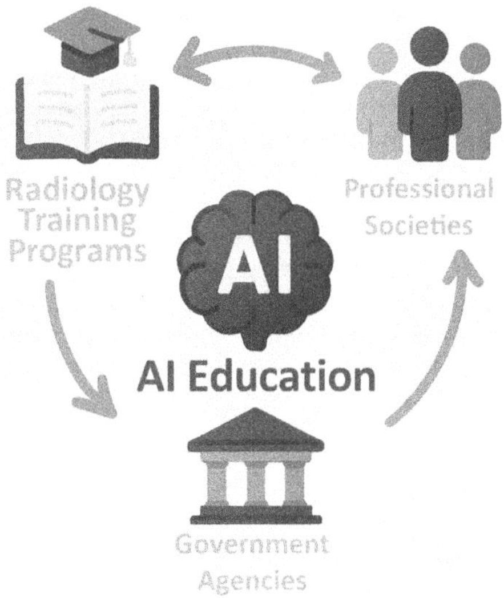

Figure 7.2 Representation of the agencies most commonly responsible for providing AI education resources for radiologists: radiology training programs, radiology professional societies, and government agencies.

lectures into the general resident education curriculum, such as the University of Alabama at Birmingham where a recurring one-week AI education series is held each year [36]. A number of training programs integrate AI education with informatics education, offering informatics pathways and fellowships that at least partially include special topics in AI, specifically as it relates to AI deployment [37–40]. Lower-resource programs may not have the personnel or expertise to develop their own on-site AI education programming or facilitate AI research. For lower-resource programs without on-site AI education programming, a number of paid and free courses are available for residents looking to develop competency in the fundamentals of AI [27, 31].

AI-related topics are tested on the U.S. Radiology board certification exam (the Qualifying [Core] Exam), particularly in the Non-Interpretive Skills (NIS) section. In 2025, the NIS study guide included basic topics on methods in algorithm training, natural language processing, deep learning for image reconstruction, deployment challenges, and bias in AI [41]. The inclusion of these topics could be considered fundamental competencies in AI literacy for U.S. radiology trainees; however, no true core curriculum currently exists for AI education. The high variability in terms of length of AI courses and depth of the content can make it difficult to determine which education strategy best serves the needs of the typical radiology trainee. The 6- to 12-month intensive AI/informatics-focused resident pathways and resident fellowships more often include topics in coding and computer science, database management, and data preparation, advanced statistical methods, and lessons in developing algorithms. Shorter courses that last one week to one month typically focus on fundamental AI topics and basic terms and methods before moving on to more practical, clinical applications of AI in different radiology subspecialties. Between the different course types, there are a number of common themes, including fundamental terms and methods of AI, data preparation and algorithm training, recognizing AI pitfalls such as algorithmic bias, algorithm drift, and "black box" results, and ethical considerations for AI integration [27, 35, 42, 43]. There has been a growing push for radiology trainees to have access to AI tools during training so that they gain hands-on experience with the types of tools they will use in their future clinical practice; however, there is continued debate on how and when this should occur.

Increasingly, fundamental topics in AI are being taught in U.S. medical schools. In a 2023–2024 survey, 77% of medical students in the United States reported that they covered AI in their curricula to some extent; however, much like the variability seen between radiology training programs, the material covered, length of courses, and depth of content differ between institutions [42]. These topics include fundamental terms and methods of AI but also cover topics relevant to the broader practice of medicine including large language models (LLMs) and clinical decision support (CDS) tools [44, 45].

7.3.2 The Netherlands

Radiology residency in the Netherlands is a five-year competency-based training overseen by the national radiology society (Nederlandse Vereniging van Radiologie [NVvR]) conducted in academic and non-academic hospitals, and at least two of five years must be completed in an academic center. Radiology is one of the most competitive specialties in the Netherlands with an acceptance rate around 2.3% of newly graduated doctors per year. In response to increasing utilization of medical imaging and the increasing demand on a limited pool of radiologists, the Dutch capacity agency advised an increase in radiologist training capacity from 2024 to 2027 [46].

Basic knowledge of medical imaging informatics is included in the common trunk education. The NVvR committee of medical techniques of the national society published a literature list of AI resources to expand knowledge in this field [47–49]. Despite the role of AI-innovation in the program, AI education is not yet uniformly integrated into the residency program. At the national level, courses and workshops have been organized by several universities and also AI masterclasses by the junior section of the national radiology society since 2019 [50].

A framework has been proposed to explore the integration of AI into radiology education, but there is a lack of opportunity for clinical practice and education leaders to develop these skills and guide the transformation of radiology training programs into AI incubators [51]. The Netherlands faces several of the same obstacles that have been described in the United States as impediments for created, tailored AI curricula, such as access to mentorship, lack of time, limited trainee interest or experience, and rapidly evolving technologies [52]. The most recent five-step framework to implement and evaluate a three-day AI-curriculum in radiology residency programs has been proposed by a multidisciplinary team of AI engineers from the University of Twente, data scientists of the Data Science Center in Health, and radiologists from the Department of University Medical Center Groningen [51]. They designed a framework consisting of five steps: to gather a multidisciplinary team of AI experts, to assess the knowledge levels and needs of residents, to define learning goals, to match these goals with effective methods, and to execute and evaluate this pilot program. The AI curriculum consisted of three days with lectures elaborating on the fundamentals of AI algorithms, quantitative approaches on data and imaging quality, use of AI in clinical care and research, basic integration of AI and billing, and legal and ethical issues. They also executed pre- and post-curriculum surveys to evaluate the course, with most participants supporting the idea that the pilot AI curriculum should be incorporated into the existing radiology training program. Lectures on AI fundamentals and group-based discussions were evaluated as the most useful, whereas hands-on laboratory sessions and building algorithms were assessed as less useful. For future iterations of the course, participants noted that topics on AI integrated workflow, legal and insurance-related issues, and cost-effectiveness of AI tools in healthcare should be included.

Radiologists in the Netherlands demonstrate a relatively high rate of AI adoption into clinical practice, with 33% of radiologists reporting use of AI in 2022 [53]. In general, the attitude toward AI in practice in the Netherlands is positive, and radiology residents and radiologists are enthusiastic about AI education and implementation in residency training and clinical practice [6]. Some centers like the University of Groningen have used the preceding framework to integrate AI into radiology training, while others, such as Leiden University and Erasmus University, have leveraged industry partnerships to develop research and education opportunities for their radiology residents [54, 55].

Medical education in the Netherlands consists of a six-year medical training program, which includes a three-year "Bachelor phase" with a focus on preclinical studies and a three-year "Masters phase," which includes internships, electives, and scientific research. University Medical Centers (UMCs) are increasingly integrating AI into general medical education, primarily in the Bachelor phase. In 2024, Leiden University Medical Center became the first medical program to include AI in its curriculum [56]. Despite the opportunities that exist within individual universities, no national standards for AI education exist, and radiology residents in the Netherlands continue to report that AI education in radiology training is lacking [51, 57].

7.3.3 South Korea

In South Korea, after graduating from medical school, trainees complete a one-year internship followed by four years of radiology training [58]. Radiology is considered one of the most competitive residency specialties in the country, having experienced a significant increase in applications between the 1990s and 2000s, into the 2010s and 2020s [59]. Radiology trainees typically rotate through different subspecialties for one to two months and may participate in supplemental education programs through the Korean Society of Radiology (KSR) during their residency training [59, 60]. AI education is not yet widely included in radiology residency programs. A 2020 survey of South Korean radiologists reported that only 16% had prior experience with AI-related studies and that 90% expressed support for incorporating AI education into radiology training in the future [61]. A subsequent publication in 2023 drew attention to the continued lack of widespread AI integration in radiology training and laid out a road map for core AI education competencies, including fundamental concepts of AI and machine learning, overview of AI applications in medicine and radiology, clinical validation and application of AI models, and development of machine learning models to solve clinical problems [62]. Korean radiologists find themselves in a similar position as radiologists in the United States and in the Netherlands, in that integration of AI into radiology practice has steeply outpaced education, with 60% of South Korean radiologists reporting use of AI in their clinical practice in 2023 [63]. The Korean Society of Radiology has made efforts to fill some of the gaps in AI education by offering supplemental educational programs and by featuring AI prominently in their annual meeting for practicing radiologists and radiology trainees [64].

Despite the relatively low level of AI education included in radiology training, South Korean medical schools have successfully instituted AI education initiatives that provide some of the most comprehensive medical student-level AI education in the world. The government project Support for Medical AI Education and Overseas Expansion was launched in 2022 and served as a catalyst for the integration of AI into medical education throughout South Korea [65]. There is a general consensus among medical graduates about the need for AI education in medical schools, and as of 2023, 75% of medical schools in Korea have incorporated AI into their curricula, mostly as part of the essential coursework [66].

Since nearly all medical schools in Korea follow a structure divided into preclinical (two years) and clinical phases (two years of pre-clerkship and two years of clerkship), AI courses are mainly offered during the preclinical phase. For example, at Dong-A University, first-year preclinical students take a 15-week course titled Medical Big Data Machine Learning Basics and Practice, which covers the history of medical AI, machine learning concepts, medical big data analysis, and AI ethics, with hands-on coding sessions for R (a computer programing language). In the second year of the preclinical phase, students take another 15-week course titled Medical Deep Learning Basics and Practice, which focuses on deep learning—ranging from basic mathematics to reinforcement learning. At Korea University, several elective courses are offered during the preclinical phase, such as AI and Future Medicine, Introduction to Digital Pathology Image Analysis, and AI in Medicine. AI and Future Medicine introduces basic AI concepts and provides hands-on experience using MATLAB (a programming and numeric computing platform).

7.3.4 United Kingdom

Radiology training in the United Kingdom (UK) occurs after completion of medical school, taking four to five years, and typically requires five years of postgraduate training. The first three years of radiology training are dedicated to a core, or generalist, curriculum. The last two years are dedicated to subspecialty training, which includes preparation for the Fellowship of the Royal College of Radiologists (FRCR) exams. Radiology is a highly competitive specialty in the UK, historically drawing strong applicants from a broad pool of junior doctors [67].

The UK is one of the global leaders in AI research and publication [8]; however, integration of AI into radiology training has been sluggish. There is a high level of interest in AI education among radiology trainees in the UK, and the broad consensus among trainees is that AI is underrepresented in radiology education. In a survey published in 2023, 83.7% of trainees expressed interest in AI use in radiology, and nearly all (98.7%) believed AI should be taught during training, but only one out of 149 (0.7%) radiology trainees surveyed reported that they received AI education during their radiology training [68].

Currently, AI topics are not included in the FRCR board certification exams, and there is no standardized national AI curriculum for radiology training. For radiologists in practice, professional societies provide the most robust opportunities for AI education. The Royal College of Radiologists (RCR) is offering structured continued professional development (CPD) through a Clinical Radiology Artificial Intelligence blended-learning course, combining online modules and live workshops [69]. Although there is limited structured AI education for radiologists in training in the UK at present, familiarity with fundamental AI and machine learning techniques is listed as a core competency for radiographers/technologists in the UK and could serve as a model for future radiology AI education curricula [70]. Additionally, UK medical schools have shown a more concerted effort in recent years to define a curriculum and core competencies for AI education during medical training [71]. The proposed medical school curriculum covers broad topics such as data governance and management, privacy and security, evaluating and implementing an AI application, and ethics of healthcare AI. A greater presence of fundamental AI education within the medical school curriculum could serve to fill the gaps in radiology training, similar to the system seen in South Korea. However, while this curriculum provides a solid foundation for healthcare AI, radiology training programs would still need to develop programming to cover the specialty-specific topics and special considerations of AI in medical imaging and clinical radiology practice.

7.3.5 International Radiology AI Education Initiatives: The Artificial Intelligence Literacy Course

Opportunities for formal radiology AI education are difficult to come by for the majority of the global radiology community. Even in high-resource settings and high-income countries, AI education infrastructure can be lacking and highly variable from institution to institution, and this trend becomes even more pronounced in low- and middle-income countries. Global health-focused radiology organizations, such as RadAID and Health4TheWorld have made strides in bridging this gap by providing free, remote radiology courses for their partner programs around the world.

The Artificial Intelligence in Radiology Education (AIRE) initiative was founded in 2020 to deliver accessible, scalable programming for radiology trainees [72, 73]. Its flagship offering, the AI Literacy Course, began as a single-institution program at the University of Alabama at Birmingham and has since grown into the world's largest free AI education resource for radiology. Delivered as a one-week course, it introduces fundamental AI concepts, clinical applications, and critical pitfalls. For most participants, it represents their first structured encounter with AI in radiology [73].

The course goals are to provide a foundational knowledge of AI terms and methods, set realistic expectations for AI's role in clinical practice, demonstrate common use cases, and discuss important ethical considerations for ethical AI implementation. Course directors aim to show participants what AI can do but, more importantly, what it cannot do by discussing key pitfalls, including narrowness (AI only being able to perform a single specific task in a specific setting), brittleness (AI failing to perform its task when conditions are even minorly changed), and risk for bias (AI demonstrating different outcomes for different demographics and patient populations) in clinical AI applications. Of particular importance to the global health community are the sessions on AI ethics and mitigating the risks of algorithm bias, as health systems in LMICs could stand to benefit the most from clinical AI integration, but these communities may have fewer data security and privacy protections and could be at higher risk of AI errors due to the historical underrepresentation of imaging data from these communities during algorithm training [22].

The curriculum includes ten lectures delivered over five days, beginning with fundamental terms and methods of AI. Subspecialty applications are covered on a rotating biennial basis—such as neuroradiology, breast imaging, pediatric imaging, and musculoskeletal imaging—alongside special topics like The AI Marketplace, ethics, and quality assurance. A hands-on industry collaboration on the final day enables learners to engage directly with AI tools integrated into radiology workflows. The course also introduces categories of AI applications, such as computer-aided detection (CADe), computer-aided triage (CADt), and computer-aided diagnosis (CADx), as well as workflow tools like medical image management and processing systems (MIMPS).

The program's growth and partnerships have been central to its international reach. Its remote, no-cost model allowed it to scale quickly to institutions lacking in-house AI expertise. Collaborations with NGOs such as RadAID and Health4TheWorld have extended access to trainees in more than 30 countries, addressing disparities in AI education, particularly between high-income regions

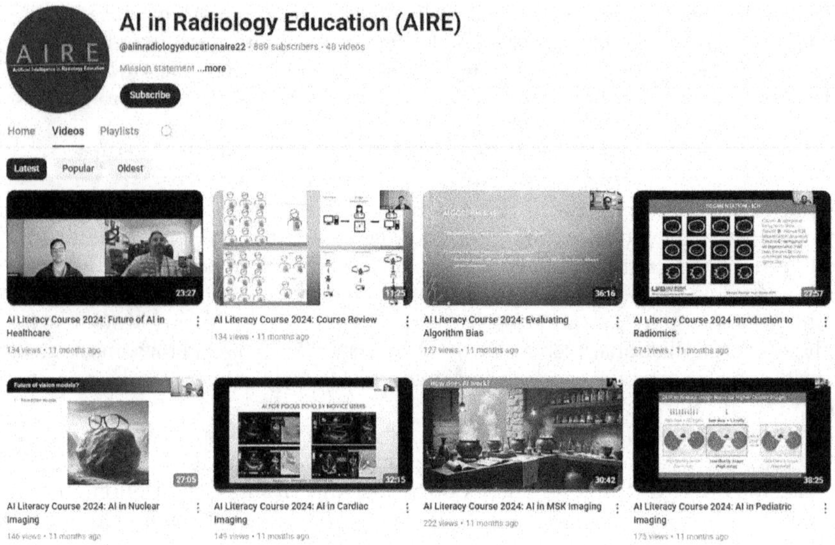

Figure 7.3 Home page for the AI in Radiology Education YouTube channel.

and LMICs [73]. The course has had an enduring effect with participants who repeat the program, demonstrating improved evaluation scores from year to year and over 90% expressing interest in continued participation.

Challenges remain for this remote AI education format. The course is offered only in English and previously was only provided in a live format. Since 2023, the course has offered an asynchronous format with recorded lectures for international participants in time zones not amenable to live participation (Figure 7.3) [74]. This format also allows for accessibility features such as closed captioning and translation into other languages; however, the use of medical and technical jargon can result in errors in transcription and translation [75]. AIRE led a Spanish language AI Literacy Course in 2022. The organization plans to collaborate with international radiology associations to provide additional non-English language courses to address the needs of international learners with content catered to the individual host regions [76–79]. Future initiatives also include (1) building partnerships with AI developers to provide hands-on demonstrations of different radiology AI applications currently in the marketplace and (2) developing an algorithm training/testing database to allow learners to experience how algorithms can be trained from a set of imaging data.

7.4 CONCLUSION

Radiology is likely the most advanced specialty for AI integration in the healthcare field; however, the corresponding educational infrastructure has not yet achieved comparable maturity. Even within high-resource settings, where AI curricula are increasingly incorporated into residency training, the lack of a core AI curriculum, disparities in educational resources between institutions, and limited opportunities for meaningful, hands-on experience with clinical AI tools will continue to serve as barriers to AI education. In countries with strong existing AI development infrastructure, such as the Netherlands, South Korea, and the UK, integration of formal AI education continues to be an unmet need for radiology trainees. Emerging initiatives at the undergraduate medical education level provide a useful foundation, yet they frequently lack sufficient emphasis on the unique challenges and applications of imaging-based AI. To prepare radiologists for practice, specialty-level instruction must address fundamental terminology, data curation, privacy and security considerations, ethical implications, and algorithmic bias, while also equipping trainees with the skills to evaluate performance metrics, identify false positives and false negatives, and critically appraise the clinical utility of AI tools.

Recent international efforts to democratize access to AI education have underscored the feasibility of scalable and equitable training models. Nevertheless, enduring barriers related to linguistic accessibility, geographic distribution, and applicability to local health systems highlight the need for continued evolution to ensure a more equitable AI future. Notably, participation from learners across more than 30 countries has demonstrated that radiology-specific AI education provides both foundational knowledge and practical value, whether as a supplement to existing curricula or as a primary source of training. The broader lesson from these initiatives is that enhancing accessibility for learners in resource-limited settings ultimately strengthens the global educational environment, underscoring the imperative to design AI education in radiology that is comprehensive, equitable, and internationally relevant.

ABBREVIATIONS

AI	artificial intelligence
FDA	Food and Drug Administration
IT	information technology
EHR	electronic health record
PACS	picture archiving and communication systems
DICOM	digital imaging storage and communications in medicine
CE	European Conformity
SaMD	software as a medical device
CAD	computer-aided detection
LMIC	low- and middle-income country
LLM	large language model
NVvR	Netherlands Society of Radiology
UMC	University Medical Center
KSR	Korean Society of Radiology
FRCR	Fellowship of the Royal College of Radiologists

REFERENCES

1. Driver, C. N., Bowles, B. S., Bartholmia, B. J., & Greenberg-Worisek, A. J. (2019, October 30). *Artificial intelligence in radiology: A call for thoughtful application. Clinical and translational science.* https://doi.org/10.1111/cts.12704
2. Thrall, J. H. (2005). Reinventing radiology in the digital age Part 1: The all-digital department. *Radiology, 236*(2), 382–385. https://doi.org/10.1148/radiol.2362050257
3. Kohl, M., Dreyer, K. J., & Geis, J. R. (2015). Rethinking radiology informatics. *American Journal of Roentgenology, 204*(4), 716–720. https://doi.org/10.2214/AJR.14.13840
4. Kahn, C. E., et al. (2007). Toward best practices in radiology reporting. *Journal of the American College of Radiology.* https://www.jacr.org/article/S1546-1440(07)00322-5/fulltext
5. Fazal, M. I., Patel, M. E., Tye, J., & Gupta, Y. (2018). The past, present and future role of artificial intelligence in imaging. *European Journal of Radiology, 105*, 246–250. https://www.sciencedirect.com/science/article/pii/S0720048X18302250

6. Nensa, F., Demircioglu, A., & Rischpler, C. (2025). Artificial intelligence in nuclear medicine. *European Journal of Radiology Open, 26*, 100512. https://www.sciencedirect.com/science/article/pii/S305057712500012X
7. U.S. Food and Drug Administration. (2025, August 29). *Artificial intelligence and machine learning (AI/ML)-enabled medical devices.* https://www.fda.gov/medical-devices/software-medical-device-samd/artificial-intelligence-and-machine-learning-aiml-enabled-medical-devices
8. Perera, N., Perchik, J. D., Perchik, M. C., & Tridandapani, S. (2022). Trends in medical artificial intelligence publications from 2000–2020: Where does radiology stand? *Open Journal of Clinical Medical Images, 2(2), 1052.*
9. Rajpurkar, P., Chen, E., Banerjee, O., & Topol, E. J. (2022). AI in health and medicine. *Nature Medicine, 28*, 31–38. https://doi.org/10.1038/s41591-021-01614-0
10. Willemink, M. J., et al. (2020, February 18). Preparing medical imaging data for machine learning. *Radiology*. https://doi.org/10.1148/radiol.2020192224
11. Tang, A., et al. (2018). Canadian Association of Radiologists white paper on artificial intelligence in radiology. *Canadian Association of Radiologists Journal, 69*(2), 120–135. https://doi.org/10.1016/j.carj.2018.02.002
12. Chockley, K., & Emanuel, E. (2016). The end of radiology? Three threats to the future practice of radiology. *Journal of the American College of Radiology, 13*(12 Pt A), 1415–1420. https://doi.org/10.1016/j.jacr.2016.07.010
13. Wang, S., Summers, R. M. (2012). Machine learning and radiology. *Medical Image Analysis, 16*(5), 933–951. https://www.sciencedirect.com/science/article/pii/S1361841512000333
14. Mukherjee, S. (2017, March 27). A.I. versus M.D.: What happens when the diagnosis is automated? *The New Yorker*. https://www.newyorker.com/magazine/2017/04/03/ai-versus-md
15. Gong, B., et al. (2019). Influence of artificial intelligence on Canadian medical students' preference for radiology specialty: A national survey study. *Academic Radiology, 26*(4), 566–577. https://doi.org/10.1016/j.acra.2018.08.018
16. Siegel, E. (2017). Rest assured, João, you are safe from artificial intelligence. *Applied Radiology*. Retrieved June 5, 2024, from https://appliedradiology.com/articles/rest-assured-jo-o-you-are-safe-from-artificial-intelligence
17. Gichoya, J. W., Nuthakki, S., Maity, P. G., & Purkayastha, S. (2018). Phronesis of AI in radiology: Superhuman meets natural stupidity. *arXiv*. https://doi.org/10.48550/arXiv.1803.11244
18. Langlotz, C. P. (2019, May 15). Will artificial intelligence replace radiologists? *Radiology: Artificial Intelligence*. https://doi.org/10.1148/RYAI.2019190058
19. Chan, H. P., Samala, R. K., & Hadjiiski, L. M. (2020). CAD and AI for breast cancer—Recent developments and challenges. *British Journal of Radiology, 93*(1108), 20190580. https://doi.org/10.1259/bjr.20190580
20. Allen, B., Agarwal, S., Coombs, L., Wald, C., & Dreyer, K. (2021). 2020 ACR Data Science Institute artificial intelligence survey. *Journal of the American College of Radiology, 18*(8), 1153–1159. https://doi.org/10.1016/j.jacr.2021.04.002
21. Li, D., Morkos, J., Gage, D., & Yi, P. H. (2022). Artificial intelligence educational and research initiatives and leadership positions in academic radiology departments. *Current Problems in Diagnostic Radiology, 51*(4), 552–555. https://doi.org/10.1067/j.cpradiol.2022.01.004
22. Mollura, D. J., et al. (2020). Artificial intelligence in low- and middle-income countries: Innovating global health radiology. *Radiology, 297*(3), 513–520. https://doi.org/10.1148/radiol.2020201434

23. Huisman, M., et al. (2021). An international survey on AI in radiology in 1,041 radiologists and radiology residents part 1: Fear of replacement, knowledge, and attitude. *European Radiology, 31*(9), 7058–7066. https://doi.org/10.1007/s00330-021-07781-5
24. Abuzaid, M. M., Elshami, W., McConnell, J., & Tekin, H. O. (2021). An extensive survey of radiographers from the Middle East and India on artificial intelligence integration in radiology practice. *Health and Technology, 11*, 1045–1050. https://doi.org/10.1007/s12553-021-00583-1
25. Yang, L., Ene, I. C., Belaghi, R. A., Koff, D., Stein, N., & Santaguida, P. L. (2022). Stakeholders' perspectives on the future of artificial intelligence in radiology: A scoping review. *European Radiology, 32*, 1477–1495. https://doi.org/10.1007/s00330-021-08214-z
26. Salastekar, N. V., Maxfield, C., Hanna, T. N., Krupinski, E. A., Heitkamp, D., & Grimm, L. J. (2023). Artificial intelligence/machine learning education in radiology: Multi-institutional survey of radiology residents in the United States. *Academic Radiology, 30*(7), 1481–1487. https://doi.org/10.1016/j.acra.2023.01.005
27. Perchik, J. D., et al. (2023). Artificial intelligence literacy: Developing a multi-institutional infrastructure for AI education. *Academic Radiology, 30*(7), 1472–1480. https://doi.org/10.1016/j.acra.2022.10.002
28. Yang, L., Ene, I. C., Belaghi, R. A., Koff, D., Stein, N., & Santaguida, P. L. (2022). Stakeholders' perspectives on the future of artificial intelligence in radiology: A scoping review. *European Radiology, 32*, 1477–1495. https://doi.org/10.1007/s00330-021-08214-z
29. Lindqwister, A. L., Hassanpour, S., Lewis, P. J., & Sin, J. M. (2021). AI-RADS: An artificial intelligence curriculum for residents. *Academic Radiology, 28*(12), 1810–1816. https://doi.org/10.1016/j.acra.2020.09.017
30. Wiggins, W. F., Caton, M. T., Magudia, K., Rosenthal, M. H., & Andriole, K. P. (2021). A conference-friendly, hands-on introduction to deep learning for radiology trainees. *Journal of Digital Imaging, 34*, 1026–1033. https://doi.org/10.1007/s10278-021-00492-9
31. Radiological Society of North America. (2024). *The RSNA imaging AI certificate program.* Oak Brook, IL: Author. https://www.rsna.org/ai-certificate
32. Hu, R., Rizwan, A., Hu, Z., Li, T., Chung, A. D., & Kwan, B. Y. M. (2023). An artificial intelligence training workshop for diagnostic radiology residents. *Radiology: Artificial Intelligence, 5*(2). https://doi.org/10.1148/ryai.220170
33. Ng, F. Y., et al. (2023). Artificial intelligence education: An evidence-based medicine approach for consumers, translators, and developers. *Cell Reports Medicine, 4*(10), 101230. https://doi.org/10.1016/j.xcrm.2023.101230
34. Deng, F., & Moy, L. (2023). The U.S. radiology residency match: Update and multidecade trends. *Radiology, 308(3), e232064.* https://doi.org/10.1148/radiol.232064
35. Imagedeep.io. (2025). *AI education and imaging platform.* Retrieved September 4, 2025, from https://imagedeep.io
36. University of Alabama at Birmingham. (2025). *Perchik directs artificial intelligence literacy course.* Retrieved September 4, 2025, from https://www.uab.edu/medicine/radiology/news-events/perchik-directs-artificial-intelligence-literary-course/
37. Mayo Clinic College of Medicine and Science. (2025). *Radiology informatics and artificial intelligence fellowship (Minnesota).* Retrieved September 4, 2025, from https://college.mayo.edu/academics/residencies-and-fellowships/radiology-informatics-and-artificial-intelligence-fellowship-minnesota/

38. University of Maryland Medical System. (2025). *Diagnostic radiology residency curriculum.* Retrieved September 4, 2025, from https://www.umms.org/ummc/pros/gme/residency/diagnostic-radiology/curriculum
39. Emory University School of Medicine. (2025). *Imaging informatics and quality.* Retrieved September 4, 2025, from https://med.emory.edu/departments/radiology/quality-informatics/imaging-informatics.html
40. Gerard, R., et al. (2022). Imaging informatics fellowship curriculum consensus: A survey of program directors. *Journal of Digital Imaging.* https://doi.org/10.1007/s10278-022-00702-y
41. American Board of Radiology. (2025). *2025 NIS study guide (Version 2).* https://www.theabr.org/wp-content/uploads/2025/01/2025-NIS-Study-Guide-v2.pdf
42. Volin, J., van Assen, M., Bala, W., Safdar, N., & Balthazar, P. (2025). Artificial intelligence and its effect on radiology residency education: Current challenges, opportunities, and future directions. *Journal of the American College of Radiology.* Advance online publication. https://doi.org/10.1016/j.jacr.2025.07.004 PubMed
43. Lindqwister, A. L., Hassanpour, S., Lewis, P. J., & Sin, J. M. (2021). AI-RADS: An artificial intelligence curriculum for residents. *Academic Radiology, 28*(12), 1810–1816. https://doi.org/10.1016/j.acra.2020.09.017
44. Boyle, P. (2024, April 10). Medical schools move from worrying about AI to teaching it. *Association of American Medical Colleges (AAMC) News.* https://www.aamc.org/news/medical-schools-move-worrying-about-ai-teaching-it
45. American Medical Association. (2024). *How AI is being incorporated into medical school.* https://www.ama-assn.org/practice-management/digital-health/how-ai-being-incorporated-medical-school
46. Neutel, K., Righolt, A., & Joldersma, C. (2024). Zo berekent het Capaciteitsorgaan het aantal opleidingsplaatsen. *In MemoRad: Jaargang 29, Nummer 1* (Vol. 29, No. 1, pp. 22–25). Nederlandse Vereniging voor Radiologie. https://radiologen.nl/system/files/bestanden/publicaties/nvvr_mr_29.1_web_volledige_bestand
47. van Ooijen, P. M. A. (Ed.). (2021). *Basic knowledge of medical imaging informatics: Undergraduate level and level I* (Imaging Informatics for Healthcare Professionals). Springer Cham. https://doi.org/10.1007/978-3-030-71885-5
48. Nederlandse Vereniging voor Radiologie. (n.d.). *AI resources for residents in radiology* [PDF]. https://radiologen.nl/sites/default/files/OenO/aios_info/ai_resources_for_residents_in_radiology_003
49. Nederlandse Vereniging voor Radiologie. (n.d.). *Radiologen.nl* [Website]. Retrieved September 25, 2025, from https://radiologen.nl/
50. Nederlandse Vereniging voor Radiologie. (n.d.). *NVvR MemoRad, 24*(3). https://radiologen.nl/system/files/bestanden/publicaties/nvvr_mr_24.3_web
51. van Kooten, M. J. T., de Boer, W. J. A., van der Zant, F., van de Schoot, R., van Ginneken, B., Vos, F. M., & van Hillegersberg, R. (2024). A framework to integrate artificial intelligence training into radiology residency programs. *Radiology: Artificial Intelligence.* Advance online publication. https://pubmed.ncbi.nlm.nih.gov/38228800/
52. Tejani, A. S., Elhalawani, H., Moy, L., Kohli, M., & Kahn, C. E. (2022). Artificial intelligence and radiology education. *Radiology: Artificial Intelligence, 5*(1), e220084. https://doi.org/10.1148/ryai.220084
53. van Leeuwen, K. G., de Wit, G. A., Broeders, M. J. M., Reijerink, J., Boellaard, R., Rombouts, S. J.,. . . Zijlstra, F. (2023). Clinical use of artificial intelligence products for radiology: Adoption in the Netherlands. *European Radiology.* https://www.ncbi.nlm.nih.gov/pmc/articles/PMC10791748/

54. Qure.ai & Erasmus MC. (n.d.). *Qure.ai and Erasmus MC launch AI innovation centre for medical imaging*. Retrieved September 25, 2025, from https://www.qure.ai/news_press_coverages/qure-ai-and-erasmus-mc-launch-ai-innovation-centre-for-medical-imaging
55. Leiden University Medical Center. (n.d.). *Artificial intelligence–based innovations in radiotherapy*. Retrieved September 25, 2025, from https://www.lumc.nl/en/afdelingen/radiotherapie/artificial-intelligence-based-innovations/
56. Leiden University. (2024, August). *LUMC first medical programme to include AI in curriculum*. Retrieved September 25, 2025, from https://www.universiteitleiden.nl/en/news/2024/08/lumc-first-medical-programme-to-include-ai-in-curriculum
57. Quantib. (n.d.). *Radiology residents have strong confidence in the future of radiology*. Retrieved September 25, 2025, from https://www.quantib.com/blog/radiology-residents-have-strong-confidence-in-the-future-of-radiology#:~:text=The%20Dutch%20residents%20rank%20%E2%80%9CUnclear,have%20on%20their%20desktops%20now
58. Lee, J. H., Park, J. S., Lee, A. L., Lim, Y. J., & Jung, S. E. (2025, April). Training of radiology residents in Korea. *Korean Journal of Radiology, 26*(4), 291–293. https://doi.org/10.3348/kjr.2024.1151
59. Ministry of Health and Welfare. (2022, February 24). *Residency Program Curriculum by Year of Training* [Official notification]. Korea: Ministry of Health and Welfare.
60. Chung, Y. E., et al. (2014). How are radiologists trained in South Korea? *Quantitative Imaging in Medicine and Surgery*. https://www.ncbi.nlm.nih.gov/pmc/articles/PMC4256247/
61. Lee, H., Park, S. H., Kim, C., Kim, S., & Cha, J. (2020). Survey of the knowledge of Korean radiology residents on medical artificial intelligence. *Journal of the Korean Society of Radiology*. https://doi.org/10.3348/jksr.2019.0179
62. Ng, F. Y., et al. (2023). Call to action: Integrating AI education into radiology training in South Korea. *Korean Journal of Radiology*. https://doi.org/10.3348/kjr.2022.1023
63. Hwang, S., et al. (2023). Survey on user experience of artificial intelligence systems in South Korea. *Radiology: Artificial Intelligence*. https://pubmed.ncbi.nlm.nih.gov/38942455/
64. Korean Cancer Radiology Association. (n.d.). *Program sessions*. Retrieved September 5, 2025, from https://kcr4u.org/program/session
65. National Academy of Medicine of Korea. (2023). *Curriculum guidelines and development for the application of medical AI competencies in undergraduate medical education* (Research Paper). Seoul: National Academy of Medicine of Korea.
66. Lee, Y. M., et al. (2024). Defining medical AI competencies for medical school graduates: Outcomes of a Delphi survey and medical student/educator questionnaire of South Korean medical schools. *Academic Medicine, 99*(5), 524–533. https://doi.org/10.1097/ACM.0000000000000561
67. Kassamali, R. H., & Hoey, E. T. (2014). Radiology training in United Kingdom: Current status. *Quantitative Imaging in Medicine and Surgery*, 4(6), 447–448. https://www.ncbi.nlm.nih.gov/pmc/articles/PMC4256234/
68. Hashmi, O. U., et al. (*2023*). Artificial intelligence in radiology: Trainees want more. *Clinical Radiology*. Advance online publication. https://www.clinicalradiologyonline.net/article/S0009-9260(23)00022-3/fulltext
69. Royal College of Radiologists. (n.d.). *Clinical radiology: Artificial intelligence (AI) blended learning course, 20 May* [Web page]. Retrieved September 4, 2025, from https://my.rcr.ac.uk/event/a2GKB000000kKMP2A2/clinical-radiology-artificial-intelligence-ai-blended-learning-course-20-may?utm_source=chatgpt.com

70. Health and Care Professions Council. (n.d.). *Radiographers—standards of proficiency: (reviewing radiographers—SOP changes)* [PDF]. Retrieved August 15, 2025, from https://www.hcpc-uk.org/globalassets/standards/standards-of-proficiency/reviewing/radiographers—sop-changes
71. Medical Schools Council. (2025, January 31). *Medical schools to prepare students with AI and data science skills.* Retrieved September 25, 2025, from https://www.medschools.ac.uk/latest/news/medical-schools-to-prepare-students-with-ai-and-data-science-skills/#:~:text=Education%2031.01.2025-,Medical%20schools%20to%20prepare%20students%20with%20AI%20and%20data%20science,increasingly%20technology%2Ddriven%20healthcare%20system
72. University of Alabama at Birmingham. (n.d.). *AirRad-Ed.* Retrieved September 25, 2025, from https://sites.uab.edu/airad-ed/
73. Perchik, J. D., et al. (2024, May 24). Going global: Scaling the artificial intelligence literacy course to an international audience. *Journal of Global Radiology.* https://doi.org/10.7191/jgr.783
74. YouTube. (n.d.). *AI in radiology education channel* [YouTube channel]. Retrieved September 6, 2025, from https://www.youtube.com/@aiinradiologyeducationaire22
75. Lanier, M. H., Wheeler, C. A., & Ballard, D. H. (2021). A new normal in radiology resident education: Lessons learned from the COVID-19 pandemic. *RadioGraphics, 41*(3). Advance online publication. https://doi.org/10.1148/rg.2021210030
76. Saxena, A., & Khamis, S. (2020). "I'll See You on Zoom!" International educators' perceptions of online teaching amid, and beyond, COVID–19. *Arab Media & Society, 30,* 1–21.
77. Parton, B. S. (2016). Video captions for online courses: Do YouTube's auto-generated captions meet deaf students' needs? *Journal of Open, Flexible and Distance Learning, 20*(1), 8–18.
78. Ciecierski-Holmes, T., et al. (2022). Artificial intelligence for strengthening healthcare systems in low- and middle-income countries: A systematic scoping review. *npj Digital Medicine, 5*(162). https://doi.org/10.1038/s41746-022-00692-7
79. Abuzaid, M. M., Elshami, W., McConnell, J., & Tekin, H. O. (2021). An extensive survey of radiographers from the Middle East and India on artificial intelligence integration in radiology practice. *Health and Technology, 11,* 1045–1050. https://doi.org/10.1007/s12553-021-00583-1

8 Artificial Intelligence in Course Design and Curriculum

A Medical Education Perspective

Neria Sebastien, Ashley Kingon

8.1 INTRODUCTION

Medical educators face an increasingly untenable challenge: healthcare's evolution demands continuous curriculum updates (1), yet the human resources required for rigorous curriculum development remain fixed or in short supply. Meanwhile, artificial intelligence tools promise to revolutionize learning design, but implementation without pedagogical grounding risks compromising the very educational principles that ensure physician competence. This tension between innovation and integrity defines the current moment in medical education.

The question is not whether AI will transform medical curriculum development, but how to harness its capabilities without sacrificing pedagogical rigor. Educators have spent decades establishing robust curriculum design frameworks that guide effective teaching and learning. Understanding by Design (UbD), developed by Wiggins and McTighe, provides an accessible starting point for curriculum development through its three-stage backward design process (2). Stage 1 begins with identifying desired results, the learning outcomes that specify what learners should know, do, or value by the end of an educational experience. Stage 2 determines acceptable evidence that demonstrates learners have achieved the desired outcomes (assessments). In Stage 3, educators plan the learning experiences and instruction that will support learners in reaching these goals (pedagogy). This backward design process applies across all levels of curriculum design, from four-year medical student educational programs to individual lectures.

While Dee Fink's Integrated Course Design model aligns with UbD, it incorporates two additional steps, one before and the other after the UbD framework. Before approaching the backward design process, Integrated Course Design introduces the consideration of situational factors (the real-world constraints and opportunities) that shape curriculum possibilities. These include, but are not limited to, the number of learners, teaching modality (such as in-person, online, simulation), learner characteristics (life situation, goals) and prior knowledge, available resources, and institutional context. For example, a learning objective to develop critical thinking skills will require a different approach for first-year medical students compared to third-year residents. Understanding these situational factors ensures that curriculum goals remain realistic and achievable within specific contexts. Then, following the UbD process, Integrated Course Design emphasizes the integrated nature of the three distinct steps, with decisions about each component impacting the others. Thus even though assessment is the second stage, decisions here will not only impact the teaching and learning activities (Step 3), but also the learning objectives from Step 1 (3).

Kern's Six-Step Approach to Curriculum Development (4) adds essential elements particularly relevant to medical education: beginning with a general need and then targeted needs assessment, establishing goals and objectives (aligns with UbD Step 1), selecting educational strategies (aligns with UbD Step 3), planning implementation, and conducting evaluation and feedback (UbD Step 2). This framework prioritizes identifying a specific challenge or need within the healthcare system that the educational unit aims to address, such

DOI: 10.1201/9781003617167-8

as a new treatment for a disease that learners in the field need to know how to utilize. Or when a new technology, such as AI, is rapidly changing the nature of the profession, there is a need for healthcare professionals entering the field to be prepared with these new skills. By dedicating a step to implementing a new curriculum, Kern's approach acknowledges the complexity of generating buy-in and support for making curricular changes. Lastly, evaluation examines both individual learners and program outcomes, encouraging reflection on curriculum effectiveness—a critical skill for both clinicians and educators.

Competency-based medical education (CBME) differs from the preceding frameworks, as it is less of a curriculum design process and more of a philosophical shift in how we think about educational progression (5). While traditional curricula assess learners' achievement of defined learning outcomes, they are time-centric and often rigid in their design. CBME shifts this thinking to recognize learners may reach learning objectives, or competencies, at different rates. In other words, Learner 1 might take six weeks to reach competency A, while Learner 2 takes eight weeks. For competency B, Learner 1 might take three weeks, while Learner 2 takes one week. The emphasis of CBME is on the observation of a learner competently performing a skill and not on spending a prescribed amount of time on learning that skill (6). CBME introduces the possibility, and challenge, of developing a curriculum that is responsive to the time variability inherent in learners' achievement of competency (6). This time variability, or variable progression, presents the opportunity for personalized learning pathways to support learners as they progress through the curriculum. These Personalized Learning Pathways (PLPs) prioritize the areas where each individual learner needs support, while de-emphasizing areas where they are already competent, optimizing the individual's progression toward competency (7).

These established frameworks provide the pedagogical infrastructure upon which artificial intelligence can be strategically integrated. This chapter argues that successful AI integration in medical curriculum development requires three essential conditions: adherence to established pedagogical frameworks, rigorous human oversight at every stage, and institutional readiness across technical, pedagogical, and ethical domains. When these conditions are met, AI serves as an efficiency multiplier rather than a substitute for educational expertise. Rather than replacing proven educational approaches, AI technologies offer capabilities to enhance curriculum development efficiency, enable data-driven decision-making, and support personalized learning pathways while maintaining the human judgment and pedagogical expertise essential to excellence in medical education. Table 8.1 provides an overview of the four major curriculum design frameworks discussed in this chapter, highlighting their origins, core principles, and applications to medical education.

This chapter proceeds in five parts. First, we examine the current state of AI applications in curriculum development, establishing both capabilities and limitations. Second, we demonstrate how AI enhances specific components within UbD, Kern's framework, and competency-based models. Third, through a case study, we illustrate systematic AI integration across the full curriculum development cycle. Fourth, we address three critical enabling conditions: teaching students about AI, integrating AI-enhanced learning experiences, and developing faculty capacity for pedagogical AI integration. Finally, we provide an institutional readiness assessment framework, enabling leaders to evaluate preparedness before embarking on AI-enhanced curriculum initiatives.

Table 8.1 Comparison of Major Curriculum Design Frameworks in Medical Education

Framework	Origin/ Authors Primary Source	Core Principles	Process/Steps	Strengths	Limitations/ Challenges
Understanding by Design (UbD)	Grant Wiggins and Jay McTighe (1998) (2)	Also referred to as backward design, the principal idea is to begin with the end in mind, what are the learner outcomes desired at the end of the learning event (course, module, lecture)	1. Identify desired results (learning outcomes) 2. Determine acceptable evidence (assessments) 3. Plan learning experiences and instruction	Clear alignment of goals, assessment, and teaching Promotes deep understanding ("big ideas" and transfer) Widely used in K–12 and higher education	Time-intensive Requires skill in defining meaningful outcomes May seem rigid if outcomes are too narrowly defined
Integrated Course Design (ICD)	L. Dee Fink (2003) (3)	Complements UbD by incorporating situational factors such as the educational context, learner and teacher characteristics, the nature of the subject, etc.	1. Analyze situational factors 2. Formulate learning goals (UbD step 1) 3. Design feedback and assessment (UbD step 2) 4. Select teaching/ learning activities (UbD step 3) 5. Integrate the three (goals, assessment, activities)	Emphasizes active learning Considers context and learner needs Promotes significant, lasting learning across cognitive, affective, and interpersonal domains	Complexity of integration Requires substantial planning and creativity May be challenging for large courses or rigid curricula

(Continued)

Table 8.1 Comparison of Major Curriculum Design Frameworks in Medical Education (Continued)

Framework	Origin/ Authors Primary Source	Core Principles	Process/Steps	Strengths	Limitations/ Challenges
Kern's Six-Step Approach	Curriculum development for medical education: A six-step approach (4)	Developed explicitly for medical education curriculum development; incorporates needs assessment before defining learner outcomes and emphasizes implementation as a standalone step	1. Problem identification and general needs assessment 2. Needs assessment of targeted learners 3. Goals and objectives (UbD step 1) 4. Educational strategies (UbD step 3) 5. Implementation 6. Evaluation and feedback (UbD step 2)	Practical and systematic Explicit focus on learner needs and context Well-suited to healthcare/competency-based fields Encourages continuous improvement	Perceived as linear, though steps are iterative Resource intensive Implementing may be challenging in less flexible institutions
Competency-Based Medical Education (CBME)	Frank et al. Competency-based medical education: theory to practice (5)	Focus on the demonstration of achievement of competencies (knowledge, skills, attitudes) rather than time spent on a task	Common features: Define competencies and milestones (UbD step 1) Develop assessment methods for competence (UbD step 2) Tailor learning to progression of each learner Focus on outcomes, rather than time spent or required	Learner-centered, flexible progression Directly tied to patient care and professional standards Strong accountability through observable outcomes	Assessment heavy; requires robust systems Risk of reducing learning to checklists Challenges with Implementation (faculty development, resources, culture change)

8.2 THE ROLE OF AI IN CURRICULUM DEVELOPMENT

Generative AI systems, including large language models like ChatGPT and Claude, as well as domain-specific tools, are actively reshaping curriculum development workflows in medical education. Their capabilities extend far beyond simple text generation: AI can draft learning objectives aligned with Bloom's taxonomy, generate clinically plausible patient scenarios, map curricula against accreditation standards, create assessment items with psychometric rigor, and analyze performance data to identify learning gaps (8). These capabilities address a fundamental tension in medical education: healthcare's accelerating pace of change demands continuous curriculum updates, yet the faculty time and expertise required for rigorous curriculum development remain constrained. However, their effectiveness depends critically on human oversight and pedagogical expertise (9), with recent research demonstrating that medical educators must serve as the essential "human in the room," bringing professional judgment, clinical experience, and educational wisdom to interpret, validate, and refine AI-generated outputs (9).

Traditional curriculum development relies on human resources (time) and expertise to develop, implement, evaluate, and iteratively update (10). As healthcare continues to evolve, our curricula must evolve to keep pace, putting a strain on our human resources. One-on-one mentoring represents the gold standard for medical education (11), but resource constraints make this approach impractical for large-scale implementation (12). The shift toward competency-based medical education (CBME) amplifies this challenge. CBME introduces personalized learning pathways (PLPs) that adapt to individual learner progression rates, creating both pedagogical opportunity and administrative complexity. Where traditional curricula assume uniform pacing, PLPs require content tailored to individual needs and systems to track variable student progression (13). AI technologies offer capabilities to support this complexity, not by replacing educational expertise, but by amplifying human capacity for personalization and data-driven optimization while preserving the pedagogical rigor essential to physician preparation. AI technologies offer capabilities to amplify human educational capacity rather than replace it, enabling personalization and data-driven curriculum optimization while preserving the pedagogical rigor essential to providing excellent medical education (14).

8.2.1 How AI Currently Enhances Curriculum Development

The University of Cincinnati College of Medicine, for instance, utilizes AI-powered curriculum mapping to ensure alignment across instructional methodologies, assignments, content, and learning objectives. Meanwhile, AI question generators create practice items tailored to individual learning gaps identified through quiz analysis (15). The University of Miami Miller School of Medicine utilizes trained AI tools to synthesize narrative assessments from multiple faculty members within minutes, a task that previously required hours of staff time (15). Harvard Medical School has developed LLM-augmented clinical training companions providing students with simulation-based practice opportunities when access to standardized patients is limited by cost or scheduling constraints (16). These applications highlight AI's potential to streamline administrative burdens and enhance learning experiences in medical education by providing scalable solutions to common resource limitations.

These implementations share common characteristics: they accelerate technical curriculum development tasks, reduce administrative burden, and enable personalization at scale. Critically, they succeed because institutions deploy AI within clear pedagogical frameworks with rigorous human oversight. AI generates initial drafts; faculty validate clinical accuracy, ensure pedagogical appropriateness, and make final determinations about educational value. This division of labor—AI handling content generation and pattern recognition, humans providing clinical judgment and educational wisdom—defines effective integration.

8.2.2 The Essential Human–AI Partnership

Recent research confirms what pioneering institutions demonstrate: AI's effectiveness depends fundamentally on human oversight and pedagogical expertise (17). Medical educators serve as the essential "human in the room," bringing professional judgment, clinical experience, and educational wisdom to interpret, validate, and refine AI-generated outputs. This partnership model recognizes that, while AI excels at rapid iteration (18), comprehensive coverage, and systematic organization, it cannot replace the contextual understanding, clinical currency, or ethical reasoning that expert educators provide.

The measure of successful AI integration is not adoption rates but improved educational outcomes achieved through thoughtful technology deployment (19). Institutions must ask not "Are we using AI?" but rather "Does AI deployment enhance learning while maintaining pedagogical integrity?" This framework-aligned approach ensures that AI serves educational goals rather than driving them, amplifying human educational capacity without compromising the standards essential to excellent medical education.

The following section discusses how AI capabilities align with and enhance established pedagogical frameworks: Understanding by Design, Kern's Six-Step Approach, and competency-based models, when deployed with appropriate human oversight and institutional support.

8.2.3 AI Enhancement within Pedagogical Frameworks

Effective AI integration requires alignment with established pedagogical frameworks rather than ad hoc technology adoption. This section demonstrates how generative AI enhances specific components of Understanding by Design, Kern's Six-Step Approach, and Integrated Course Design when deployed with appropriate human oversight. The pattern across frameworks is consistent: AI accelerates technical tasks (such as content generation, alignment checking, and gap analysis), while educators maintain control over pedagogical decisions that require clinical expertise and professional judgment.

8.2.3.1 Understanding by Design (UbD) and Generative AI

Large language models can significantly streamline the backward design process while maintaining pedagogical integrity (20). When developing learning outcomes, educators are leveraging generative AI to brainstorm comprehensive competency statements, generate multiple variations of learning objectives, and align outcomes with established frameworks (21). While AI can support curriculum development through content generation and analysis, educators must balance the incorporation of new technologies with learners' preservation of core medical competencies to ensure graduates are equipped with the knowledge, skills, and attitudes necessary to join the healthcare profession (without being reliant on AI) (22).

For assessment design, UbD's second stage, AI systems demonstrate practical value in generating test items and evaluation frameworks. However, research consistently emphasizes that human expertise remains essential for validating the accuracy of these assessments (23). The AI-generated materials serve as starting points that require educator review to ensure clinical accuracy, appropriate level of difficulty, and alignment with learning objectives. For instance, AI can rapidly generate diverse case scenarios for clinical reasoning assessments, but faculty must critically evaluate these scenarios for medical plausibility and educational efficacy (24).

Similarly, for teaching and learning activities, AI is being utilized for brainstorming possible activities, verifying alignment between activities, assessments, and learning objectives, as well as providing detailed instructions for implementation of activities and support for incorporating situational factors into activity design. AI excels in this ideation and logistic support for educational activities, but still the "human in the room" is essential to ensure the feasibility and accuracy of all output (25).

8.2.3.2 Dee Fink's Situational Factors and AI

Generative AI proves particularly valuable when considering situational factors that shape curriculum design. When facing constraints such as large class sizes or limited teaching time, educators can query AI for evidence-based strategies tailored to specific contexts. Ideas might include utilizing virtual tutors and AI-driven feedback systems, while maintaining face-to-face interaction, to facilitate the development of skills of higher complexity. Alternatively, it could involve introducing experiential learning, case-based curricular components, or simulations that enhance students' critical thinking abilities (26).

8.2.4 Integrated Course Design: Situational Factors and Contextual AI Use

Dee Fink's emphasis on situational factors highlights both AI's utility and limitations. When educators face constraints—such as large class sizes, limited teaching time, or diverse learner backgrounds—AI can generate evidence-based strategies adapted to specific contexts (27). For a 200-student pharmacology course with limited contact hours, AI might suggest flipped classroom approaches, peer teaching structures, or adaptive online modules with face-to-face time reserved for complex skill development.

The critical limitation: Situational analysis remains fundamentally human and must be provided to AI as context. AI cannot independently assess institutional culture, political dynamics affecting curriculum change, faculty resistance patterns, or the subtle resource constraints that make theoretically sound suggestions practically infeasible. Educators must evaluate whether AI-generated strategies align with their institutional reality while preserving the human elements of medical education—patient interaction, ethical reasoning, empathy, and professional identity formation (28).

8.2.4.1 Kern's Six-Step Approach and Current AI Tools

Each step of Kern's framework (Table 8.1) offers specific opportunities for AI enhancement using currently available technologies:

- **Problem/needs assessment:** AI systems can identify areas of curriculum requiring improvement by comparing educational outcomes to global health trends, accreditation standards, and student competency frameworks through sophisticated gap analysis (29).
- **Goals and objectives:** Generative AI can draft objectives, map them to competency frameworks, and identify potential gaps or redundancies across a curriculum, though human review remains essential for ensuring clinical relevance and appropriate scope (30).
- **Educational strategies:** AI systems can reduce the time required to develop content and strategies optimal for supporting student learning. AI can support

the development of activities from content creation to developing detailed implementation strategies (31).

- **Implementation:** AI systems can generate communication strategies, materials, and resources supporting buy-in for the new curriculum, while also strategizing solutions to potential challenges raised by stakeholders (24).
- **Evaluation:** Automated performance dashboards can track faculty and student performance in real time. Data can be compiled to support development of personalized learning pathways and to identify students requiring additional support, curricular gaps and shortcomings, and overall performance of the curriculum (32).

The pattern across UbD, Integrated Course Design, and Kern's Approach reveals a fundamental division of labor: AI excels at content generation, systematic organization, and pattern recognition; humans excel at clinical validation, contextual interpretation, and adaptive problem-solving. Successful integration maintains this boundary, deploying AI where it amplifies efficiency while preserving human expertise where it remains irreplaceable. This synthesis highlights the necessity of thoughtful adaptation in educational methodologies to leverage AI effectively, particularly in preparing medical educators for guiding AI-assisted learning while preserving core competencies.

8.2.5 Practical Applications for Curriculum Developers

Medical educators can leverage generative AI across the full spectrum of curriculum development tasks when guided by three essential principles: clear pedagogical purpose, rigorous quality control, and systematic documentation. These applications share a critical characteristic: They succeed because institutions treat AI as a collaborative partner that accelerates technical work, while educators maintain control over substantive pedagogical decisions requiring clinical expertise, institutional knowledge, and professional judgment. Table 8.2 synthesizes current AI applications across curriculum development tasks, detailing both AI capabilities and required human oversight, with evidence from pioneering institutions and practical prompt examples for immediate implementation.

8.2.5.1 Key Implementation Principles

- **Start with clear prompts:** Provide AI with specific context, including learner level, course objectives, and institutional constraints.
- **Iterate and refine:** Use AI-generated outputs as first drafts that require expert review and modification.
- **Maintain quality control:** Validate all AI suggestions for clinical accuracy, pedagogical appropriateness, and alignment with accreditation standards.
- **Document the process:** Keep records of prompts used and modifications made to build institutional knowledge.

8.2.5.2 Getting Started: A Staged Approach

For institutions beginning AI integration, evidence suggests a staged implementation approach:

- **Stage 1 (months 1–3)—Low-stakes ideation:** Start with brainstorming applications: generating activity ideas, drafting initial learning objectives, exploring assessment formats. These low-risk applications build faculty comfort

Table 8.2 AI-Enhanced Curriculum Development

Application	Generative AI Capabilities	Required Human Oversight	Implementation Evidence	Example Prompt Starter
Learning objectives and competencies	• Generate comprehensive outcome statements • Align with Bloom's taxonomy • Map to Accreditation Council for Graduate Medical Education (ACMGE) and Liaison Committee on Medical Education (LCME) standards • Identify gaps in coverage	• Validate clinical relevance • Ensure appropriate scope for learner level • Confirm institutional alignment	Arabian Gulf University: AI successfully generated pharmacology objectives with appropriate action verbs (33).	"Create learning objectives for [topic] aligned with [standard] for [learner level] . . . "
Clinical cases and scenarios	• Generate diverse patient presentations • Vary demographics and complexity • Include rare conditions • Create branching scenarios	• Verify medical accuracy • Check clinical plausibility • Review for bias • Ensure educational value	Empirical studies indicate that about 23% of AI cases require expert modification before use (33). For example, physician reviewers found 97% of AI-generated vignettes usable after confirmation/revision, and item-writing studies report that ~30% of AI-generated MCQs are unsuitable without further changes (34).	"Generate a clinical case of [condition] for [level] students including [specific elements] . . ."
Assessment design	• Create multiple-choice questions (MCQs), short answer questions (SAQs), and objective structured clinical examinations (OSCEs) • Generate rubrics • Produce varied difficulty levels • Map items to objectives	• Check against current evidence • Validate answer keys • Pilot test with learners • Psychometric analysis	University of Cincinnati: AI generates personalized practice questions based on individual learning gaps (35).	"Create assessment items testing [concept] at [Bloom's level] for [context] . . ."

(Continued)

Table 8.2 AI-Enhanced Curriculum Development (Continued)

Application	Generative AI Capabilities	Required Human Oversight	Implementation Evidence	Example Prompt Starter
Curriculum mapping and alignment	• Compare against accreditation requirements • Identify curricular redundancies and gaps • Track competency coverage and progression • Generate compliance reports	• Interpret standards contextually • Make strategic decisions • Plan substantive improvements	University of Cincinnati: AI-powered mapping aligns all curricular elements with learning outcomes (36).	"Map curriculum against [accreditation standard] and identify gaps . . ."
Content integration and compression	• Analyze for optimal placement points • Suggest consolidation strategies • Identify essential versus supplementary content • Propose efficient sequencing	• Balance competing priorities • Preserve core competencies • Consider resource constraints • Maintain educational quality	Authors' independent evaluation shows GenAI can reduce lesson planning time.	"Integrate [new content] into existing curriculum without adding contact hours . . ."
Framework transitions	• Restructure objectives for new frameworks • Convert traditional to competency-based formats • Generate milestone progressions • Create assessment criteria	• Provide pedagogical vision • Ensure clinical applicability • Design valid assessments • Lead faculty development	Limited published data; primarily institutional pilots	"Convert traditional objectives to competency-based milestones with progression criteria . . ."

with AI tools while developing prompt engineering skills without impacting learner outcomes.

- **Stage 2 (months 4–6)—Supervised content development:** Progress to content creation under close oversight: clinical cases reviewed by multiple faculty, assessment items pilot-tested before deployment, curriculum maps validated against official standards. Establish quality control protocols during this phase.
- **Stage 3 (months 7–12)— Systematic integration:** Expand to complex applications: curriculum alignment, personalized learning pathway development, performance analytics. By this stage, faculty possess the expertise to integrate AI effectively while maintaining pedagogical rigor.
- **Stage 4 (year 2 and onward)—Innovation and scholarship:** Conduct implementation research, contribute to evidence base, mentor other institutions, and advance the field through systematic study of AI's educational impact.

These practical applications demonstrate AI's capacity to enhance curriculum development efficiency and enable personalization at scale. However, successful implementation requires more than technical deployment; it demands attention to ethical frameworks, data quality, institutional readiness, and faculty development. The following section examines these critical prerequisites for sustainable AI integration.

8.2.6 Critical Prerequisites for Success

Successful AI integration in medical curriculum development rests on four interdependent foundations: ethical governance with human oversight, technical infrastructure ensuring data quality and security, clear understanding of current AI capabilities and limitations, and institutional readiness through faculty development. These prerequisites are not optional enhancements but essential conditions, deploying AI without establishing these foundations risks compromising educational quality, violating ethical standards, or wasting institutional resources on failed implementation attempts.

Ethical framework and human oversight: The integration of AI into medical education presents challenges, particularly around ethical considerations, requiring a balanced approach that includes faculty development to ensure AI serves as a supplement to, rather than a replacement for, core medical competencies (37). All AI-generated content requires expert validation for clinical accuracy, pedagogical appropriateness, and alignment with professional values. Educators must establish explicit review processes and maintain transparency about AI use with learners and colleagues (30).

Data quality and prompt engineering: The principle of data in/data out is particularly relevant to generative AI in educational contexts. As we have demonstrated, context is critical in curriculum development. The "human in the room" must provide the context for AI to produce meaningful outputs. Further, many of the aforementioned ideas rely on AI accessing personal material (with the prompt "Map curriculum against [accreditation standard] and identify gaps . . ." AI can do this only with access to your curriculum and to the defined accreditation standards.). If your data in is poor, the data out will also be poor. In addition, poor quality prompts yield poor quality outputs. Educators must develop skills in crafting clear, specific requests that provide necessary context and constraints while remaining vigilant about potential biases in AI training data or clinically outdated information (38).

Understanding current capabilities and limitations: While evidence highlights a wide range of applications, including curriculum analysis, curriculum redesign, enhanced assessment development, and streamlined administrative tasks. Most generative AI applications in medical education remain in the early stages, with sophisticated predictive analytics and fully adaptive learning systems still largely experimental rather than widely validated for routine use (39).

Current AI limitations educators must recognize:

- **Clinical knowledge currency:** AI training data has cutoff dates; emerging treatments, updated guidelines, or new evidence may not appear in outputs.
- **Context blindness:** AI cannot assess institutional politics, resource constraints, or cultural factors affecting implementation feasibility.
- **Bias amplification:** Training data biases (demographic, geographic, linguistic) can manifest in the generated content.
- **Inconsistent quality:** Output reliability varies unpredictably; identical prompts may yield either excellent or problematic results.
- **No pedagogical judgment:** AI cannot determine whether an "accurate" assessment item actually measures the intended competency.

These limitations don't preclude effective use. They demand informed integration with appropriate oversight.

8.2.6.1 Institutional Readiness and Faculty Development

Successful AI implementation requires coordinated, multidisciplinary capacity building combining expertise in educational technology, clinical medicine, instructional design, and ethics (40). Training programs must emphasize not just technical skills (using AI tools, crafting prompts) but critical evaluation frameworks (assessing output quality, recognizing limitations, maintaining pedagogical primacy) and ethical considerations (transparency, bias recognition, appropriate use boundaries).

8.2.6.2 Staged Faculty Development Approach

- **Phase 1—Foundation building:** Educators need reliable access to approved AI tools, training in effective prompting and output validation, and clear institutional guidelines about appropriate use cases. Starting with low-stakes applications (brainstorming, initial draft generation) allows competency building before tackling complex curriculum challenges (41).
- **Phase 2—Supervised application:** Faculty progress to creating content under collegial oversight, peer review of AI-enhanced materials, collaborative prompt refinement, shared learning from both successes and failures. This phase establishes quality standards and builds institutional expertise.
- **Phase 3—Independent integration:** Experienced faculty deploy AI within their curriculum development workflows while maintaining rigorous self-assessment and documentation. Champions emerge to mentor colleagues and guide institutional expansion.
- **Global Context Considerations:** International variation in AI readiness highlights the need for context-sensitive implementation. Surveys in Pakistan revealed high enthusiasm but limited infrastructure and institutional support, underscoring challenges in resource-constrained settings (42). Conversely, Singapore's coordinated investment in AI-enhanced adaptive learning as part of its national workforce strategy demonstrates how aligned health systems and

educational policies can accelerate innovation (43). These examples illustrate that successful AI integration depends not just on technology access but on institutional capacity, policy support, and contextual adaptation.

Having established the critical prerequisites for AI integration, we now turn to practical applications across three essential domains: developing curriculum content with AI assistance, preparing learners to practice in AI-enhanced healthcare environments, and integrating AI-powered tools directly into learning experiences. Each domain builds upon these foundational prerequisites while presenting distinct implementation challenges and opportunities.

8.2.7 Practical Applications: Leveraging Generative AI for Curriculum Development

While previous sections demonstrated AI's capacity to enhance curriculum development processes, medical educators must also address three additional challenges: preparing students to practice in AI-enhanced healthcare environments, engaging students as partners in AI curriculum design, and integrating AI-powered tools directly into learning experiences. These applications extend beyond using AI to build curricula, they represent AI as both a competency domain and a learning modality within medical education itself.

The most immediate and impactful application of generative AI in medical education lies in streamlining the labor-intensive processes of curriculum design and course material development. This section demonstrates how educators can harness LLM tools to enhance efficiency while maintaining pedagogical quality across three critical domains: developing and refining curricula, preparing learners to use AI effectively, and integrating AI-enhanced learning experiences into educational programs.

8.2.8 Teaching about AI: Preparing Learners for AI-Enhanced Practice

As AI technologies become increasingly prevalent in healthcare delivery, medical curricula must prepare learners to practice effectively in AI-enhanced clinical environments. Recent scoping work mapping AI in medical education underscores substantial growth in publications alongside persistent gaps in curricular design, implementation quality, and rigorous outcomes evaluation, particularly a reliance on low-level measures (such as satisfaction) rather than competency development or behavior change (14). Complementing this, a dedicated scoping review of AI ethics teaching finds the literature to be recent and largely conceptual, with a scarcity of empirical evaluations and a pressing need for clearer learning objectives, assessment strategies, and faculty development to ensure safe, effective, and ethically grounded use of AI in clinical training (44). Collectively, these reviews indicate that preparing graduates for AI-enhanced practice requires intentional curricular frameworks, robust assessment of competencies, and explicit attention to ethical reasoning and professional responsibilities.

Students' attitudes toward AI education are generally positive. A large, cross-national survey spanning 48 countries and 192 faculties found that most students support integrating AI-related coursework into existing curricula and report actively learning—or planning to learn—about AI applications in medicine (45). Nevertheless, a multicountry survey of 642 health professions students reported that 66.4% had low AI knowledge, underscoring a persistent gap between enthusiasm and actual integration (46). As AI becomes integral to healthcare delivery, medical students require structured competency development across five domains. Table 8.3 outlines core competencies for AI literacy in medical education, including foundational concepts, clinical applications, critical evaluation skills, ethical practice, and prompt engineering. These competencies integrate throughout preclinical and clinical training, progressing from conceptual understanding to practical application in clinical contexts.

Table 8.3 Core Competencies for AI Literacy in Medical Education

Competency Domain	Learning Objectives	Teaching Methods	Assessment Approaches	Implementation Level
Foundational AI concepts	• Define machine learning, neural networks, LLMs • Explain how AI systems learn from data • Recognize validation and testing • Discuss AI limitations	• Interactive lectures with demonstrations • Hands-on tool exploration • Case-based discussions • Guest speakers from AI field	• Knowledge tests • Concept maps • Reflective essays • Group presentations	Preclinical curriculum (years 1–2)
Prompt engineering and tool use	• Craft effective AI prompts • Iterate and refine outputs • Validate AI-generated content • Document AI assistance appropriately	• Hands-on workshops • Supervised practice • Peer review activities • Portfolio development	• Practical assessments • Output quality review • Documentation audits • Competency checklists	Clinical rotations (years 3–4)
Clinical AI applications	• Identify appropriate AI use cases • Interpret AI-generated outputs • Integrate AI into clinical workflow • Recognize when AI may be inappropriate	• Clinical case scenarios • Simulation exercises • Structured AI tool use • Supervised clinical practice	• OSCE stations with AI tools • Clinical reasoning exercises • Portfolio documentation • Direct observation	Clinical rotations (years 3–4)
Critical evaluation skills	• Assess AI tool validity and reliability • Identify algorithmic bias • Evaluate evidence quality • Question AI recommendations	• Journal club on AI studies • Bias identification exercises • Error analysis workshops • Comparative tool evaluation	• Critical appraisal assignments • Debate participation • Error identification tests • Peer teaching	Integrated throughout curriculum
Ethical AI practice	• Apply ethical frameworks to AI use • Protect patient data privacy • Maintain human oversight • Communicate AI role to patients	• Ethics case discussions • Role-playing scenarios • Policy analysis • Patient communication practice	• Ethics OSCEs • Written case analysis • Communication assessments • Professionalism evaluation	Integrated throughout curriculum

A cross-sectional needs assessment of 3,018 medical students found that most perceived AI as assistive technology, and it could facilitate access to information (85.8%) and reduce errors (70.5%). Half of students worried about a possible reduction in physician services. Students expressed a clear need for curriculum updates to equip future physicians with knowledge and skills to effectively use AI while ensuring professional values are protected (47).

The curriculum must balance technical literacy with critical thinking about AI's role in medicine—emphasizing the ability to determine when and why human intervention is essential. Students need hands-on experience with tools they will encounter in practice, combined with frameworks for ethical decision-making and skills to maintain professional judgment when using AI-assisted systems.

8.2.9 Student Agency and Codesign in AI Curriculum Development

Incorporating student agency in AI curriculum design enhances relevance and trust while ensuring that educational innovations serve learner needs. Rather than positioning students solely as recipients of AI-enhanced education, emerging models engage them as active partners in curriculum development and tool evaluation (48). Within health professions education is a rich history of student involvement in curriculum development. As AI is a "new to the masses" rapidly evolving innovation, learners often have more experience with AI than seasoned faculty. Collaborating to codesign AI curricula will yield superior results to either group working alone.

Participatory design studies show that medical students can cocreate AI tutors and curricular elements alongside faculty and developers, ensuring outputs are pedagogically appropriate and learner-centered (49). Similarly, exploratory codesign workshops with students in project-based learning settings highlight how learners help define appropriate assessment strategies and ethical boundaries for AI use (50). These collaborative approaches produce educational tools that better address authentic learning needs while fostering student investment in AI integration outcomes.

8.2.9.1 Practical Implementation of Student Codesign

Practical implementation of student codesign includes establishing student representation on AI curriculum advisory boards, involving learners in cocreation for AI-enhanced assessments and rubrics, engaging students in pilot testing of AI-generated resources, and creating structured feedback mechanisms for ongoing refinement. This participatory approach not only enriches educational quality but also develops students' critical evaluation skills and prepares them for collaborative practice in AI-enhanced healthcare environments (51).

8.2.10 Integrating AI-Enhanced Learning Experiences

Beyond using AI to develop curriculum and teaching about AI as a competency, educators can strategically integrate AI-powered tools directly into learning experiences to support attainment of existing competency requirements. A comprehensive BEME (best evidence medical education) scoping review mapped AI applications across medical education, categorizing implementations using the SAMR framework (substitution, augmentation, modification, redefinition) to understand how AI transforms rather than merely replicates traditional teaching (45). While AI can enhance curriculum development, it also enables direct integration into learning experiences. Table 8.4 maps current AI educational technologies to tested applications, known limitations, and implementation requirements, helping educators make evidence-based decisions about technology adoption.

Table 8.4 AI-Enhanced Learning Experiences—Current Capabilities and Limitations

Technology Type	Current Evidence	Applications	Known Limitations	Implementation Requirements
AI clinical simulations	Harvard developed LLM-augmented clinical training companions providing practice opportunities when standardized patients were unavailable due to cost/time constraints (16).	• Communication skills practice • Clinical reasoning development • History taking exercises • Diagnostic reasoning	• Cannot replicate physical exam • Limited emotional nuance • May lack cultural context • Requires human validation	• Robust LLM platform and significant development of appropriate AI agents • Clinical oversight • Integration with curriculum • Student orientation
Adaptive learning systems	Research shows improvement in knowledge retention and faster competency progression (52).	• Personalized content sequencing • Real-time difficulty adjustment • Individualized practice • Gap-based remediation	• Requires extensive data • May reduce peer learning • Risk of educational fragmentation • Expensive to implement	• Specialized learning management system • Data infrastructure • Faculty training • Ongoing refinement
Performance analytics	Harvard Medical School (HMS) pilot project uses EHR data to identify learning gaps by comparing curriculum objectives with patients whom students actually encountered, enabling personalized learning recommendations (53).	• Personalized early identification of where learners need more support • Pattern recognition • Intervention targeting • Longitudinal tracking	• Data privacy concerns • Risk of false predictions • May miss contextual factors • Requires interpretation	• EHR integration • Analytics platform • Privacy safeguards • Clinical context integration
AI-powered assessment	HMS developed an AI grading system for short-answer questions that summarizes strengths/weaknesses and suggests teaching strategies, reducing grading time from 8 hours to minutes (54),	• Rapid feedback provision • Pattern identification • Consistency in scoring • Large-scale application	• May miss nuanced responses • Requires careful calibration of AI system • Cannot assess all competencies • Needs human oversight	• Validated AI tools • Faculty review process • Calibration studies • Student transparency
Virtual patients	Virtual reality/augmented reality (VR/AR) combined with AI shows improvement in diagnostic accuracy and increase in procedural confidence (55).	• Rare condition exposure • Emergency scenario practice • Unlimited repetition • Safe error-based learning	• High development costs • Technical complexity • Cannot replace all clinical experience • Maintenance intensive	• VR/AR infrastructure • Content development • Technical support • Faculty buy-in

The successful integration of AI-enhanced learning experiences requires discerning when technology adds value and when traditional approaches remain preferable. A recent BEME scoping review argues that, as AI reshapes medical practice, medical education must adapt by coupling technical proficiency with explicit ethical and professional formation so learners can harness AI responsibly while safeguarding the human elements of care (14). Human instruction remains indispensable for cultivating nuanced judgment, complex ethical reasoning, cultural competency, and interpersonal skills that current AI cannot replicate (56). Consequently, curricula should emphasize preservation of clinical reasoning alongside technological fluency, ensuring that future physicians can function effectively when AI tools are unavailable and can critically appraise AI-generated recommendations (57). Overall, educators must balance AI integration with core medical competencies and undertake thoughtful pedagogical redesign rather than mere tool adoption (58).

8.3 AI INTEGRATION ACROSS CURRICULUM DEVELOPMENT FRAMEWORKS

The following hypothetical application of AI for curriculum development, mapped across UbD, ICD, and Kern's frameworks demonstrates that AI integration principles transcend specific methodologies, supporting various approaches to systematic curriculum development. Success depends not on the framework chosen but on maintaining pedagogical primacy while leveraging AI as an efficiency multiplier. The critical distinction remains between tasks where AI excels—rapid content generation, systematic organization, pattern recognition—and those requiring irreplaceable human judgment—clinical validation, contextual interpretation, and adaptive problem-solving.

8.3.1 Case Study Introduction: AI-Enhanced Curriculum Development in Practice

Dr. Sarah Ellis, a faculty member in infectious disease at a 500-bed academic medical center, was tasked with developing a new antimicrobial stewardship curriculum for internal medicine (IM) trainees. With 48 IM trainees across three training years, limited protected curriculum time (4 hours total), and the urgent need to address rising rates of inappropriate antibiotic prescribing documented in recent institutional audits, Dr. Ellis faced the classic medical education challenge: comprehensive learning objectives constrained by practical realities. Her systematic approach to AI integration within curriculum design illustrates both the technology's power and its limitations. While Table 8.2 demonstrated AI applications across specific tasks, Table 8.5 traces this development process through six phases, showing the complementary roles of AI capabilities and human judgment at each stage.

Dr. Ellis's experience illustrates the essential partnership between AI efficiency and human expertise. AI accelerated content generation, literature synthesis, and initial assessment development, tasks that would have otherwise required substantial faculty time. However, every phase demanded her clinical judgment, institutional knowledge, and pedagogical expertise. AI could not interpret local resistance patterns, recognize politically sensitive implementation barriers, assess resource availability, or distinguish curriculum design flaws from learner performance issues. Most critically, AI generated technically correct outputs that often missed the educational mark, confusing accuracy with appropriateness, compliance with engagement, and performance metrics with meaningful learning. The technology proved invaluable for scaffolding and acceleration but was

Table 8.5 AI Integration across Curriculum Development Frameworks

Curriculum Development Phase	Framework Alignment	AI Capabilities	Essential Human Expertise	Quality Assurance and Implementation	Dr. Ellis's Practical Application
Phase 1: Needs and Context Analysis					
Problem Identification and Situational Factors	Kern Step 1: Problem identification Kern Step 2: Targeted needs assessment Fink ICD Step 1: Situational factors	• Synthesize literature on healthcare trends • Generate comprehensive issue lists • Organize priorities systematically • Draft needs assessment surveys • Analyze data patterns • Identify knowledge gaps	• Interpret local patient populations • Determine institutional priorities • Identify stakeholder concerns • Validate clinical accuracy • Interpret learner feedback • Discern cohort characteristics and institutional context	*Quality control:* Cross-reference AI analysis with local epidemiological data and institutional antibiograms *Implementation note:* AI provides comprehensive starting points but cannot replace contextual understanding of institutional culture and constraints.	Dr. Ellis used AI to synthesize national resistance patterns from the Centers for Disease Control and Prevention (CDC) reports and generate draft needs assessment surveys, reducing literature review time from an estimated 12 hours to 3. However, interpreting the institution's local antibiogram data required her infectious disease expertise—AI suggested empiric vancomycin for methicillin-resistant *Staphylococcus aureus* (MRSA) coverage rates that her clinical knowledge recognized as outdated for their specific patient population. She also identified through direct observation (not AI) that trainees' real barrier was not knowledge deficits but workflow integration challenges that surveys alone wouldn't capture.

Phase 2: Defining Outcomes and Objects					
Learning Outcomes and Competencies	Kern Step 3: Goals and objectives UbD Stage 1: Identify desired results Fink ICD Step 2: Learning goals	• Generate comprehensive outcomes statements • Align with Bloom's taxonomy • Map to ACGME/LCME standards • Identify gaps in coverage • Create "essential questions" for topics • Map outcomes to competency levels	• Determine enduring understandings (what truly matters long term) • Prioritize competing outcomes • Ensure clinical relevance • Balance breadth versus depth • Refine for clinical precision • Ensure measurability	*Transformation strategy:* Convert generic objectives to specific, measurable outcomes (such as "Understand antimicrobial resistance" → "Demonstrate appropriate antibiotic selection for resistant organisms in clinical scenarios with 85% accuracy"). *Framework alignment:* Focus on what trainees retain years post-training versus transient knowledge	AI-generated comprehensive antimicrobial stewardship objectives aligned with ACGME milestones, but Dr. Ellis personally refined them to emphasize enduring principles (stewardship frameworks, resistance mechanisms) rather than specific drug dosages that change frequently. When AI suggested "Demonstrate appropriate antibiotic selection for resistant organisms with 85% accuracy," she recognized that this focused on performance metrics without addressing the underlying clinical reasoning. She revised it to: "Apply antimicrobial stewardship principles to develop evidence-based treatment plans for complex infections, articulating the rationale for antibiotic selection, duration, and de-escalation strategies."

(Continued)

Table 8.5 AI Integration across Curriculum Development Frameworks (Continued)

Phase 3: Assessment Design					
Evidence of learning	UbD Stage 2: Determine acceptable evidence Fink ICD Step 3: Feedback and assessment Kern Step 6 (partial): Learner Evaluation	• Generate diverse assessment formats (MCQs, SAQs, OSCEs) • Create rubrics with performance levels • Suggest authentic assessment tasks • Draft case-based scenarios • Map items to objectives • Produce varied difficulty levels	• Validate assessment-outcome alignment • Ensure assessment authenticity • Design meaningful feedback mechanisms • Determine acceptable performance levels • Check against current evidence • Pilot test with learners	*Validation protocol:* 25% of AI-generated assessment items typically require expert modification; pilot test all rubrics with faculty reviewers before implementation *Psychometric requirement:* Conduct inter-rater reliability checks and item analysis	AI-generated assessment rubrics for antibiotic selection cases and drafted 15 clinical scenarios of varying complexity. Dr. Ellis pilot-tested these with three faculty colleagues who identified that 5 scenarios (33%) contained subtle clinical inaccuracies, one case suggested fluoroquinolone use for a patient population where resistance rates made this inappropriate. The rubrics distinguished surface knowledge from clinical competence well but required modification of approximately 30% of criteria based on trial assessments to ensure they captured trainees' reasoning processes, not just final antibiotic choices.

Phase 4: Educational Strategies					
Learning experiences and teaching methods	Kern Step 4: Educational Strategies UbD Stage 3: Plan Learning Experiences Fink ICD Step 4: Teaching/learning activities	• Suggest evidence-based teaching methods • Generate learning activities • Sequence content logically • Create practice opportunities • Generate case frameworks • Propose active learning strategies	• Select methods matching learner needs • Evaluate practical feasibility • Match to faculty strengths • Scaffold complexity appropriately • Respond to learner feedback • Refine for educational value	*Resource alignment:* Modify AI suggestions based on available resources, faculty capabilities, and time constraints *Adaptive implementation:* Adjust difficulty progression during implementation based on observed performance patterns	When institutional stakeholders raised concerns about adding another curriculum requirement to already overwhelmed trainees, AI generated multiple integration strategies: embedding content in the morning report, using asynchronous modules, creating point-of-care tools. Dr. Ellis's institutional knowledge was crucial for selecting approaches, she knew that the morning report was already overprogrammed, but recognized an opportunity to integrate with the existing quality improvement curriculum. AI could not anticipate that the simulation center had just acquired new funding, enabling her to propose case-based simulations that AI had initially ranked as "resource-prohibitive."

(Continued)

Table 8.5 AI Integration across Curriculum Development Frameworks (Continued)

Phase 5: Implementation					
Deployment and Faculty Development	Kern Step 5: Implementation	• Draft communication materials for stakeholders • Create session templates and schedules • Generate scheduling frameworks • Develop faculty resources • Strategize solutions to anticipated barriers	• Navigate institutional barriers • Lead faculty development • Adapt to resistance • Manage change processes • Build stakeholder buy-in	*Customization requirement:* Tailor all AI-generated materials for stakeholder-specific messaging and institutional cultural appropriateness *Change management:* Faculty expertise essential for relationship building and addressing concerns AI cannot anticipate	AI-drafted faculty development materials, session templates, and even anticipated objections from busy clinicians. However, when infectious disease faculty expressed concern about curriculum time competing with clinical duties, Dr. Ellis drew on her understanding of departmental politics and relationships to position the curriculum as addressing a quality gap that affected faculty's own patient care. AI's suggested talking points were factually accurate but politically tone-deaf; they emphasized regulatory compliance rather than patient outcomes, which she knew would create resistance rather than buy-in.

Phase 6: Evaluation and Continuous Improvement					
Program and Learner Assessment	Kern Step 6: Evaluation and Feedback Fink ICD Step 5: Integration UbD: Iterative Refinement	• Generate assessment instruments and rubrics • Analyze performance patterns • Track outcome achievement • Identify statistical trends • Evaluate program outcome achievement • Suggest modifications based on data	• Validate assessment criteria • Interpret data contextually • Design targeted interventions • Determine significance of findings • Prioritize improvements • Balance multiple considerations	*Diagnostic distinction*: Differentiate between learner performance issues versus curricular emphasis gaps to determine appropriate responses (remediation versus teaching strategy revision) *Validation requirements*: Ensure rubric validity through pilot testing, inter-rater reliability checks, and stakeholder feedback	Six months post-implementation, AI analysis of resident performance data revealed lower diagnostic stewardship scores than expected. AI suggested increasing remediation and adding more didactic content. However, Dr. Ellis recognized this pattern reflected inadequate curricular emphasis on diagnostic stewardship principles rather than learner deficiencies, a contextual judgment AI could not make. She revised teaching strategies to incorporate more diagnostic reasoning cases and decision-making frameworks. This required understanding that the problem was curriculum design, not learner ability, a distinction requiring the educational expertise AI lacks.

fundamentally unable to replace the "human in the room," who brought contextual understanding, clinical wisdom, and adaptive problem-solving to curriculum development.

The parallel structure across UbD, ICD, and Kern's frameworks demonstrates that AI integration principles are framework-agnostic. Success depends not on the framework chosen but on maintaining pedagogical primacy while leveraging AI as an efficiency multiplier for appropriate tasks. This hypothetical example demonstrates that AI integration principles transcend specific frameworks, supporting various approaches to systematic curriculum development when implemented with appropriate human oversight and pedagogical grounding.

If educators like Dr. Ellis are to effectively integrate AI into their educational practice, they require more than technical training in prompt engineering and output validation. They need sophisticated understanding of when AI enhances versus when it potentially compromises educational objectives. The following section examines how to develop this pedagogical AI integration expertise among medical educators.

8.4 DEVELOPING AI-READY MEDICAL EDUCATORS

The successful integration of AI into curriculum development depends fundamentally on faculty preparedness. Educators require not merely technical proficiency with AI tools, but sophisticated understanding of how to integrate these technologies pedagogically while maintaining educational excellence and professional judgment. This distinction between technical use and pedagogical integration represents the critical challenge in faculty development.

8.4.1 Essential Competencies: Beyond Technical Skills

Medical educators need competencies spanning multiple domains to effectively leverage AI in curriculum development. Technical skills (such as understanding how LLMs work, crafting effective prompts, interpreting AI outputs) provide a necessary foundation but prove insufficient without complementary pedagogical expertise (59).

Technical competency domain includes understanding AI capabilities and limitations, developing prompt engineering skills, evaluating output quality, and troubleshooting common issues. However, educators must balance incorporation of new technologies with preservation of core medical competencies to provide comprehensive education, requiring sophisticated interpretation of when AI enhances versus when it potentially compromises educational objectives (58).

Pedagogical integration competency represents the more challenging domain, requiring educators to determine when AI use aligns with learning objectives, to maintain educational quality standards, to preserve the human elements of teaching, and to critically evaluate AI's educational impact. Recent national survey reporting indicates that only 28% of U.S. physicians feel prepared to manage AI-related risks in practice, and many voice concerns about appropriate-use boundaries, signaling gaps in clinical AI literacy that parallel the challenges of educational AI integration (60).

The critical question becomes not "Can faculty use AI?" but rather "Are faculty successfully integrating AI to improve educational outcomes while maintaining pedagogical principles?" This requires assessment approaches that examine implementation quality rather than merely adoption rates (14).

8.4.2 Assessing Pedagogical Integration: Moving Beyond Usage Metrics

Traditionally, evaluation of faculty development focuses on participation rates and satisfaction scores. However, effective AI integration requires deeper assessment of pedagogical competence. Evidence-based selection of AI tools demands that educators critically evaluate whether technology serves educational goals or merely provides technological novelty (61).

8.4.2.1 Pedagogical Integration Assessment Framework

- **Level 1—Basic technical use:** Faculty can operate AI tools and generate outputs but may not critically evaluate quality or educational appropriateness. Assessment indicators include:
  - generates AI content, uses basic prompts, obtains outputs.
- **Level 2—Quality-controlled application:** Faculty critically evaluate AI outputs for clinical accuracy and pedagogical value. Assessment indicators include:
  - validates AI content against evidence, modifies outputs for educational context, identifies errors or limitations.
- **Level 3—Strategic pedagogical integration:** Faculty deploy AI purposefully within established frameworks to enhance specific educational objectives. Assessment indicators include:
  - selects appropriate use cases, maintains framework alignment, preserves human teaching elements, documents rationale for AI use.
- **Level 4—Pedagogical innovation and scholarship:** Faculty advance the field through systematic study of AI's educational impact and dissemination of effective practices. Assessment indicators include:
  - conducts implementation research, shares evidence-based practices, mentors colleagues, contributes to educational scholarship.

This framework enables institutions to assess faculty development beyond simple technology adoption, focusing on pedagogical sophistication in AI integration (62).

8.4.3 Professional Development Strategies

Effective faculty development requires tiered programming that accommodates varying expertise levels while advancing all educators toward pedagogical integration competence (63).

Foundational tier addresses educators new to AI, focusing on: understanding AI capabilities and limitations, developing basic prompt engineering skills, learning quality control processes, and recognizing appropriate use cases. Workshop format includes hands-on practice with curriculum development tasks: generating learning objectives, creating assessment items, drafting clinical cases, with immediate expert feedback on output quality and pedagogical appropriateness (64).

Applied integration tier serves educators comfortable with AI basics, emphasizing: systematic integration within pedagogical frameworks, advanced prompt strategies for complex tasks, collaborative AI use in curriculum committees, and documentation of effective practices. Activities include case-based learning, analyzing successful and unsuccessful AI implementations, peer review of AI-enhanced curricula, and structured mentorship pairing experienced users with those developing expertise (60).

Advanced scholarship tier supports educators ready to advance the field through: implementation research design, outcomes assessment methodology, dissemination strategies, and leadership in institutional AI integration. This tier produces the evidence base for effective practices while developing institutional experts who guide ongoing development efforts (65).

8.4.4 Integration with Existing Faculty Development

Rather than creating parallel AI training programs, successful institutions integrate AI competency development within existing faculty development structures. Grand Rounds on educational innovation incorporate AI applications, teaching skills workshops include AI-enhanced methods, and curriculum development programs address AI integration as a standard component rather than separate topics (63).

Peer learning communities and mentorship models prove particularly effective. Faculty learning communities focused on curriculum innovation provide safe spaces for experimentation, sharing failures alongside successes, and collaborative problem-solving around AI integration challenges. Structured mentorship pairs early adopters with colleagues beginning their AI journey, providing personalized guidance contextualized to specific educational roles and responsibilities (64).

Continuous emphasis on pedagogical judgment remains the critical success factor. Faculty development must reinforce that AI serves educational goals, not vice versa. The measure of success is not AI adoption rates but rather improved educational outcomes achieved through thoughtful technology integration guided by pedagogical expertise (62).

8.5 INSTITUTIONAL READINESS SELF-ASSESSMENT

Before embarking on AI integration initiatives, institutions should assess their preparedness across multiple dimensions. Table 8.6 provides a comprehensive framework for evaluating institutional readiness across six critical domains, enabling leadership teams to identify strengths, prioritize areas requiring development, and establish baseline measures for ongoing AI integration efforts.

Interpretation: Institutions with predominantly "Strong" ratings (4 or more domains) are well positioned to begin comprehensive AI integration, though they should still address remaining gaps during early implementation. Those with mixed ratings should prioritize developing "Needs Work" areas before extensive deployment, beginning with low-stakes pilot projects in 1–2 strong domains while building capacity in weaker areas. Institutions with primarily "Needs Work" ratings should focus on foundational development, particularly in faculty competence, pedagogical framework, and ethical governance, before pursuing AI-enhanced curriculum initiatives. Regardless of current readiness level, all institutions should treat this as a dynamic, iterative process requiring regular reassessment as both institutional capacity and AI technologies evolve rather than as a one-time achievement.

8.6 CONCLUSION

The integration of AI into medical curriculum development represents both unprecedented opportunity and significant responsibility for medical educators. The evidence presented throughout this chapter demonstrates that AI technologies can enhance curriculum development efficiency, support personalized learning, and enable data-driven educational improvements when implemented within established pedagogical frameworks with requisite human oversight.

Table 8.6 Institutional Readiness for AI-Enhanced Curriculum Development

Readiness Domain	Assessment Questions	Current Status
Strategic vision	• Do institutional leaders articulate clear educational rationale for AI integration? • Are AI initiatives aligned with educational mission and values? • Is there commitment to evidence-based implementation? • Are success metrics defined beyond technology adoption?	☐ Strong ☐ Developing ☐ Needs Work
Technical infrastructure	• Do faculty have access to reliable AI tools? • Is there adequate IT support for implementation? • Are data privacy and security protocols established? • Can AI systems integrate with existing educational technologies?	☐ Strong ☐ Developing ☐ Needs Work
Faculty competence	• Have educators received training in AI fundamentals? • Can faculty critically evaluate AI outputs for quality? • Do educators understand pedagogical integration principles? • Are mentorship/support systems available?	☐ Strong ☐ Developing ☐ Needs Work
Pedagogical framework	• Is AI integration guided by established educational frameworks? • Are quality control processes defined and implemented? • Is there emphasis on maintaining human oversight? • Are educational outcomes prioritized over technological novelty?	☐ Strong ☐ Developing ☐ Needs Work
Ethical governance	• Are policies established for appropriate AI use? • Is there transparency with learners about AI deployment? • Are bias recognition and mitigation strategies in place? • Do guidelines address data privacy and student consent?	☐ Strong ☐ Developing ☐ Needs Work
Evaluation capacity	• Are mechanisms established to assess educational impact? • Can the institution track both benefits and challenges? • Is there commitment to continuous improvement? • Are findings shared to advance the field?	☐ Strong ☐ Developing ☐ Needs Work

AI enhances, not replaces: The most important finding across all applications is that AI functions optimally as an amplifier of human educational expertise rather than as a replacement for pedagogical judgment. From generating learning objectives to analyzing assessment data, AI provides valuable starting points and analytical capabilities, while educators supply the clinical expertise, contextual understanding, and educational wisdom essential to quality curriculum development.

Framework alignment ensures success: Systematic integration within proven frameworks—Understanding by Design, Fink's Integrated Course Design, Kern's Six-Step Approach, competency-based medical education models—provides the pedagogical infrastructure necessary for effective AI deployment. Technology introduced without this grounding risks becoming a distraction rather than enhancement.

Quality control remains paramount: Every AI-generated output requires expert validation. Current generative AI tools produce clinically inaccurate information, pedagogically inappropriate suggestions, and contextually irrelevant content with sufficient frequency that rigorous review processes are non-negotiable. Educators must function as the essential "human in the room" throughout all AI-assisted curriculum development processes.

Faculty development determines impact: The distinction between technical AI competence and pedagogical integration expertise is essential. Successful implementation requires faculty who cannot merely use AI tools but who understand when, how, and why to deploy them within sound educational practice. Assessment must focus on pedagogical sophistication rather than simple adoption metrics.

GLOSSARY

Academic integrity in AI contexts: Policies and practices ensuring appropriate, transparent use of AI tools by learners and faculty, including disclosure, attribution, and limits on generative assistance.

Accreditation Council for Graduate Medical Education (ACGME): Sets residency/fellowship standards, including competencies relevant to clinical training.

Adaptive assessment: Testing approach that adjusts item difficulty based on examinee responses to estimate ability efficiently (for example, computerized adaptive testing).

Bias (algorithmic): Systematic error in models that leads to unfair or disparate outcomes across groups; can arise from data, labels, features, or deployment context.

Bloom's taxonomy: Hierarchical framework for cognitive learning objectives (remember to create), frequently used to scaffold outcomes and assessments.

Competency-based medical education (CBME): An outcomes-oriented approach emphasizing demonstration of competencies rather than time-based training.

Generative AI: Models that produce new content (text, images, code) conditioned on prompts or context (such as LLMs for clinical case drafts).

Liaison Committee on Medical Education (LCME): Accredits U.S. and Canadian MD programs; competencies and standards shape curricular design.

Learning outcomes: Specific, measurable statements describing what learners should know or be able to do at the end of instruction.

LLM (large language model): Neural network trained on large corpora for next-token prediction; supports tasks such as summarization, question-answering, and feedback generation.

Learning management system(LMS): Platform for course administration, content delivery, and assessment (such as Canvas).

Prompt engineering: Techniques for crafting inputs, instructions, and context to elicit accurate, useful, and reproducible model outputs.

Reliability (assessment): Consistency of measurement across items/raters/occasions (for example, internal consistency, inter-rater reliability).
Rubric: Criterion-referenced scoring guide articulating performance levels aligned to outcomes; supports transparency and consistency.
Understanding by Design (UbD): Backward-design approach: identify desired results → determine evidence/assessment → plan learning experiences.
Validity (assessment): The degree to which evidence and theory support the interpretations of test scores for intended uses (content, construct, and consequential validity).

ABBREVIATIONS

ACGME	Accreditation Council for Graduate Medical Education
AI	artificial intelligence
CBME	competency-based medical education
CDC	Centers for Disease Control and Prevention
EHR	electronic health record
LCME	Liaison Committee on Medical Education
LLM	large language model
LMS	learning management system
MCQ	multiple-choice question
MRSA	methicillin-resistant *Staphylococcus aureus*
OSCE	objective structured clinical examination
PLP	personalized learning pathway
SAMR	substitution, augmentation, modification, redefinition
SAQ	short answer question
UbD	Understanding by Design

REFERENCES

1. Schubert T, Oosterlinck T, Stevens RD, Maxwell PH, van der Schaar M. AI education for clinicians. *EClinicalMedicine*. 2025;79:102968. Available from: http://dx.doi.org/10.1016/j.eclinm.2024.102968
2. Wiggins G, McTighe J. *Understanding by Design*. 2nd ed. Alexandria, VA: Association for Supervision and Curriculum Development; 2005.
3. Fink LD. *Creating Significant Learning Experiences: An Integrated Approach to Designing College Courses*. San Francisco: Jossey-Bass; 2003.
4. Schneiderhan J, Guetterman TC, Dobson ML. Curriculum development: A how-to primer. *Fam Med Community Health*. 2019;7(2):e000046. Available from: http://dx.doi.org/10.1136/fmch-2018-000046
5. Bhattacharya S. Competency-based medical education: An overview. *Annals of Medical Science & Research*. 2023;2(3):132–8. Available from: http://dx.doi.org/10.4103/amsr.amsr_27_23
6. Magzoub ME, Taha MH, Waller S, Al Eissa AM, Hamdy H, Norcini J, et al. Going beyond competencies: Building blocks for a patient- and population-centered medical curriculum. *Med Teach*. 2024;46(12):1568–74. Available from: http://dx.doi.org/10.1080/0142159X.2024.2412786
7. Thomas PA, Kern DE, Hughes MT, Chen BY, editors. *Curriculum Development for Medical Education: A Six-Step Approach*. 3rd ed. Baltimore: Johns Hopkins University Press; 2016.
8. Blanco MA, Nelson SW, Ramesh S, Callahan CE, Josephs KA, Jacque B, et al. Integrating artificial intelligence into medical education: A roadmap informed by a survey of faculty and students. *Med Educ Online*. 2025;30(1):2531177. Available from: http://dx.doi.org/10.1080/10872981.2025.2531177

9. Patil NG, Kou NL, Baptista-Hon DT, Monteiro O. Artificial intelligence in medical education: A practical guide for educators. *MedComm Futur Med.* 2025;4(2). Available from: http://dx.doi.org/10.1002/mef2.70018
10. Charow R, Jeyakumar T, Younus S, Dolatabadi E, Salhia M, Al-Mouaswas D, et al. Artificial intelligence education programs for health care professionals: Scoping review. *JMIR Med Educ.* 2021;7(4):e31043. Available from: http://dx.doi.org/10.2196/31043
11. Ong YT, Quek CWN, Pisupati A, Loh EKY, Venktaramana V, Chiam M, et al. Mentoring future mentors in undergraduate medical education. *PLoSOne.* 2022;17(9):e0273358. Available from: http://dx.doi.org/10.1371/journal.pone.0273358
12. Ali M. The role of AI in reshaping medical education: Opportunities and challenges. *Clin Teach* [Internet]. 2025;22(2):e70040. Available from: http://dx.doi.org/10.1111/tct.70040
13. Fariani RI, Junus K, Santoso HB. A systematic literature review on personalised learning in the higher education context. *Technol Knowl Learn.* 2023;28(2):449–76. Available from: http://dx.doi.org/10.1007/s10758-022-09628-4
14. Gordon M, Daniel M, Ajiboye A, Uraiby H, Xu NY, Bartlett R, et al. A scoping review of artificial intelligence in medical education: BEME Guide No. 84. *Med Teach.* 2024;46(4):446–70. Available from: http://dx.doi.org/10.1080/0142159X.2024.2314198
15. Boyle P. *AI in Medical Education: 5 Ways Schools are Employing New Tools* [Internet]. Washington, DC: AAMC; 2025 [cited 2025 Sep 30]. Available from: https://www.aamc.org/news/ai-medical-education-5-ways-schools-are-employing-new-tools (Section on University of Miami narrative-assessment summarization.)
16. Gehrman E. *How Generative AI is Transforming Medical Education* [Internet]. Boston, MA: Harvard Medicine Magazine; 2024 Mar [cited 2025 Mar 15]. Available from: https://magazine.hms.harvard.edu/articles/how-generative-ai-transforming-medical-education
17. Ouyang F, Jiao P. Artificial intelligence in education: The three paradigms. *Computers and Education Artificial Intelligence.* 2021;2:100020. Available from: http://dx.doi.org/10.1016/j.caeai.2021.100020
18. Dong C, Aw DCW, Lee DWC, Low SC, Yan CC. Generative AI in healthcare: Insights from health professions educators and students. *International Medical Education.* 2025;4(2):11. Available from: http://dx.doi.org/10.3390/ime4020011
19. Delello JA, Sung W, Mokhtari K, Hebert J, Bronson A, De Giuseppe T. AI in the classroom: Insights from educators on usage, challenges, and mental health. *Educ Sci (Basel).* 2025;15(2):113. Available from: http://dx.doi.org/10.3390/educsci15020113
20. Yadav G. Scaling evidence-based instructional design expertise through Large Language Models. *arXiv* [cs.CL]. 2023. Available from: http://arxiv.org/abs/2306.01006
21. Alasadi EA, Baiz CR. Generative AI in education and research: Opportunities, concerns, and solutions. *J Chem Educ.* 2023;100(8):2965–71. Available from: http://dx.doi.org/10.1021/acs.jchemed.3c00323
22. Lee H. The rise of ChatGPT: Exploring its potential in medical education. *Anat Sci Educ.* 2024;17(5):926–31. Available from: http://dx.doi.org/10.1002/ase.2270
23. Turner L, Knopp MI, Mendonca EA, Desai S. Bridging artificial intelligence and medical education: Navigating the alignment paradox. *ATS Sch.* 2025;6(2):135–48. Available from: http://dx.doi.org/10.34197/ats-scholar.2024-0086PS

24. Almansour M, Soliman M, Aldekhyyel R, Binkheder S, Temsah M-H, Malki KH. An academic viewpoint (2025) on the integration of generative artificial intelligence in medical education: Transforming learning and practices. *Cureus.* 2025;17(3):e81145. Available from: http://dx.doi.org/10.7759/cureus.81145
25. Swiecki Z, Khosravi H, Chen G, Martinez-Maldonado R, Lodge JM, Milligan S, et al. Assessment in the age of artificial intelligence. *Computers and Education: Artificial Intelligence.* 2022;3:100075. Available from: http://dx.doi.org/10.1016/j.caeai.2022.100075
26. Sriram A, Ramachandran K, Krishnamoorthy S. Artificial intelligence in medical education: Transforming learning and practice. *Cureus.* 2025;17(3):e80852. Available from: http://dx.doi.org/10.7759/cureus.80852
27. Schaekermann M, Jhun P. *How Google's AI Can Help Transform Health Professions Education* [Internet]. Mountain View, CA: Google Research. 2025 Aug [cited 2025 Sep 30]. Available from: https://research.google/blog/how-googles-ai-can-help-transform-health-professions-education/
28. Kasneci E, Sessler K, Küchemann S, Bannert M, Dementieva D, Fischer F, et al. ChatGPT for good? On opportunities and challenges of large language models for education. *Learn Individ Differ.* 2023;103:102274. Available from: http://dx.doi.org/10.1016/j.lindif.2023.102274
29. Sharma M, Murphy R, Doody GA. Do we need a core curriculum for medical students? A scoping review. *BMJ Open.* 2019;9(8):e027369. Available from: http://dx.doi.org/10.1136/bmjopen-2018-027369
30. Varma JR, Fernando S, Ting BY, Aamir S, Sivaprakasam R. The global use of artificial intelligence in the undergraduate medical curriculum: A systematic review. *Cureus.* 2023; Available from: http://dx.doi.org/10.7759/cureus.39701
31. Mir MM, Mir GM, Raina NT, Mir SM, Mir SM, Miskeen E, et al. Application of artificial intelligence in medical education: Current scenario and future perspectives. *J Adv Med Educ Prof.* 2023;11(3):133–40. Available from: http://dx.doi.org/10.30476/JAMP.2023.98655.1803
32. Sposato M. Artificial intelligence in educational leadership: A comprehensive taxonomy and future directions. *Int J Educ Technol High Educ.* 2025;22(1). Available from: http://dx.doi.org/10.1186/s41239-025-00517-1
33. Yanagita Y, Yokokawa D, Uchida S, Li Y, Uehara T, Ikusaka M. Can AI-generated clinical vignettes in Japanese be used medically and linguistically? *J Gen Intern Med.* 2024;39(16):3282–9. Available from: http://dx.doi.org/10.1007/s11606-024-09031-y
34. Ahmed A, Kerr E, O'Malley A. Quality assurance and validity of AI-generated single best answer questions. *BMC Med Educ.* 2025;25(1):300. Available from: http://dx.doi.org/10.1186/s12909-025-06881-w
35. Sridharan K, Sequeira RP. Artificial intelligence and medical education: Application in classroom instruction and student assessment using a pharmacology & therapeutics case study. *BMC Med Educ.* 2024;24(1):431. Available from: http://dx.doi.org/10.1186/s12909-024-05365-7
36. Artificial Intelligence at University of Cincinnati [Internet]. Ai-qa.uc.edu. [cited 2025 Oct 7]. Available from: https://ai-qa.uc.edu/
37. Shoaib M, Sayed N, Singh J, Shafi J, Khan S, Ali F. AI student success predictor: Enhancing personalized learning in campus management systems. *Comput Human Behav. 2024;158:108301.* Available from: http://dx.doi.org/10.1016/j.chb.2024.108301
38. Hamilton A. Artificial intelligence and healthcare simulation: The shifting landscape of medical education. *Cureus.* 2024;16(5):e59747. Available from: http://dx.doi.org/10.7759/cureus.59747

39. Wu Q, Wang Y, Lu L, Chen Y, Long H, Wang J. Virtual simulation in undergraduate medical education: A scoping review of recent practice. *Front Med (Lausanne)*. 2022;9:855403. Available from: http://dx.doi.org/10.3389/fmed.2022.855403
40. Plackett R, Kassianos AP, Mylan S, Kambouri M, Raine R, Sheringham J. The effectiveness of using virtual patient educational tools to improve medical students' clinical reasoning skills: A systematic review. *BMC Med Educ*. 2022;22(1):365. Available from: http://dx.doi.org/10.1186/s12909-022-03410-x
41. Youm J, Dabzadeh Z. *Twelve Tips to Guide the Use of Data with Generative AI for Accreditation and Continuous Quality improvement* [Internet]. Irvine, CA: UCI School of Medicine; 2024 Mar 30 [cited 2025 Oct 6]. Available from: https://www.aamc.org/media/82576/download
42. Naseer MA, Saeed S, Afzal A, Ali S, Malik MGR. Navigating the integration of artificial intelligence in the medical education curriculum: A mixed-methods study exploring the perspectives of medical students and faculty in Pakistan. *BMC Med Educ*. 2025;25(1):273. Available from: http://dx.doi.org/10.1186/s12909-024-06552-2
43. *National AI Strategy* [Internet]. Singapore: Smart Nation Singapore. [cited 2025 Oct 7]. Available from: https://www.smartnation.gov.sg/initiatives/national-ai-strategy
44. Weidener L, Fischer M. Teaching AI ethics in medical education: A scoping review of current literature and practices. *Perspect Med Educ*. 2023;12(1):399–410. Available from: http://dx.doi.org/10.5334/pme.954
45. Busch F, Hoffmann L, Truhn D, Ortiz-Prado E, Makowski MR, Bressem KK, et al. Global cross-sectional student survey on AI in medical, dental, and veterinary education and practice at 192 faculties. *BMC Med Educ*. 2024;24(1):1066. Available from: http://dx.doi.org/10.1186/s12909-024-06035-4
46. Issa WB, Shorbagi A, Al-Sharman A, Rababa M, Al-Majeed K, Radwan H, et al. Shaping the future: Perspectives on the integration of artificial intelligence in health profession education: A multi-country survey. *BMC Med Educ*. 2024;24(1):1166. Available from: http://dx.doi.org/10.1186/s12909-024-06076-9
47. Civaner MM, Uncu Y, Bulut F, Chalil EG, Tatli A. Artificial intelligence in medical education: A cross-sectional needs assessment. *BMC Med Educ*. 2022;22(1):772. Available from: http://dx.doi.org/10.1186/s12909-022-03852-3
48. Ambrosetti É, Gaudin C, Flandin S, Poizat G. Students as co-designers in health professional education: A scoping review. *BMC Med Educ*. 2025;25(1):645. Available from: http://dx.doi.org/10.1186/s12909-025-07110-0
49. Wang A, Ruparel R, Iurchenko A, Jhun P, Séguin JA, Strachan P, et al. Generative AI for medical education: Insights from a case study with medical students and an AI tutor for clinical reasoning. In: *Proceedings of the Extended Abstracts of the CHI Conference on Human Factors in Computing Systems*. New York, NY, USA: ACM; 2025. p. 1–8. Available from: https://doi.org/10.1145/3706599.37212
50. Martin AF, Tubaltseva S, Harrison A, Rubin GJ. Participatory co-design and evaluation of a novel approach to generative AI-integrated coursework assessment in higher education. *Behav Sci (Basel)*. 2025;15(6):808. Available from: http://dx.doi.org/10.3390/bs15060808
51. Sethi I, Dine CJ. Exploring the landscape of student representation in medical curriculum development across U.S. MD schools: A comparative analysis. *BMC Med Educ*. 2025;25(1):747. Available from: http://dx.doi.org/10.1186/s12909-025-07114-w

52. Kerfoot BP, DeWolf WC, Masser BA, Church PA, Federman DD. Spaced education improves the retention of clinical knowledge by medical students: A randomised controlled trial. *Med Educ*. 2007;41(1):23–31. Available from: http://dx.doi.org/10.1111/j.1365-2929.2006.02644.x
53. Tang B, Lam ACL, Wong B, Ginsburg S. *Shaping the Future of Medical Education through Data-Driven Learning* [Internet]. Harvard.edu. [cited 2025 Oct 7]. Available from: https://learn.hms.harvard.edu/insights/all-insights/shaping-future-medical-education-through-data-driven-learning
54. Grévisse C. LLM-based automatic short answer grading in undergraduate medical education. *BMC Med Educ*. 2024;24(1):1060. Available from: http://dx.doi.org/10.1186/s12909-024-06026-5
55. Tene T, Vique López DF, Valverde Aguirre PE, Orna Puente LM, Vacacela Gomez C. Virtual reality and augmented reality in medical education: An umbrella review. *Front Digit Health*. 2024;6:1365345. Available from: http://dx.doi.org/10.3389/fdgth.2024.1365345
56. Montemayor C, Halpern J, Fairweather A. In principle obstacles for empathic AI: Why we can't replace human empathy in healthcare. *AI Soc*. 2022;37(4):1353–9. Available from: http://dx.doi.org/10.1007/s00146-021-01230-z
57. Schwartzstein RM. Clinical reasoning and artificial intelligence: Can AI really think? *Trans Am Clin Climatol Assoc*. 2024;134:133–45. Available from: https://pubmed.ncbi.nlm.nih.gov/39135584/
58. Russell RG, Lovett Novak L, Patel M, Garvey KV, Craig KJT, Jackson GP, et al. Competencies for the use of artificial intelligence-based tools by health care professionals. *Acad Med*. 2023;98(3):348–56. Available from: http://dx.doi.org/10.1097/ACM.0000000000004963
59. Tolentino R, Baradaran A, Gore G, Pluye P, Abbasgholizadeh-Rahimi S. Curriculum frameworks and educational programs in AI for medical students, residents, and practicing physicians: Scoping review. *JMIR Med Educ*. 2024;10:e54793. Available from: http://dx.doi.org/10.2196/54793
60. Littrell A. *Physicians See AI as a Tool—and a Threat* [Internet]. MedicalEconomics. 2025 [cited 2025 Oct 7]. Available from: https://www.medicaleconomics.com/view/physicians-see-ai-as-a-tool-and-a-threat
61. Ng FYC, Thirunavukarasu AJ, Cheng H, Tan TF, Gutierrez L, Lan Y, et al. Artificial intelligence education: An evidence-based medicine approach for consumers, translators, and developers. *Cell Rep Med*. 2023;4(10):101230. Available from: http://dx.doi.org/10.1016/j.xcrm.2023.101230
62. Fernandez N, Audétat M-C. Faculty development program evaluation: A need to embrace complexity. *Adv Med Educ Pract*. 2019;10:191–9. Available from: http://dx.doi.org/10.2147/AMEP.S188164
63. Steinert Y, Mann K, Anderson B, Barnett BM, Centeno A, Naismith L, et al. A systematic review of faculty development initiatives designed to enhance teaching effectiveness: A 10-year update: BEME Guide No. 40. *Med Teach*. 2016;38(8):769–86. Available from: http://dx.doi.org/10.1080/0142159X.2016.1181851
64. Kochhar K, Longtin K, Wilson S, Ho M, Brokaw J, Wallach P. Implementation of Faculty Learning Communities to support medical education scholarship in a regional campus system. *Journal of Regional Medical Campuses*. 2023;6(2). Available from: http://dx.doi.org/10.24926/jrmc.v6i2.4886
65. Benjamin J, Masters K, Agrawal A, MacNeill H, Mehta N. Twelve tips on applying AI tools in HPE scholarship using Boyer's model. *Med Teach*. 2025;47(6):949–54. Available from: http://dx.doi.org/10.1080/0142159X.2024.2445058

9 Using AI to Enhance Recruitment of Trainees in Residency and Fellowship

Arlene Ruiz de Luzuriaga, Grace Wei

9.1 INTRODUCTION

Every year, tens of thousands of applications from senior medical students and resident physicians are submitted to training programs nationwide in the hopes of securing a coveted residency or fellowship position, respectively. During the inaugural cycle of the National Resident Matching Program (NRMP) in 1976, there were 16,700 active applicants applying for 16,000 residency positions [1]. Fifty years later, that number has nearly tripled. The most recent data from the 2025 Main Residency Match reveals the highest number of applications of any year thus far, with 47,000 applicants vying for 43,000 available residency positions [2]. Similarly, applications to post-residency fellowship training programs have experienced a similar trend, growing from an average of 4,000 in 1993 to 15,000 in 2025 [3].

Depending on the specialty, program size, and geographic location, residency programs may receive 500 to over 4,000 applications per cycle, and individual reviewers may find themselves responsible for evaluating applications in the tens to hundreds [4]. The substantial growth in the volume of applicants to residency and subspecialty fellowship programs is only one of the many changes graduate medical education (GME) recruitment has experienced. Additionally, residency and subspecialty fellowship training recruitment has undergone a digital transformation over the past 30 years. Applications were previously paper-based, handwritten, and significantly shorter. The creation, in 1996, of the Electronic Residency Application Service (ERAS) was a pivotal point, enabling applicants to submit materials electronically, faster, and more securely [5] and, perhaps inadvertently, allowing for longer applications and a growing number of metrics used to evaluate and stratify applicants.

While these changes have allowed for the creation of an exceptional candidate pool and ability to better evaluate applicants holistically, the sheer volume and associated workload for training program leadership and other recruitment faculty members pose a challenge for programs aiming to conduct thorough reviews of each applicant. As the number of programs to which each candidate applies has risen in parallel, it has become increasingly difficult for applicants to explore and identify programs of best fit. Artificial intelligence (AI) presents a promising tool with a wide breadth of possible functions to support the recruitment process for both applicants and training programs alike, ranging from candidate engagement, to application review, to interview coordination for the residency and fellowship match processes.

9.2 PRESENT LANDSCAPE OF RECRUITMENT IN RESIDENCY AND FELLOWSHIP

Building a competitive application to residency and fellowship programs begins many months prior to recruitment season, often on day one of medical school or residency training. Additionally, the application cycle itself also stretches nearly 12 months, typically running from spring-to-spring of any given year. Here, we break this down into five core periods of the application cycle: pre-submission, submission and application review, interview season, the match process, and the post-match experience (Table 9.1). For simplicity, we will focus on the timeline of

DOI: 10.1201/9781003617167-9

Table 9.1 Residency Match Process

Core Period	Timeline	Components
Pre-submission	Months prior to application deadline	Applicant database resources
Submission and application review	Application deadline and immediate subsequent period	Applications are submitted electronically through centralized online application systems (Electronic Residency Application Service [ERAS] being the most widely used [6]. Packet comprised of multiple components, including the MyERAS Application (demographic information, educational background, extracurricular activities, and research experiences) and personal statement and supporting documents, including letters of recommendation, transcripts and medical student performance evaluations (MSPE or Dean's Letters), and USMLE and/or COMLEX scores
Interview season	Typically, 1–5 months following application deadline	Coordination of schedules for applicants and interviewers Scheduling software: Directly through ERAS or via third-party platforms (such as Thalamus Core and Itinerary Wizard (https://www.thalamusgme.com/), RezRate (https://www.rez-rate.com/), Interview Broker (https://www.interviewbroker.com/), and 3rd Friday (https://3rdfriday.com/) [7–10]
Match process	Typically, early spring following application deadline	Applicant rank order list Residency program rank order list
Post-match	Following Match Day	Roughly 10% of applicants may remain unmatched. Supplemental Offer and Acceptance Program (SOAP) process [12,13] Applicants may choose to reach out to programs directly or choose different specialties or geographic locations than originally applied for.

the Main Residency Match for prospective applicants entering residency training; however, most of the discussion can also be applied to subspecialty fellowship recruitment.

Pre-submission: Many months prior to the deadline for residency application submissions, prospective applicants begin exploring and identifying the programs to which they are interested in applying. This process is influenced by many factors, including but not limited to, individual applicant characteristics, specialty competitiveness, geographic preferences, program features, and long-term career goals.

Submission and application review: Applications are submitted electronically through centralized online application systems, with the Electronic Residency Application Service (ERAS) being the most widely used [6]. The residency application packet is extensive and comprises multiple components, including the MyERAS Application (demographic information, educational background, extracurricular activities, and research experiences), personal statement, supporting documents, which include letters of recommendation, transcripts and medical student performance evaluations (MSPEs or Dean's Letters), and USMLE and/or COMLEX scores.

Interview season: A variety of software platforms is available to training programs for extending and scheduling interviews. Interview coordination can be done directly through ERAS or via third-party platforms such as Thalamus Core and Itinerary Wizard (https://www.thalamusgme.com/), RezRate (https://www.rezrate.com/), Interview Broker (https://www.interviewbroker.com/), and 3rd Friday (https://3rdfriday.com/) [7–10]. The interview season is logistically highly complex as both applicants and training programs must navigate invitations, faculty availability, scheduling conflicts, rescheduling, and cancellations; the entire process requires an extensive amount of coordination and flexibility from both sides.

The match process: At the close of interview season, applicants create a rank order list of programs where they are interviewed from the most to least preferred. Similarly, residency programs create a list of applicants to be interviewed in order of preference. Whether a candidate ultimately matches at a particular program depends not only on their preferences and the program's preferences but also on the rank order list of every other applicant ahead of them on the program's rank list. This intricate process is carried out by the NRMP, an independent nonprofit organization that uses a proprietary algorithm to pair applicants with available training positions [11].

The post-match experience: Due to a greater number of applicants compared to available positions and the inherent mathematical structure of the Match algorithm, roughly 10% of the applicant pool remains unmatched. An unmatched applicant may take several paths. Many enter the Supplemental Offer and Acceptance Program (SOAP) process, a highly condensed version of the Match, that attempts to pair unmatched applicants with remaining unfilled residency positions [12, 13]. For those who remain unmatched after SOAP, aside from waiting until the next application cycle, other options to obtain a training position could include reaching out to programs directly to seek any remaining unfilled spots, though this often may be in an entirely different specialty or geographic location than was originally sought.

9.3 ROLE OF AI AND REAL-WORLD APPLICATIONS

Artificial intelligence (AI) is becoming an increasingly dominant technology across many industries, and medical recruitment for residency and fellowship is no exception [14, 15]. In the context of resident and fellow recruitment, important areas of AI being leveraged include:

- **Machine learning (ML):** Algorithmic models that enable computer systems to independently learn from data and improve their performance without programming [16].
- **Natural language processing (NLP):** Algorithmic models that enable computer systems to recognize, understand and interpret, and communicate via human language [17–19].
- **Predictive analytics (PA):** The integration of historical data, mathematical models, and machine learning to predict future outcomes [20, 21].
- **Generative AI (GAI):** The integration of preexisting content (written text, images, photos, videos, music, etc.) with machine learning to create new content [22, 23].
- **Autonomous systems (AS):** Operational systems that use AI-driven algorithms and models, such as those just noted, to function independently, without human oversight.

9.3.1 Pre-Submission

AI tools can be especially valuable for applicant engagement during the months leading up to submission, a critical period when candidates are actively deciding to which programs to apply. Applicants frequently utilize online databases—such as Residency Explorer, FREIDA, Texas STAR, and Residency Navigator—to gather information about prospective programs. However, there are challenges with using these tools. First, the information available within these databases is often fragmented or outdated, limiting their utility, in part because the data are often self-reported by either applicants or programs without a standardized timeline or uniform method for data collection.

Utilizing AI-driven data management tools for streamlining and standardizing data collection from applicants and programs could improve the accuracy and completeness of these databases. Many widely used survey platforms have already begun integrating AI into survey creation and analytics, such as SurveyMonkey's AI Insights (https://www.surveymonkey.com/) and Qualtrics's AI (https://www.qualtrics.com/) [24, 25]. Furthermore, the presence of multiple, separate databases can be cumbersome and time-consuming to navigate. Generative AI and autonomous systems could be leveraged to create a single, centralized platform that consolidates historical and current applicant and program data for more efficient and streamlined access.

In addition to information and impressions that can be uniquely gathered on an interview day, this may offer a "one-stop shop" resource for program information, particularly to help address gaps or unanswered questions. Currently, applicants gather information about training programs via several databases, program websites, social media outlets, and word of mouth. Many programs also host live informational sessions, offering the opportunity for applicants to engage directly with faculty and current trainees. However, due to time limitations and scheduling, most programs are usually only able to host one or two sessions, making it difficult to accommodate the schedules of all interested candidates.

Further, with a limited number of sessions, there is often a high turnout per session. While this serves to positively promote networking, it may also hinder the ability of individual applicants from asking questions or engaging with the group. An AI-driven platform offers greater availability and flexibility of access to applicants juggling a busy schedule and may allow for more timely and personalized engagement with programs.

In 2023, Yi et al. launched a novel AI-based chatbot for the Duke University Medical Center Department of Anesthesiology Pain Management Fellowship website, providing prospective applicants on-demand, 24/7 access to question-and-answer (Q&A) services [26]. The chatbot was also piloted to coordinate event logistics for live Q&A sessions, including managing attendee registration, calendar invites, and event reminders. Positive feedback regarding the experience included the chatbot being quick, helpful, and friendly to use. Most applicants utilized the chatbot to learn about specific fellowship training program information, the broader department or university, and the surrounding geographic area. Limitations with the chatbot included difficulty with answering highly specific or uncommon questions and failing to understand certain user inquiries. Still, while these chatbots are not intended to replace human-to-human communication, they may provide a promising supplementary means of engagement especially when direct interaction with the program is unavailable.

In summary, there are many avenues by which AI can help streamline access to residency and fellowship program information and aid applicants with more effectively identifying programs that best meet their training goals.

9.3.2 Submission and Application Review

The prospective role of AI in the application submission and review process is perhaps one of the most promising areas of innovation in graduate medical education (GME) recruitment. With the continued growth in volume of applications comes an equally urgent need for practical solutions to improve the efficiency of application review without compromising attention to detail. Under the current system, the mismatch between reviewer burden and time availability lends limitations to the requisite comprehensive approach to application review. Suppose, for example, that each application required at least 20 minutes to evaluate the essential components; this would equate to nearly 170 hours of continuous review time for a program that reviews 500 applications. This number of hours escalates quickly for larger programs reviewing substantially more applications [27].

Several third-party software platforms have developed AI-driven tools to address the challenges associated with high volumes of application reviews, including reviewer fatigue and reliance on traditional parameter cutoff-based screening. Among the most prominent is Thalamus, a growing and increasingly adopted software platform in the GME recruitment space [7]. As previously noted, Thalamus Core and Itinerary Wizard have traditionally been used for interview scheduling and management. In 2020, the company added Thalamus Cortex to its lineup, an AI-powered application review tool. Thalamus Cortex utilizes algorithms such as ML, NLP and optical character recognition (OCR), among others, to extract and consolidate data from residency application packets. This platform presents data in an organized reviewer-friendly interface designed to facilitate more efficient, holistic reviews, and it claims to reduce application screening times by 50%. In the upcoming 2026 match cycle, the AAMC and Thalamus have launched a partnership allowing complimentary access to pilot all Thalamus software platforms for all programs participating in ERAS. A similar platform, 3rd Friday, initially developed for interview scheduling, has also developed an AI-driven application analysis tool to assist programs with identifying candidates of best fit [10].

Many residency and fellowship training programs have started employing AI-driven tools to assist with applicant screening and holistic review. Several pilot studies utilizing such tools are summarized next.

Burk-Rafel et al. developed, piloted, and validated a machine learning decision support tool (DST) to assist with holistic application reviews for an internal medicine residency training program [16]. They trained an ML model with historical data, comprising 8000 applications from the 2018 to 2020 application cycles, to predict the probability of an applicant receiving an interview invitation, with a sensitivity of 91% and specificity of 85%. These performance metrics remained stable when test scores were removed from the training model, highlighting that the model was using more than objective test scores to predict interview invitation success rates. The model was also validated via real-world pilot testing and demonstrated a 93% concordance rate with faculty reviewer decisions. Upon further review, the 7% divergent selections were actually deemed promising candidates that may have been overlooked amid a very large application pool.

Sarraf et al. leveraged an established AI tool in natural language processing (NLP) and sentiment analysis, the IBM Watson™'s Natural Language Understanding™ (NLU) and Tone Analyzer™ (TA), to assess letters of recommendations (LORs) for potential gender bias in applications to their general surgery residency training program [19]. These NLP tools analyzed two decades' worth of LORs and were able to identify disparate patterns in the use of gendered wording and degree of positivity in LORs stratified by applicant sex. The ability of NLP to analyze language patterns and identify subtle nuances in written text, such as sentiment and tone, may serve as a valuable tool in assisting training programs with review of LORs.

Drum et al. built an ML model to support holistic application review at their combined internal medicine–pediatrics residency training program [18]. The model was trained on four years of historical data, from the 2015 to 2019 application cycles, using over 10,000 pieces of text extracted from narrative sections of ERAS. These excerpts were then annotated and linked to program-specific values associated with predicted resident success metrics, including both objective measures such as academic strength and more subjective qualities such as leadership, self-awareness, and adaptability. Their ML model achieved a sensitivity and specificity of 0.64 and 0.97, respectively. Prospective model validation demonstrated that both the number and specific type of annotations assigned to applicants by the ML model were predictive of interview-invitation success.

At their large urban internal medicine residency training program, Mahtani et al. developed an NLP tool to enhance the efficiency of evaluating the narrative experiences section of the ERAS application, which comprises up to 20 combined volunteer and research experiences per applicant [17]. The algorithm was trained on nearly 200,000 experience entries from 65,000 applications over three years of residency application cycle data. The NLP tool effectively condensed these lengthy sections into key words and phrases that were then used to predict the likelihood of receiving an interview invitation. Terminology related to leadership, research, and volunteer service in social justice and health disparities emerged as the most predictive of interview invitations.

Vasan et al. integrated both NLP and ML tools to create an AI model capable of analyzing LORs to predict the likelihood of interview success at their otolaryngology residency training program [20]. The algorithm was trained on 1600 vectorized LORs from a single application cycle and tested on five different pre-built ML models (Logistic Regression, Naive Bayes, Decision Tree, Random Forest, and Support Vector Machine). The Decision Tree ML model was the most effective in extracting and correlating meaningful information from LORs to interview success.

At their general surgery residency training program, Markow et al. utilized ChatGPT 4.0 to evaluate medical student performance evaluations (MSPE, also known as Dean's Letters). AI-based evaluations were then compared to manual review by experienced faculty on the residency selection committee [28]. On average, the scores assigned by manual review were significantly lower and more variable than those generated by the AI. In comparison, ChatGPT-based scores were typically higher and more similar across students as compared to faculty review.

Notably, not all studies showed congruence between AI-driven models and human selection. Hassan et al. also evaluated the utility of commercial AI screening tools in applicant review for their general surgery residency training program. This tool was preconfigured with weighted preferences for specific applicant characteristics set directly by the program director and compared to their own review of the same candidate pool during a single application cycle [29]. While many of the previously discussed studies have shown promising results with AI-driven tools, this study found only a 7% overlap in interview candidates selected by the program director compared to AI-based screening. These results raise a number of critical questions and considerations. Given the current early stages of AI development, would the model have performed better with further training? Was the tool effectively preconfigured? It's important to emphasize that the use of AI in application screening may serve best as a supportive adjunct tool, not as a replacement for human review.

9.3.3 Interviews

For many candidates, interview season is one of the most stressful periods of the application cycle, and AI-driven tools have considerable potential to streamline this process. Several tools are being developed to help applicants prepare more effectively for interviews. Software platforms such as BigInterview (https://www.biginterview.com/) and MatchAResident (https://www.matcharesident.com) now offer on-demand virtual mock interviews powered by AI-generated feedback [30, 31]. These services offer convenient interview practice, accessible at any time and place, to help applicants improve their communication skills and confidence, well in advance of the scheduled interview day.

AI technologies may also assist with reducing the administrative burdens of interview coordination. While many interview platforms now allow applicants to self-schedule, a significant amount of manual coordination still occurs. Important deadlines and logistics, including important forms and interview day schedules, must be communicated clearly to candidates in a timely fashion. Further, managing rescheduling requests and last-minute cancellations adds considerably to the workload; much of this labor-intensive process is handled by email or phone communication with small teams of program coordinators. AI tools could reduce these administrative burdens by automating scheduling and repetitive tasks.

9.3.4 The Match Process

While many of the early pilot studies, as previously discussed, have primarily focused on application screening and holistic review to support interview invitation decisions, there have also been efforts to apply AI technology to the creation of rank order lists. In a 2023 study, Rees and Ryder employed the Random Forest (RF) ML model to analyze candidate data and tested its ability to predict ranked versus unranked status and matriculant versus non-matriculant status of applicants to their internal medicine residency training program [21]. The algorithm was trained on 5000 residency applications from 2016 to 2019. When tested against retrospective outcomes, the RF model demonstrated impressive predictive accuracy in distinguishing ranked from unranked applicants, though only modest accuracy in predicting matriculation status at that program. Nevertheless, these findings suggest AI could serve as a valuable tool in supporting training programs as they create their rank order lists.

9.3.5 The Post-Match Experience

Many of the AI tools discussed in prior sections of the application cycle can similarly prove useful in helping unmatched applicants navigate their options, particularly during the SOAP process. From an applicant standpoint, AI-optimized program informational databases can assist applicants with identifying unfilled programs to which to apply, especially as many of these programs may not have initially been under their consideration. Conversely for programs, AI-integrated holistic review and interview coordination platforms, such as Thalamus Cortex and 3rd Friday, can help with rapidly reviewing new candidate applications and coordinating interview scheduling within the SOAP's compressed timeline.

9.4 LIMITATIONS AND FUTURE DIRECTIONS

The use of AI technology is becoming increasingly integrated into many fields in healthcare, including GME. It remains critical to consider the limitations and challenges associated with AI as we navigate how best to incorporate this technology into residency and fellowship recruitment. These tools should be implemented thoughtfully and with clear human oversight to ensure that GME recruitment processes remain fair and equitable.

9.4.1 Technical Limitations

Core to AI is that it is built on data. While seemingly obvious, it follows that the effectiveness of an AI system depends directly on the quality and quantity of data by which it was trained. The majority of ML models piloted in training programs thus far have utilized limited datasets, comprising at most a few years of single institution applicant data. Thus these models may not be widely generalizable, and they may struggle when applied to other institutions, specialties, or future application cycles, especially as candidate profiles and selection criteria evolve from year to year. It will be critical for systems to continuously retrain their ML models with the most relevant applicant data to ensure that their algorithms represent the most up-to-date trends in recruitment. Naturally, larger datasets for training are also needed to improve the quality of AI algorithms in this space. The newly established partnership between the AAMC and Thalamus represents an opportunity for ML models to train and learn from vastly larger datasets than previously available.

Another limitation of AI of utmost importance revolves around data regulation and management, particularly regarding privacy and confidentiality. The nature of any software-based technology renders it inherently susceptible to the risk of data breaches and unauthorized access. The integration of AI tools into recruitment efforts involves widespread access to sensitive applicant data, raising concerns over the security of confidential candidate information. As AI technology continues to advance, the parallel development of secure safeguards and data security oversight are needed to minimize risks of cybersecurity breaches and misuse.

9.4.2 Risk of Bias

While the uses of AI tools in recruitment are designed to reduce bias in applicant reviews, inherent limitations of data-driven systems are also associated with the risk of propagating existing biases. As discussed previously, AI models are largely trained on historical data and designed to replicate patterns of success. As aptly described by Gottlieb-Smith et al., these models may overlook or undervalue newer applicant qualities or attributes that have not been previously represented in past training datasets [32]. Along similar lines, any existing biases present within these datasets may be learned by the AI model and carried forward [32–34]. For example, if in a particular training dataset, older applicants tended to have a higher interview success rate—regardless of the actual qualifications by which they were selected—the model may tend to favor older applicants, even if age was not a significant factor during the actual selection process. AI models and the historical datasets by which they were trained should be thoroughly reviewed and perhaps routinely audited to assess for biased algorithms.

9.4.3 Ethical Concerns

Substantial ethical concerns have been raised regarding the use of AI in residency and fellowship recruitment. First, there exists the potential for applicants to shape their application based on what they think the AI tools are looking for in order to replicate the patterns or terminology flagged as successful by prior interviewed or matched candidates. Second, there is also increasing concern over utilization of generative AI tools by applicants in preparing application materials, particularly narrative components such as personal statements and LOR [22]. In a 2024 survey of medical students, over 50% reported having used or planned to use AI to assist with writing their personal statements [23].

From the program perspective, there has been growing concern involving AI-generated personal statements and LORs; some have attempted to evaluate the ability of human reviewers to recognize AI-based written products. Koleilat et al. found that experienced attending physicians from a residency selection committee were able to discern AI versus human written personal statements with 87% sensitivity but only 37% specificity and with 55% accuracy, underscoring the growing difficulty in differentiating between the two [35]. Others have attempted to assess the perceived quality of statements written by AI versus human-written work. In a blinded survey of radiology program directors, Gordon et al. found that AI-generated personal statements were typically rated lower quality compared to naturally written works [36]. In this study, the reviewers were also able to discern which statements were AI-generated with relative accuracy. Pilot studies employing AI tools in writing LORs have also been conducted. Mansour et al. evaluated the ability of an AI model to produce well written letters [37]. Interestingly, they found that AI-generated letters were selected by reviewers only 30% of the time, and they also identified a large discrepancy in reviewer ability to recognize AI-generated products, ranging from 15 to 90%. In a similar study, Simister et al. found that reviewers struggled to recognize AI-produced letters, correctly identifying them only 60% of the time [38]. Notably and importantly, human-generated letters were overall more highly rated across reviewers. Rising concerns over the authenticity of narrative written statements and LORs also brings into question the weight that will be placed on these application components in future cycles. It is possible that more emphasis will be placed on interpersonal interactions—such as interviews, networking, and elective rotations—within the recruitment process compared to prior years.

The incorporation of AI into GME recruitment remains new and largely uncharted territory. Further research is needed to evaluate the efficiency of AI-based tools in supporting applicant reviews on larger, prospective scales and their effectiveness in identifying candidates that best align with the unique values and goals of individual programs. To address the technical challenges, risks of bias, and ethical concerns surrounding the integration of AI into this space, most can agree that judicious use by both applicants and programs with regulatory oversight is essential. National governing bodies, such as the ACGME and NRMP, and specialty-specific organizations, such as the Association of Program Directors (APD) within each field, and specialty societies, are in important positions to develop and communicate clear guidelines regarding the appropriate use of AI tools in the recruitment process [32, 33, 35]. From a program standpoint, improved transparency regarding the use of AI tools in applicant screening and holistic review are needed to establish trust and preserve the overall integrity of the recruitment process [33]. Important factors, including which ML models are employed, how they were trained, and what efforts have been made to reduce the risk of model bias, should be disclosed. Similarly, from a candidate perspective, it is equally important to establish authenticity and accountability safeguards to ensure that all submitted materials are reflective of an applicant's own and original work.

9.5 CONCLUSION

The landscape of recruitment in GME has changed immensely since the first NRMP Match cycle nearly 50 years ago. By 2075, it may be entirely unrecognizable as applicant competitiveness continues to climb, as the priorities of training programs continue to evolve with increasing efforts toward optimizing holistic review and as AI technology continues to rapidly advance. AI has the potential to positively impact residency and fellowship recruitment across multiple domains, from helping applicants better identify target programs to helping programs reduce reviewer fatigue and improve the processing of large volumes of applications. Importantly, human thought and communication should not be minimized or lost in this process. While not meant to replace human review, AI may serve as a promising supportive tool in the recruitment process to optimize the strongest matches between trainees and training programs.

GLOSSARY

Accreditation Council for Graduate Medical Education: Governing body overseeing the accreditation for all graduate medical education training programs.

American Association of Medical Colleges: National nonprofit organization that serves to represent medical schools and academic healthcare systems in the United States.

American Medical Association: National professional organization that serves to advance and advocate for the interests of physicians and medical trainees.

Artificial intelligence: Concept of computer systems able to perform tasks that traditionally require human intelligence.

Association of Program Directors: National professional organizations that serves to support residency and fellowship program directors within each respective specialty.

Authenticity: An overarching characteristic that implies honesty, truth, and integrity.

Autonomous systems: Operational systems that use AI-driven algorithms and models, such as those previously noted, to function independently without human oversight.

Bias: A disproportionate tendency, inclination, or prejudice against a person, group, or thing.

Blinded: Practice in research studies and projects in which knowledge of the study intervention is withheld from participants to prevent undue influence or bias.

Chatbot: An automated software program designed to simulate and engage with normal human conversation.
Concordance: The concept of shared agreement or consistency.
Decision support tool: Products designed to assist individuals in making informed choices.
Divergent: The concept of moving in different or opposing directions.
Ethical: Relating to the concept of moral principles.
Electronic Residency Application Service: An online application service used to apply for medical residency and fellowship training programs.
Fellowship: A post-residency training program to pursue additional specialized medical training in a particular subspecialization (such as cardiology, gastroenterology, etc.)
Generalizable: The concept of being widely applicable to a larger population.
Generative artificial intelligence: Integration of preexisting content (written text, images, photos, videos, music, etc.) with machine learning to create new content.
Graduate medical education: Formal hands-on medical training following graduation from medical school to specialize, prepare for, and achieve qualifications for independent practice.
Holistic: The concept of utilizing multiple relevant contributing components to evaluate a thing, person, group, or system.
Machine learning: Algorithmic models that enable computer systems to independently learn from data and improve their performance without programming.
Main Residency Match: The algorithm carried out by the National Residency Matching Program to pair medical residency programs with incoming resident physician trainees.
Medical Student Performance Evaluations: A standardized letter of evaluation prepared by all medical schools for each medical student that summarizes their performance in training.
National Board of Medical Examiners and National Board of Osteopathic Medical Examiners: National governing bodies that oversee the development, revision, and administration of medical licensing examinations.
National Resident Matching Program: A national nonprofit organization that oversees systems to pair medical residency programs with incoming resident physician trainees.
Natural language processing: Algorithmic models that enable computer systems to recognize, understand, interpret, and communicate via human language.
Natural language understanding: A subset of natural language processing focused primarily on the comprehension and interpretation of human language.
Optical character recognition: The ability of software programs to identify printed text.
Predictive analytics: Integration of historical data, mathematical models, and machine learning to predict future outcomes.
Qualitative: The concept using non-numeric descriptive characteristics to describe things, people, concepts, and experiences.
Quantitative: The concept using numeric, measurable data to describe things, people, concepts, and experiences.
Random Forest: A machine learning model that utilizes decision trees to make predictions.
Residency: A post–medical school training program to establish competency and qualifications in a medical specialty.

Sensitivity: The ability of a test to correctly identify true positive cases.
Specificity: The ability of a test to correctly identify true negative cases.
Supplemental Offer and Acceptance Program: A system to pair unfilled residency training program positions with unmatched applicants.
United States Medical Licensing Examination: A three-step medical licensing examination in the United States.

ABBREVIATIONS

ACGME	Accreditation Council for Graduate Medical Education
MD	allopathic
AOA	Alpha Omega Alpha
AAMC	American Association of Medical Colleges
AMA	American Medical Association
AI	artificial intelligence
APD	Association of Program Directors
AS	autonomous systems
DST	decision support tool
ERAS	Electronic Residency Application Service
FREIDA	Fellowship and Residency Electronic Interactive Database Access
GAI	generative artificial intelligence
LORs	letters of recommendation
ML	machine learning
MSPE	Medical Student Performance Evaluations
NBME	National Board of Medical Examiners
NBOME	National Board of Osteopathic Medical Examiners
NIH	National Institutes of Health
NRMP	National Resident Matching Program
NLP	natural language processing
NLU	natural language understanding
OCR	optical character recognition
PA	predictive analytics
Q&A	question and answer
RF	Random Forest
SOAP	Supplemental Offer and Acceptance Program
USMLE	United States Medical Licensing Examination
Texas STAR	University of Texas Southwestern Seeking Transparency in Application to Residency

REFERENCES

1. Signer M. *Results and Data: 2005 Main Residency Match* [Internet]. Washington, DC: National Resident Matching Program; 2005 Apr [cited 2025 Jul 12]. Available from: https://www.nrmp.org/match-data/2005/04/results-and-data-2005-main-residency-match/
2. *NRMP Releases 2025 Main Residency Match Results and Data Report, Providing In-Depth Insight into the Largest Residency Match in History* [Internet]. NRMP; 2025 [cited 2025 Jul 12]. Available from: https://www.nrmp.org/about/news/2025/05/nrmp-releases-2025-main-residency-match-results-and-data-report-providing-in-depth-insight-into-the-largest-residency-match-in-history/
3. Lamb D. *Results and Data: Specialties Matching Service, 2025 Appointment Year* [Internet]. Washington, DC: National Resident Matching Program; 2025 Feb [cited 2025 Jul 12]. Available from: https://www.nrmp.org/match-data/2025/02/results-and-data-specialties-matching-service-2025-appointment-year/

4. Lamb D. *Results and Data: 2025 Main Residency Match* [Internet]. Washington, DC: National Resident Matching Program; 2025 May [cited 2025 Jul 12]. Available from: https://www.nrmp.org/match-data/2025/05/results-and-data-2025-main-residency-match/
5. Mandel LP, Spadoni LR, Hewitson LA, Vontver LA. One residency's experience with the electronic residency application service. *Fam Med.* 1997 Mar;29(3):209–12.
6. *Apply to Residencies with the ERAS® System* [Internet]. Students & Residents. [cited 2025 Jul 31]. Available from: https://students-residents.aamc.org/applying-residencies-eras/apply-residencies-eras-system
7. *Thalamus | GME Residency Interview Scheduling Software* [Internet]. [cited 2025 Jul 31]. Available from: https://www.thalamusgme.com/
8. *Interview Broker* [Internet]. [cited 2025 Jul 31]. Available from: https://www.interviewbroker.com/interview/
9. *RezRATE: Recruitment Software for Graduate Medical Educators* [Internet]. RezRATE. [cited 2025 Jul 31]. Available from: https://www.rezrate.com/
10. *AI—3rdFriday* [Internet]. [cited 2025 Jul 21]. Available from: https://3rdfriday.com/ai/
11. *How it Works: The Matching Algorithm* [Internet]. NRMP. [cited 2025 Jul 31]. Available from: https://www.nrmp.org/intro-to-the-match/how-matching-algorithm-works/
12. Vance S, Figg BJ, Wagner MJ. Graduate medical education tool kit for the Supplemental Offer and Acceptance Program: Navigating the National Resident Matching Program supplemental offer assistance program. *AEM Educ Train.* 2021 Mar 17;5(2):e10588.
13. Detterline S, Ferguson R. In the SOAP: The Supplemental Offer and Acceptance Program (SOAP) from the perspective of a Community Hospital Residency. *J Community Hosp Intern Med Perspect.* 2012 Jul 16;2(2):10.3402/jchimp.v2i2.18712.
14. Gupta A, Malik P, Pathania M, Rathaur VK. Overview of artificial intelligence in medicine. *J Family Med Prim Care.* 2019 Jul;8(7):2328–31.
15. Solomonides AE, Koski E, Atabaki SM, Weinberg S, McGreevey JD, Kannry JL, et al. Defining AMIA's artificial intelligence principles. *J Am Med Inform Assoc.* 2021 Nov 2;29(4):585–91.
16. Burk-Rafel J, Reinstein I, Feng J, Kim MB, Miller LH, Cocks PM, et al. Development and validation of a machine learning-based decision support tool for residency applicant screening and review. *Acad Med.* 2021 Nov 1;96(11S):S54–61.
17. Mahtani AU, Reinstein I, Marin M, Burk-Rafel J. A new tool for holistic residency application review: Using natural language processing of applicant experiences to predict interview invitation. *Acad Med.* 2023 Sep 1;98(9):1018–21.
18. Drum B, Shi J, Peterson B, Lamb S, Hurdle JF, Gradick C. Using natural language processing and machine learning to identify internal medicine-pediatrics residency values in applications. *Acad Med.* 2023 Nov 1;98(11):1278–82.
19. Sarraf D, Vasiliu V, Imberman B, Lindeman B. Use of artificial intelligence for gender bias analysis in letters of recommendation for general surgery residency candidates. *Am J Surg.* 2021 Dec;222(6):1051–9.
20. Vasan V, Cheng CP, Lerner DK, Pascual K, Mercado A, Iloreta AM, et al. Machine learning for predictive analysis of otolaryngology residency letters of recommendation. *Laryngoscope.* 2024 Sep;134(9):4016–22.

21. Rees CA, Ryder HF. Machine learning for the prediction of ranked applicants and matriculants to an internal medicine residency program. *Teach Learn Med*. 2023;35(3):277–86.
22. Chen JX, Bowe S, Deng F. Residency applications in the era of generative artificial intelligence. *J Grad Med Educ*. 2024 Jun;16(3):254–6.
23. Smith B, Ramadoss T, D'Amario V, Shoja MM, Rajput V, Cervantes J. Utilization and perception of generative artificial intelligence by medical students in residency applications. *J Investig Med*. 2025 Apr;73(4):338–44.
24. *AI Driven Experience Management Platform—Qualtrics XM* [Internet]. Qualtrics. [cited 2025 Jul 31]. Available from: https://www.qualtrics.com/platform/
25. *SurveyMonkey AI | Generate & Analyze Surveys with AI* [Internet]. SurveyMonkey. [cited 2025 Jul 31]. Available from: https://www.surveymonkey.com/product/features/ai/
26. Yi PK, Ray ND, Segall N. A novel use of an artificially intelligent Chatbot and a live, synchronous virtual question-and answer session for fellowship recruitment. *BMC Med Educ*. 2023 Mar 11;23(1):152.
27. Ruiz de Luzuriaga AM. The potential for artificial intelligence tools in residency recruitment. *Cutis*. 2024 Feb;113(2):56–9.
28. Markow M, Jebbia M, Hasjim BJ, Nahmias J, Grigorian A, Burruss S, et al. Artificial intelligence: Reducing inconsistency in the surgical residency application review process. *Am J Surg*. 2024 Dec;238:115816.
29. Hassan M, Ayad M, Nembhard C, Hayes-Dixon A, Lin A, Janjua M, et al. Artificial intelligence compared to manual selection of prospective surgical residents. *J Surg Educ*. 2025 Jan;82(1):103308.
30. *AI Interview Software & Instant Feedback* [Internet]. [cited 2025 Jul 31]. Available from: https://www.biginterview.com/video-ai
31. *Residency Interview Preparation Services | Match A Resident* [Internet]. [cited 2025 Jul 31]. Available from: https://www.matcharesident.com/interview-prep
32. Gottlieb-Smith R, Xixis K, Martindale JM, Goldstein JHR, Rosati J. Artificial intelligence in residency recruitment. *Neurology Education*. 2024 Sep;3(3):e200150.
33. Rosenthal JT, Hafferty FW, Kulasegaram KM, Wendland CL, Taylor JS. Artificial intelligence meets holistic review: Promises and pitfalls of automating the medical education admissions process. *Acad Med*. 2025 May 1;100(5):541–6.
34. Ajmani A, Klufas T, Zhou AE, Sloan B, Grant-Kels JM. Ethical implications of artificial intelligence in residency applicant screening. *J Am Acad Dermatol*. 2025 May 23;S0190–9622(25)02198-X.
35. Koleilat I, Bongu A, Chang S, Nieman D, Priolo S, Patel NM. Residency application selection committee discriminatory ability in identifying artificial intelligence-generated personal statements. *J Surg Educ*. 2024 Jun;81(6):780–5.
36. Gordon EB, Maxfield CM, French R, Fish LJ, Romm J, Barre E, et al. Large language model use in radiology residency applications: Unwelcomed but inevitable. *J Am Coll Radiol*. 2025 Jan;22(1):33–40.
37. Mansour J, Burman M, Bernstein M, Sandman E, Yammine K, Daher M, et al. Should my recommendation letter be written by artificial intelligence? *Can J Surg*. 2024 Jun 6;67(3):E243–6.
38. Simister SK, Huish EG, Tsai EY, Le HV, Halim A, Tuason D, et al. Can artificial intelligence deceive residency committees? A randomized multicenter analysis of letters of recommendation. *JAAOS—Journal of the American Academy of Orthopaedic Surgeons*. 2025 Mar 15;33(6):e348.

10 AI Evaluation of Clinicians

Best Practices for Implementation in the Large Language Model Era

Bryce Thornton, Jeffrey R. Curtis, John D. Osborne

10.1 INTRODUCTION

The evaluation of clinicians is a foundational activity in medicine, underpinning medical education, credentialing, quality assurance, and professional accountability [1, 2]. Despite its centrality, clinician evaluation remains labor-intensive, variably applied, and difficult to scale. From grading OSCEs and assessing clinical documentation during training, to peer review, chart audits, and quality improvement in practice, most evaluation workflows depend heavily on expert human judgment. While this reliance preserves clinical nuance, it introduces well-documented challenges: limited faculty time, interrater variability, susceptibility to bias, delayed feedback, and difficulty generating longitudinal, high-resolution performance data [3, 4].

The emergence of large language models (LLMs) introduces a qualitatively new opportunity to augment and to scale the evaluation of clinicians who perform these clinical tasks. Unlike earlier generations of machine learning systems, LLMs interact naturally with unstructured clinical data such as radiology imaging, video records, free-text notes, written rationales, and narrative assessments at scale [5, 6]. They can generate explanatory judgments, identify omissions or inconsistencies, and provide formative feedback aligned with evaluation rubrics including the ability to perform "zero-shot," meaning it can produce a reasonable evaluation from instructions alone, without prior task-specific training examples. These properties align closely with how clinicians are evaluated in real-world settings, where performance is rarely reducible to a single numeric outcome and often requires interpretation, justification, and contextual reasoning [7].

Figure 10.1 illustrates the operational workflow underlying LLM-based clinician evaluation. The workflow proceeds from task definition (Section 10.2) through iterative dataset development (Section 10.3) and model adaptation (Section 10.4) to formal evaluation (Section 10.5), with feedback loops that return to earlier stages when performance criteria are not met. Key decision points include whether the task requires generative output and where development will take place. This last decision is closely tied to de-identification [8] decisions that often drive whether deployment must occur behind institutional firewalls or can occur through HIPAA-compliant cloud infrastructure. The ability to access state-of-the-art HIPAA-compliant infrastructure further impacts model availability and constrains which models are available to pursue an LLM-as-a-judge [9] strategy that is strongly advocated in this chapter.

Historically, clinical evaluation workflows have followed a linear and resource-intensive trajectory: Cases are curated, rubrics are designed, evaluators are trained and calibrated, and expert review is conducted manually at scale. This approach has proven difficult to sustain as clinical and educational demands increase. In many settings, the bottleneck is not the absence of evaluative criteria, but the limited capacity to apply them consistently and to provide timely, individualized feedback. As a result, evaluations are often delayed, overly coarse, or focused narrowly on checklist completion rather than clinical reasoning or professional judgment [2].

DOI: 10.1201/9781003617167-10

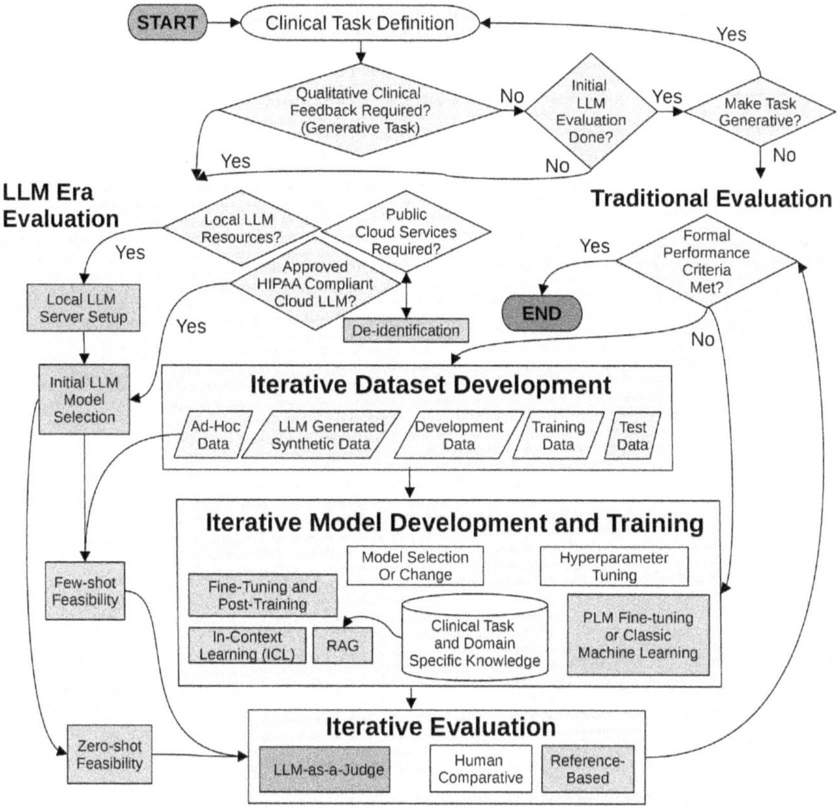

Figure 10.1 Overview of the design of AI systems for clinical evaluation, including task definition, dataset development, model optimization, and evaluation.

LLMs invert this paradigm. Because they can be deployed rapidly and operate at scale, they enable an evaluation-first workflow in which preliminary assessments can be generated immediately and compared against human standards. In some contexts—such as low-stakes formative feedback—these preliminary assessments may already meet institutional needs. In others, they serve as decision-support tools that triage cases, surface ambiguities, or prepopulate structured reviews for expert adjudication. Importantly, this inversion does not eliminate the need for human oversight; rather, it concentrates expert effort where it is most valuable [10].

Despite rapid experimentation, deployment of LLM-based clinician evaluation systems remains uneven and methodologically fragmented. Many existing studies focus on whether LLMs can perform clinical reasoning tasks, answer medical questions, or generate notes, rather than whether they can reliably evaluate human clinicians performing those same tasks. Evaluation methods are often borrowed from generic natural language processing benchmarks, emphasizing lexical similarity or task accuracy [11] without accounting for the interpretive and contextual demands of clinician assessment [4]. In high-stakes contexts like trainee remediation, professional review, or quality assurance, these gaps will limit trust and adoption [12].

This chapter addresses that gap by focusing explicitly on AI systems designed to evaluate clinicians, rather than AI systems evaluated for clinical performance. It is written for clinician informaticians and clinical educators who may be new to deep learning and large language models but who are positioned to lead evaluation initiatives at their institutions. Because the methods used to evaluate AI-generated outputs overlap substantially with those used to evaluate clinician-generated outputs, a working understanding of core machine learning practices is essential; accordingly, this chapter provides an applied overview of these methods in the context of clinician evaluation. Three dominant paradigms for assessing LLM-based evaluators are examined: reference-based evaluation, expert human comparative evaluation, and LLM-as-a-judge approaches. Across these paradigms, expert human judgment remains the epistemic anchor for clinician assessment [1, 13], and automated evaluators must be calibrated, audited, and governed accordingly [14, 15]. LLM-as-a-judge approaches, particularly when aligned with expert human knowledge, represent the most promising path toward scalable clinician assessment.

10.2 DEFINING CLINICIAN EVALUATION TASKS

Effective deployment of AI-based clinician evaluation begins with a precise task definition that determines the scope, methodology, and technical requirements of the entire pipeline. As shown in Figure 10.1, the first decision node asks whether the assessment requires qualitative clinical feedback or, rather, the task is inherently generative. This distinction is consequential as it governs whether the system must follow a large language model (LLM) evaluation pathway or traditional machine learning pathways can be evaluated. This decision shapes all downstream choices regarding data, model architecture, and evaluation strategy.

10.2.1 Application Domain

Within clinician assessment, two principal application domains can be distinguished. The first, *proxies of skill*, involves standardized simulations or structured tasks designed to isolate specific competencies. Objective structured clinical examinations (OSCEs) are representative tools used during training to assess readiness under controlled conditions [16, 17]. These afford high experimental control and relatively straightforward annotation. The second domain, *artifacts of clinical work*, encompasses authentic products of practice such as clinical notes, diagnostic justifications, and treatment plans [1]. These artifacts capture the complexities of a live clinical environment but complicate the validation process. Reconciling inconsistent annotations frequently necessitates a retrospective chart review to understand the provider's original intent [18]. Privacy constraints under the Health Insurance Portability and Accountability Act (HIPAA) further complicate work with real clinical artifacts relative to PHI-free proxy data. For teams less experienced in clinical AI, proxies of skill are generally a more tractable starting point.

10.2.2 Output Modality and the Generative Decision

The central branching logic in Figure 10.1 hinges on whether the evaluation task requires generative output (for example, open-ended narrative feedback, explanatory critique, or reasoning) or discrete outputs such as numeric scores or pass/fail determinations suffice. When both inputs and outputs are structured, traditional machine learning or encoder-based models [19] are typically preferable: They are faster, cheaper, and more straightforward to validate. If an evaluation requires only discrete outputs, and no qualitative feedback is needed, the workflow routes to a traditional evaluation pathway using pretrained language model

(PLM) fine-tuning or classical machine learning, proceeding directly to formal performance criteria assessment.

LLMs become most valuable when either the inputs or the desired outputs are inherently unstructured or explanatory. For example, in an OSCE documentation task where trainees submit free-text SOAP notes, an LLM can generate formative feedback by flagging omitted findings, critiquing reasoning gaps, and suggesting rubric-aligned improvements. When generative output is required, the system enters the LLM evaluation pathway, which introduces additional decisions around infrastructure, data handling, and iterative development (see Sections 10.3–10.5). Importantly, the figure includes a feedback loop: if a non-generative task fails to meet performance criteria, teams may reconsider whether reformulating the task as generative could improve evaluation quality.

10.2.3 Model Access and Deployment

Once the generative decision is made, model access and deployment represent the next critical dimension (Figure 10.1). Teams with local GPU resources can deploy open-weight models, such as Meta's Llama or DeepSeek R1 [20], behind institutional firewalls, maintaining data security for sensitive datasets [21, 22]. LLM servers such as vLLM [23] or Ollama [24] manage batching, memory, and concurrent access, functioning analogously to web servers. When local resources are unavailable and public cloud services are required, the workflow directs teams to HIPAA-compliant cloud LLM end points with mandatory de-identification of clinical data prior to transmission [25]. Closed-weight systems such as OpenAI's GPT or Google's Gemini offer state-of-the-art performance through API access, though at higher operational cost and with ongoing privacy considerations [26].

Unless there is strong evidence that a closed-weight system is required, beginning with open-weight models is generally advisable. The performance gap between open- and closed-weight models is narrowing, local deployment reduces costs and encourages experimentation, and switching to a closed-weight model later is straightforward when already using LLM servers. Most early evaluation systems have focused on text-based inputs, but emerging multimodal LLMs capable of processing audio and video create new opportunities to evaluate competencies including communication skills and procedural technique that are not fully captured in written documentation alone [10].

10.3 DATA AND GOVERNANCE FOR CLINICIAN EVALUATION

The development of datasets for clinician assessment is an iterative process, as shown in Table 10.1. Readers familiar with machine learning workflows will recognize the practices described in this section; they are included here because they require specific adaptation when applied to clinical evaluation, notably due to the regulatory constraints surrounding protected health information and the severe scarcity of sharable datasets. Datasets in this context may include real-world clinical documentation (for example, progress notes or discharge summaries), simulated or OSCE-style notes, or audio and video recordings of standardized patient encounters.

10.3.1 Data Governance

Data governance encompasses the ethical, legal, and operational frameworks governing clinical data use in AI development, principally regulated in the United States by HIPAA. These safeguards protect patient privacy but create barriers to reproducibility. Secondary use typically requires Institutional Review Board (IRB) review and formal data-use agreements [27]. De-identification (the process of removing Protected Health Information [PHI] and Personally Identifying

Information [PII]), can mitigate constraints, with leading systems removing 98–99% of HIPAA Safe Harbor elements [28, 29]. However, this performance remains insufficient at scale, particularly when text contains implicit identifiers not enumerated as Safe Harbor elements. Surrogate replacement systems [30, 31] further reduce risk, and it is recommended that developers apply de-identification algorithms [8] to clinical text and images where practical.

Synthetic notes have been proposed as an alternative, but LLMs may reintroduce PHI through model memorization [32] and high-quality synthetic notes exhibit comparable privacy concerns [33]. Multidisciplinary oversight committees are best positioned to navigate these challenges [34]. For production systems, every step of the AI life cycle should be documented, with a clinician-in-the-loop process integrated throughout [35].

10.3.2 Data Sourcing

Clinical text varies substantially by specialty and institution; models trained at a single site typically experience 10–20% performance drops elsewhere, whether in imaging [36] or in transformer-based clinical NLP [37] or cross-institutional LLM evaluations [38]. The MIMIC corpus remains the only readily available large-scale public clinical dataset (Table 10.1). If sourcing EHR data from one or multiple institutions, data harmonization is often required because sites often encode the same clinical concepts differently. Common data models (CDMs) such as Fast Health Interoperability Resources (FHIR) [39], Observational Medical Outcomes Partnership (OMOP) [40], and Patient Centered Outcome Research Institute (PCORnet) standardize structured fields, and NLP can normalize variables derived from clinical unstructured text for analysis [41]. In educational contexts, simulated datasets such as OSCE notes may offer greater consistency and fewer governance barriers than real-world clinical data.

10.3.3 Data Labeling and Quality Control

Labeled data remain essential: without explicit labels, evaluation is limited to ad hoc assessment rather than reproducible measurement. Labels may include expert ratings of documentation quality, pass/fail competency determinations, identification of omitted findings, categorical judgments of communication effectiveness, and other workflow outputs.

Table 10.1 Publicly Available Datasets Relevant to Clinical Evaluation Tasks

Data Types and Source	Clinical Task Evaluated	Reference
EHR histories, vitals, labs, notes from MIMIC-IV ED	Diagnosis, triage level, and specialty assignment for ED patients	Gaber et al., 2025 [42]
Curated clinical histories, labs/imaging from MIMIC-IV	Diagnostic accuracy for 4 common abdominal pathologies	Hager et al., 2024 [43]
PubMed case reports with diagnosis and reasoning trace	Final diagnosis generation from case report	Wu et al., 2025 [44]
Case text, images, captions, metadata from PubMed case reports	Imaging captioning for medical education	Nievas Offidani et al., 2025 [45]
Case text, free-text fields from MIMIC and I2B2 challenges	Problem summarization and medical question answering	Gao et al., 2023 [46]

10.3.3.1 LLM-First Evaluation

As illustrated in Figure 10.1, LLMs enable an evaluation-first workflow that fundamentally changes the economics of dataset development. Rather than investing in extensive annotation before any model is tested, developers can assess zero-shot feasibility at the outset: a small set of human-labeled exemplars is tested in a zero- or few-shot fashion across one or more LLMs to establish a baseline and gauge task difficulty. When initial performance meets user-defined criteria, only a formal test set is needed, avoiding additional costly annotation. Even when performance falls short, LLM-assisted strategies remain viable: an LLM may generate provisional labels (such as a diagnosis) subsequently reviewed by expert annotators or even fully synthetic labeled data to accelerate dataset creation. This LLM-first approach, visible in Figure 10.1's zero-shot and few-shot feasibility paths, represents a paradigm shift from the traditional supervised learning framework of label, train, and then evaluate to one of evaluate, identify gaps, and then label selectively, with or without LLM assistance.

10.3.3.2 Human Labeling and Criteria Refinement

Expert disagreement is inherent to clinical evaluation; concordance may be low even among faculty rating the same trainee's performance. A minimum of two raters evaluating shared samples is necessary to calculate inter-rater reliability (IRR). The process should begin with rubric development and calibration, followed by independent labeling of unseen data, with an acceptable IRR score (such as Cohen's kappa >0.75) as a prerequisite for proceeding [47]. When disagreement reflects rubric ambiguity, the resulting inconsistency can propagate into the model; when it reflects legitimate clinical diversity, enforcing artificial consensus risks training on a single narrow perspective [6, 48].

10.3.3.3 Data Partitioning, Class Imbalance, and Synthetic Data

Where sample size permits, labeled data should be partitioned into training, development (validation), and held-out test sets [49, 50]. The development (validation) set supports iterative refinement during development. It is used while revising prompts or rubrics, tuning hyperparameters or thresholds, selecting among models, and deciding whether synthetic data helps. Because these choices involve repeated checks on the same data, they can inadvertently overfit the system to that dataset. Using the validation set for model refinement helps minimize overfitting, leaving the test set unaffected by model development. The training set is the pool of labeled cases used to teach the system what good performance looks like. This can be done by placing selected examples directly in the prompt, as in-context examples, or by updating model parameters through fine-tuning. The held-out test set is reserved for a final estimate of performance on unseen cases and is ideally used once. When data are limited, or when no iterative optimization is planned, a separate validation set may be omitted in favor of cross-validation or a simpler train/test split, provided the prompt and evaluation plan are determined before testing. In practice, clinical datasets are often refined over time; therefore, labeling should be treated as an iterative process, and adding diverse high-quality examples is typically the most reliable path to improvement, so dataset construction should not be viewed as a "one-off" step [51].

Class imbalance is a common concern: when over 90% of examples are labeled Pass, the model may fail to learn features of the minority Fail class [52]. Mitigation strategies include oversampling [53] and LLM-generated synthetic data. As shown in Table 10.2, synthetic data generation encompasses pre-annotation, data augmentation, and dataset expansion, typically implemented through prompt-based generation, retrieval-augmented pipelines, and self-refinement

Table 10.2 LLM Synthetic Data Generation Strategies

Description	Generated Labels	Generated Data	Use Case	Example
Pre-annotation	Yes	No	Increase labeling rate	LLM prescores OSCE notes for human review
Data augmentation	No	Yes	LLM continue-training	Synthetic surgical procedure videos for rare cases
Dataset expansion	Yes	Yes	Performance improvement	Synthetic Fail-class OSCE notes to balance training data

frameworks [54–56]. Evaluators should directly test whether synthetic data improve performance before committing to a costly manual review.

10.4 MODEL SELECTION AND ADAPTATION FOR EVALUATION

10.4.1 Overall Approach and Model Selection

Building on the evaluation-first workflow described in Section 10.3.3.1, model selection and adaptation follow a path of least resistance. Clinical implementors should begin with a zero-shot evaluation using a cloud API that offers strong out-of-the-box performance [57] for a fast assessment. This preliminary evaluation can be zero-shot, where the prompt consists solely of task instructions without examples of expected output. In a clinical evaluation context, this might comprise a grading rubric and a student case history submission, allowing the model to infer rubric application from its pretrained knowledge [10, 58]. The goal at this stage is not to select a final model but to establish a performance baseline that reveals whether the task is tractable and where the primary gaps lie.

All data governance and deployment considerations discussed in Section 10.3 remain applicable to the preliminary evaluation. When handling protected health information, requests must be routed through HIPAA-compliant end points with secure institutional agreements before deployment, even during initial ad hoc chatbot validation [59].

For model selection, it is difficult to predict which specific models will outperform others given the pace of advancement; leaderboards can be informative but may overstate performance when models are optimized for a benchmark metric rather than for generalization to clinical use cases. Therefore, it is prudent to invest in a robust, model-independent evaluation framework that enables rapid comparison across candidate models as better models continually emerge. Designing this framework to be model-agnostic ensures that new models can be benchmarked against consistent criteria and references.

Following initial evaluation, in-context learning (Section 10.4.2) should be incorporated by providing the model with exemplar submissions paired with expert rubric-based evaluations. In data-rich scenarios, such as when a sufficiently large corpus of previously graded OSCE notes is available, supervised fine-tuning (Section 10.4.3) can further align model outputs with institutional grading standards. In data-poor scenarios, context engineering, including expanding rubric definitions or embedding clinical guidelines within the prompt, may prove more effective than fine-tuning. These approaches are not mutually exclusive, and agentic workflows (Section 10.4.4) represent a final option when a single LLM yields unsatisfactory performance.

10.4.2 Model Adaptation: In-Context Learning

In-context learning (ICL) refers to the ability of an LLM to adapt its behavior based on information provided in the prompt, without any parameter updates [60]. In clinical evaluation, few-shot prompting corresponds to providing graded exemplar performances alongside the rubric and student submission. Most studies report diminishing returns beyond three to five exemplars; in clinical prediction tasks such as discharge likelihood or ICU admission, one study found no noticeable advantage beyond five in-context examples [61]. Similarly, for USMLE-style examination and clinical decision support, additional examples yielded only minimal gains for GPT-4 [62].

When prompt-based adaptation does not meet performance requirements, developers may advance to fine-tuning (Section 10.4.3) or automated prompt optimization using frameworks such as DSPy [63]. More sophisticated reasoning strategies include Chain-of-Thought prompting, which elicits intermediate reasoning steps [64]; Tree-of-Thought, which explores multiple reasoning branches before selecting the best path [65] and Graph-of-Thought, which structures reasoning as a graph of interconnected ideas [66]. For example, Nachane [67] applied Chain-of-Thought to a modified MedQA-USMLE dataset containing open-ended medical questions with clinician-approved reasoned answers.

10.4.3 Model Adaptation: Supervised Fine-Tuning and Context Engineering

Supervised fine-tuning (SFT) adapts an LLM on a labeled dataset of input–output pairs to align its outputs with domain-specific standards. For open-weight models, Parameter-Efficient Fine-Tuning (PEFT) [68] techniques such as Low-Rank Adaptation (LoRA) [69] reduce computational costs by freezing most base model parameters and training only a small set of low-rank matrices. An LLM could, for example, be fine-tuned on OSCE responses paired with expert-generated grades and rationales, learning to reproduce expert scoring patterns and deliver rubric-aligned feedback. Even with modest zero- or few-shot baselines, targeted fine-tuning often enables open-weight models to match or exceed closed-weight systems on domain-specific tasks at lower cost [70, 71]. Cloud vendors also permit fine-tuning through vendor-provided services, offering limited customization while the provider hosts the adapted model.

Retrieval-augmented generation (RAG) [72] offers an alternative when fine-tuning is impractical or when contemporaneous factual grounding is required, for instance when clinical guidelines change more frequently than a model can be retrained [73, 74]. At inference, the model output is dynamically conditioned on retrieved knowledge sources, enabling evaluation of clinical reasoning against evidence-based frameworks rather than relying solely on pretraining. As shown in Figure 10.1, RAG sits alongside ICL and fine-tuning within the iterative model development and training phase.

10.4.4 AI Agents

The field is advancing rapidly toward agentic workflows, systems that function as reasoning engines capable of decomposing complex tasks, invoking external tools, and self-correcting [75–77]. For clinical evaluation, agent-based systems could orchestrate multistep assessment pipelines: retrieving relevant clinical guidelines, applying rubrics to student documentation, cross-checking for clinical safety concerns, and generating formative feedback, with each step performed by a specialized sub-component. Frameworks under active development include LangChain/LangGraph [78, 79] for developer-driven agents, AutoGen for role-based multi-agent collaborations [80] and OctoTools for tool-calling-dependent tasks [81]. This space is evolving rapidly as of early 2026.

10.5 EVALUATING EVALUATORS (LLMS)

Selecting a suitable evaluation method is a critical decision, as it defines the criteria for success and shapes the interpretation of results. Non-generative AI restricts outputs to predefined categorical or numerical values validated against ground-truth references [82], whereas generative clinical outputs are open-ended and can include detailed narrative feedback. Such outputs often lack a single definitive reference, as multiple linguistically distinct responses can express clinically equivalent meaning [83]. This challenge is amplified in clinical evaluation, where correct assessments of trainee or clinician performance may differ in emphasis, structure, and phrasing while remaining equally valid. A faculty member grading a trainee's SOAP note, for example, might focus on diagnostic reasoning while another equally qualified rater emphasizes treatment plan completeness; both assessments may be clinically sound yet lexically dissimilar.

To address these limitations, developers should adopt the subject–criteria–reference–result framework [84], which conceptualizes evaluation as a functional mapping (Figure 10.2). In this schema, developers specify the model output (subject), task-specific evaluation criteria, and, when appropriate, reference exemplars. The evaluator, which could be a computational algorithm, human expert, or auxiliary LLM acting as a judgment agent (LLM-as-a-judge) then produces a performance judgment or result. This framework is deliberately evaluator-agnostic, allowing systematic comparison across all three paradigms discussed next.

Developers should choose between two primary strategies for subject evaluation: pointwise and pairwise comparison. In pointwise evaluation, each model output is assessed independently against predefined criteria and, optionally, a reference standard (Figure 10.3). In pairwise evaluation, two or more outputs generated from the same input prompt are compared directly to determine relative quality or preference (Figure 10.4) [85]. The criteria define specific standards by which the subject is assessed, expressed through clearly defined dimensions (for example, diagnostic accuracy, completeness) and rubrics that translate those dimensions into measurable rating scales. The result is the evaluator's output, generally taking the form of quantitative ratings, qualitative rationales, or both. Following this framework, the next step is to select an appropriate evaluator from three primary paradigms.

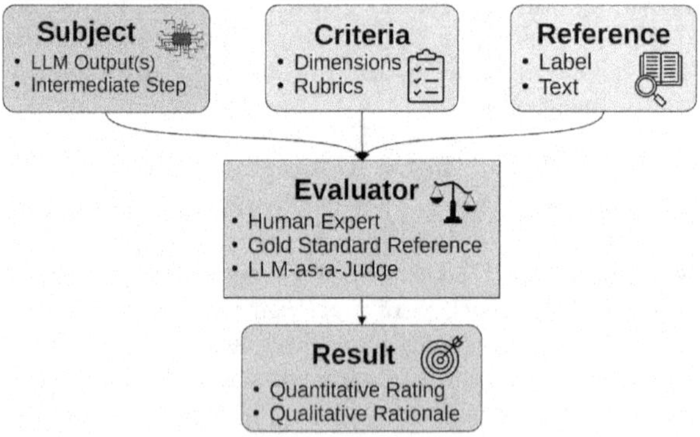

Figure 10.2 Conceptual framework for LLM evaluation using the subject–criteria–reference–result schema.

The evaluation-first workflow (Section 10.3.3.1) also informs evaluator selection. An initial LLM-as-a-judge run, for example, can reveal whether a rubric is sufficiently unambiguous for automated scoring or whether human comparative evaluation is necessary, helping developers focus expert resources on the paradigms and edge cases where they add the most value.

10.5.1 Paradigm 1: Reference-Based Evaluation

Use reference-based evaluation to measure how closely model outputs align with trusted clinical or benchmark references. This approach quantifies agreement through pointwise comparison (Figure 10.3), working best for structured, non-generative tasks such as diagnostic classification or risk prediction. To quantify agreement, use inter-rater reliability (IRR) metrics. Cohen's kappa is appropriate for categorical outputs, whereas the intraclass correlation coefficient (ICC) is commonly used for continuous predictions, consistent with how human–human reliability is typically reported [47, 86]. Values above 0.8 generally indicate strong alignment.

When evaluating generative models, apply reference-based metrics with caution. Lexical similarity metrics such as ROUGE [87], BLEU [88], and METEOR [89] reward exact token overlap but often penalize clinically valid outputs that express equivalent meaning using alternative phrasing [11]. When semantic fidelity matters more than surface matching, embedding-based metrics such as BERTScore [90] or BLEURT [91] better capture meaning-level agreement. In clinical tasks, semantic metrics should generally be prioritized over lexical ones because expert evaluators routinely accept diverse phrasings that convey the same clinical judgment. Reference-based evaluation is most effective as a first-line quantitative screen during early development. It is computationally inexpensive, fully reproducible, and well suited to rapid iteration during the LLM-first feasibility phase described in Section 10.3. However, as the evaluation system matures, reference-based metrics should be paired with human or LLM-as-a-judge assessments to capture dimensions of quality that automated metrics miss.

10.5.2 Paradigm 2: Human Comparative Evaluation

Human comparative evaluation serves as the reference standard for assessing LLM performance in clinical domains. This paradigm anchors algorithmic behavior in expert reasoning and remains essential wherever interpretive nuance or ethical accountability is required [92, 93]. Both pointwise and pairwise strategies apply here: individual raters may score a single LLM output against a rubric (pointwise) or compare two outputs side by side to determine which is superior (pairwise,

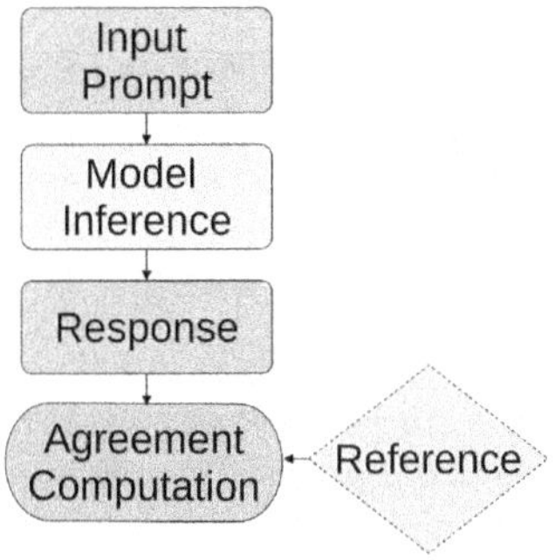

Figure 10.3 Pointwise comparison evaluation.

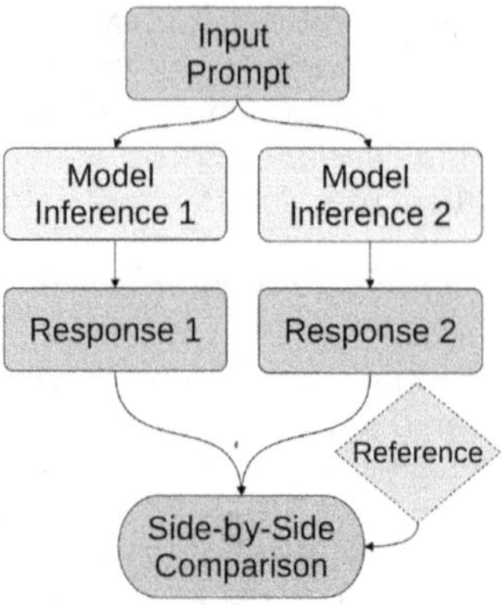

Figure 10.4 Pairwise comparison evaluation.

Figure 10.4). Engage qualified expert raters early and require explicit rationales for every decision.

The evaluation process can be structured in phases to balance rigor and efficiency. These phases include a Pilot phase to establish alignment and rubric reliability through calibration sessions and inter-rater reliability measurement; an Expansion phase to scale validated rubrics to larger datasets with periodic recalibration and random audit sampling; and a Maintenance phase to sustain reliability and traceability through documentation of rating adjustments and integration of updates into model quality assurance and regulatory records (Table 10.3). This staged workflow creates a calibrated foundation for automated or hybrid LLM-as-a-judge systems that inherit human standards and ensures that evaluation criteria are refined before scaling.

Despite the value of human evaluation, it has well-known limitations including the need for expert rater compensation and their limited availability [94]. Replacing domain experts with crowdsourced annotators, who often lack the contextual knowledge needed for accurate judgment in clinical settings, brings its own series of problems and ethical pitfalls including self-selection bias, exploitation, and other "gig economy" ethical issues [95]. These issues mean that serious consideration should be given to hybrid pipelines where LLM-as-a-judge prescreen low-complexity cases and human experts adjudicate ambiguous or high-impact outputs. Regardless of the chosen approach, audit trails to support institutional review or regulatory audits will be needed in any scenario [96].

10.5.3 Paradigm 3: LLM-Based Evaluation

Use the LLM-as-a-judge paradigm to scale and standardize evaluation. An LLM-as-a-judge is an LLM configured to act as an automated evaluator, generating assessments according to predefined criteria and rubrics [97, 98]. This paradigm operates within the same subject–criteria–reference–result framework (Figure 10.2) and supports both pointwise and pairwise strategies: an LLM-as-a-judge may score individual outputs against a rubric (Figure 10.3) or rank competing outputs side by side (Figure 10.4). The principal advantage is throughput since LLM-as-a-judge can evaluate thousands of outputs in the time required for a single human rater to score dozens, accelerating iterative model development where rapid feedback cycles are essential.

Table 10.3 Phased Workflow for Human Comparative Evaluation

Phase	Purpose	Key Actions
Pilot	Establish alignment and rubric reliability	Train raters; score a limited subset; compute IRR; resolve discrepancies through consensus sessions
Expansion	Scale validated rubrics to larger datasets	Apply criteria to broader corpora; conduct periodic recalibration and random audit sampling
Maintenance	Sustain reliability and traceability	Document rating adjustments and audit results; integrate updates into model QA and regulatory records

However, before relying on LLM-as-a-judge results, it is still recommended to calibrate its scoring against expert human raters. Measure calibration reliability using Cohen's kappa or ICC for categorical ratings and Spearman's rho or Kendall's tau for ranked comparisons [14, 99]. Define minimum acceptable thresholds (such as Cohen's kappa ≥0.8) before deployment. Running LLM-as-a-judge scoring early with minimal setup can identify systematic disagreements with human raters before scaling annotation, allowing targeted rubric revision rather than wholesale relabeling.

After the initial evaluation, it is still recommended to continuously monitor the LLM-as-a-judge for judgment drift, the gradual divergence of LLM-as-a-judge behaviors from expert consensus over time or across input distributions. Recognize common systematic biases: position bias (favoring earlier responses in pairwise comparisons), verbosity bias (preferring longer answers), self-enhancement bias (favoring outputs from similar model architectures), and prompt sensitivity [14, 99–101]. Mitigate these through position swapping, self-consistency sampling, panel-based evaluation using multiple diverse models, and in-context exemplar reinforcement [51, 102].

LLM-as-a-judge should be treated as a supplement, not a replacement, for expert human judgment. Even when quantitative reliability approaches human-level concordance, retain human oversight for all high-stakes clinical, and educational decisions. Integrate continuous auditing and ethical oversight into governance workflows to ensure that LLM-as-a-judge-based evaluation remains aligned with institutional standards and regulatory requirements. As the field matures, LLM-as-a-judge systems calibrated against expert consensus offer the most promising path toward scalable, reproducible clinician assessment, but only if their outputs remain transparent, auditable, and subject to ongoing human validation.

10.6 CASE STUDY

This section details a case study demonstrating the application of the proposed framework within medical education, focusing on the use of LLMs for assessing student performance. Conducted at UT Southwestern Medical Center's Simulation Center, this initiative examined the feasibility and performance of an LLM-based automated grading system for post-encounter notes from OSCEs [10], which measure clinical competence through live simulated patient encounters [16]. After examining the simulated patient, students completed progress notes summarizing their differential diagnosis, supporting findings, and management plan [103, 104]. Student performance in OSCEs is evaluated using predefined grading rubrics that delineate the criteria for satisfactory performance. Historically, these notes required manual grading by expert evaluators like physicians and clinical instructors, a process that was time-intensive and subject to inter-rater variability. The system's primary aim was to substantially reduce faculty grading workload while preserving the rigor and fairness of human evaluation. Specifically, the study evaluated whether a zero-shot LLM could reliably assess diagnostic reasoning and documentation quality in the absence of domain-specific fine-tuning.

In this system, both the rubric items and the student's post-encounter note are reformulated into a series of engineered prompts for automatic assessment by zero-shot prompting an LLM, thus requiring no prior task-specific fine-tuning data. Each rubric element was expressed as a discrete yes/no claim-verification task. The desired components of the student's note and the rubric were constructed into a grading prompt to generate automated evaluations. A large dataset of expert-labeled student post-encounter notes was curated from up to 4 years prior to deployment to validate the LLM system. Owing to the non-generative nature of the task, the researchers chose to evaluate their model using reference-based evaluation. GPT-4 in a zero-shot configuration demonstrated an 89.7% item-level agreement with expert graders, with Cohen's kappa of 0.79. Prospective evaluation was performed across all 245 pre-clerkship student submissions. The model achieved 82.9% agreement with human graders and a Cohen's kappa of 0.66, reflecting adequate agreement with human raters. The system achieved a 91% reduction in human grading effort and decreased turnaround time from weeks to days. Although this fell below the Cohen's kappa ≥0.8 benchmark suggested in Section 10.5.3 for autonomous deployment, it was considered sufficient for the intended faculty-supervised workflow.

The research team also fine-tuned smaller, locally hosted open-weight models through knowledge distillation from closed-weight model outputs. Specifically, they fine-tuned Llama-2–7B for the same task with GPT-4 as the teacher model to guide calibration. The training dataset was composed of GPT-4-generated outputs from the retrospective dataset that aligned with expert human grades. Testing on the prospective dataset demonstrated comparable performance to GPT-4 while offering enhanced data privacy preservation and institutional control.

This case exemplifies the successful implementation of the principles outlined in this chapter. By integrating human expertise, reproducible evaluation protocols, and diverse LLM-based methodologies, the case demonstrates how such systems can be operationalized from conceptual design through real-world deployment.

10.7 LEARNING HEALTH SYSTEMS AND FUTURE DIRECTIONS

This chapter presents a conceptual framework for the development, optimization, and evaluation of LLMs used for clinical assessment. At the core of this framework lies expert human judgment, even when LLM-as-a-judge is employed. The objective of these systems is not to replace expert judgment but to amplify and scale it as the field progresses toward increasingly autonomous evaluation workflows characterized by hybrid systems integrating human and artificial intelligence. The continued maturation of the LLM-as-a-judge framework holds the potential to reduce the barriers associated with large-scale evaluation of clinical AI systems. Realizing this vision demands engagement with methodological challenges: identification and mitigation of model biases, navigation of data governance constraints, and cultivation of institutional trust. Ethical dimensions, including fairness across demographic groups and the accountability implications of automated professional assessment, remain important areas for future work.

The integration of LLMs into clinical education and practice represents a transformative opportunity. LLM-driven evaluative systems possess the capacity to catalyze broader systemic transformation by generating the structured, high-resolution performance data necessary to advance the vision of a LHS [105–107]. Within such a system, routine clinical and educational activities continuously produce data that are rapidly analyzed, synthesized into actionable evidence, and reintegrated into practice, creating a self-sustaining feedback loop of improvement.

REFERENCES

1. Epstein, R.M. and E.M. Hundert, Defining and assessing professional competence. *JAMA*, 2002. 287(2): p. 226–235.
2. Epstein, R.M., Assessment in medical education. *New England Journal of Medicine*, 2007. 356(4): p. 387–396.
3. Boulet, J.R., et al., The use of standardized patient assessments for certification and licensure decisions. *Simulation in Healthcare*, 2009. 4(1): p. 35–42.
4. Brooks, M.A., Medical education and the tyranny of competency. *Perspectives in Biology and Medicine*, 2009. 52(1): p. 90–102.
5. Lee, J., et al., BioBERT: A pre-trained biomedical language representation model for biomedical text mining. *Bioinformatics*, 2019. 36(4): p. 1234–1240.
6. Singhal, K., et al., Toward expert-level medical question answering with large language models. *Nature Medicine*, 2025. 31(3): p. 943–950.
7. Steinmann, A.F., et al., The modern teaching physician—responsibilities and challenges: An APDIM white paper. *The American Journal of Medicine*, 2009. 122(7): p. 692–697.
8. Meystre, S.M., et al., Automatic de-identification of textual documents in the electronic health record: A review of recent research. *BMC Medical Research Methodology*, 2010. 10(1): p. 70.
9. Wang, R., et al., Can LLMs replace human evaluators? An empirical study of LLM-as-a-judge in software engineering. *Proceedings of the ACM on Software Engineering*, 2025. 2(ISSTA): p. 1955–1977.
10. Jamieson, A.R., et al., Rubrics to prompts: Assessing medical student post-encounter notes with AI. *NEJM AI*, 2024. 1(12).
11. Reiter, E., A structured review of the validity of BLEU. *Computational Linguistics*, 2018. 44(3): p. 393–401.
12. Schuwirth, L.W. and C.P. Van der Vleuten, Programmatic assessment: From assessment of learning to assessment for learning. *Medical Teacher*, 2011. 33(6): p. 478–485.
13. Hodges, B., Assessment in the post-psychometric era: Learning to love the subjective and collective. *Medical Teacher*, 2013. 35(7): p. 564–568.
14. Zheng, L., et al., Judging LLM-as-a-judge with MT-bench and chatbot arena. *arXiv e-prints*, 2023: p. arXiv:2306.05685.
15. Guidance, W., *Ethics and Governance of Artificial Intelligence for Health*. 2021, World Health Organization. p. 1–165.
16. Khan, K.Z., et al., The objective structured clinical examination (OSCE): AMEE guide no. 81. Part I: An historical and theoretical perspective. *Medical Teacher*, 2013. 35(9): p. e1437–e1446.
17. Boursicot, K.A.M., T.E. Roberts, and W.P. Burdick, Structured assessments of clinical competence, in *Understanding Medical Education*. 2018, Wiley. p. 335–345.
18. Trebble, T.M., et al., Determining doctors' views on performance measurement and management of their clinical practice. *Future Hospital Journal*, 2015. 2(3): p. 166–170.
19. Devlin, J., et al., Bert: Pre-training of deep bidirectional transformers for language understanding, in *Proceedings of the 2019 Conference of the North American Chapter of the Association for Computational Linguistics: Human Language Technologies*, Vol. 1 (long and short papers). 2019.

20. Guo, D., et al., DeepSeek-R1 incentivizes reasoning in LLMs through reinforcement learning. *Nature*, 2025. 645(8081): p. 633–638.
21. Nowak, S., et al., Privacy-ensuring open-weights large language models are competitive with closed-weights GPT-4o in extracting chest radiography findings from free-text reports. *Radiology*, 2025. 314(1): p. e240895.
22. Dennstädt, F., et al., Implementing large language models in healthcare while balancing control, collaboration, costs and security. *NPJ Digital Medicine*, 2025. 8(1): p. 143.
23. Kwon, W., et al., Efficient memory management for large language model serving with paged attention, in *Proceedings of the 29th Symposium on Operating Systems Principles*. 2023.
24. Ollama, *Run Large Language Models Locally*. 2024, Ollama.
25. Burns, M.L., et al., Generative AI costs in large healthcare systems, an example in revenue cycle. *NPJ Digital Medicine*, 2025. 8(1): p. 579.
26. Neupane, S., S. Mittal, and S. Rahimi, Towards a HIPAA compliant agentic AI system in healthcare. *arXiv preprint*, 2025: p. arXiv:2504.17669.
27. McGraw, D. and K.D. Mandl, Privacy protections to encourage use of health-relevant digital data in a learning health system. *NPJ Digital Medicine*, 2021. 4(1): p. 2.
28. Hartman, T., et al., Customization scenarios for de-identification of clinical notes. *BMC Medical Informatics and Decision Making*, 2020. 20(1).
29. Kayaalp, M., et al., De-identification of address, date, and alphanumeric identifiers in narrative clinical reports, in *AMIA . . . Annual Symposium Proceedings/AMIA Symposium. AMIA Symposium, 2014*. 2014: p. 767–776.
30. Carrell, D., et al., Hiding in plain sight: Use of realistic surrogates to reduce exposure of protected health information in clinical text. *Journal of the American Medical Informatics Association*, 2013. 20(2): p. 342–348.
31. Trotter, A., et al., *uabnlp/BRATsynthetic: 0.4*. 2025, Zenodo.
32. Li, A., et al., Memorization in large language models in medicine: Prevalence, characteristics, and implications. *arXiv preprint*, 2025: p. arXiv:2509.08604.
33. Sarkar, A.R., et al., De-identification is not enough: A comparison between de-identified and synthetic clinical notes. *Scientific Reports*, 2024. 14(1): p. 29669.
34. Wells, B.J., et al., A practical framework for appropriate implementation and review of artificial intelligence (FAIR-AI) in healthcare. *NPJ Digital Medicine*, 2025. 8(1): p. 514.
35. Price II, W.N., Clinicians in the loop of medical AI. 75 *Emory L.J.*, 2025: p. 1265.
36. Zech, J.R., et al., Variable generalization performance of a deep learning model to detect pneumonia in chest radiographs: A cross-sectional study. *PLoS Medicine*, 2018. 15(11): p. e1002683.
37. Khambete, M.P., et al., Quantification of BERT diagnosis generalizability across medical specialties using semantic dataset distance. *AMIA Summits on Translational Science Proceedings*, 2021. 2021: p. 345.
38. Keloth, V.K., et al., Social determinants of health extraction from clinical notes across institutions using large language models. *NPJ Digital Medicine*, 2025. 8(1): p. 287.
39. Ayaz, M., et al., The fast health interoperability resources (FHIR) standard: Systematic literature review of implementations, applications, challenges and opportunities. *JMIR Medical Informatics*, 2021. 9(7): p. e21929.
40. Weeks, J. and R. Pardee, Learning to share health care data: A brief timeline of influential common data models and distributed health data networks in U.S. health care research. eGEMs (Generating Evidence & Methods to Improve Patient Outcomes), 2019. 7(1): p. 4.

41. Reeves, R.M., et al., Adaptation of an NLP system to a new healthcare environment to identify social determinants of health. *Journal of Biomedical Informatics*, 2021. 120: p. 103851.
42. Gaber, F., et al., Evaluating large language model workflows in clinical decision support for triage and referral and diagnosis. *NPJ Digital Medicine*, 2025. 8(1).
43. Hager, P., et al., Evaluation and mitigation of the limitations of large language models in clinical decision-making. *Nature Medicine*, 2024. 30(9): p. 2613–2622.
44. Wu, K., et al., MedCaseReasoning: Evaluating and learning diagnostic reasoning from clinical case reports. *arXiv e-prints*, 2025: p. arXiv:2505.11733.
45. Nievas Offidani, M., et al., An open-source clinical case dataset for medical image classification and multimodal AI applications. *Data*, 2025. 10, 123. https://doi.org/10.3390/data10080123.
46. Gao, Y., et al., Dr. bench: Diagnostic reasoning benchmark for clinical natural language processing. *Journal of Biomedical Informatics*, 2023. 138: p. 104286.
47. McHugh, M.L., Interrater reliability: The kappa statistic. *Biochemia Medica*, 2012: p. 276–282.
48. Runyon, C., Using large language models (LLMs) to apply analytic rubrics to score post-encounter notes. *Medical Teacher*, 2025. 47(11): p. 1772–1780.
49. Van Der Goot, R., We need to talk about train-dev-test splits, in *Proceedings of the 2021 Conference on Empirical Methods in Natural Language Processing*. 2021.
50. Jurafsky, D. and J.H. Martin, *Speech and Language Processing: An Introduction to Natural Language Processing, Computational Linguistics, and Speech Recognition, with Language Models*. 3rd ed. 2026, Stanford, CA: Stanford University.
51. Whang, S.E., et al., Data collection and quality challenges in deep learning: A data-centric AI perspective. *The VLDB Journal*, 2023. 32(4): p. 791–813.
52. Kim, J., T. Kim, and J. Choo, EPIC: Effective prompting for imbalanced-class data synthesis in tabular data classification via large language models. *arXiv preprint*, 2024: p. arXiv:2404.12404. https://doi.org/10.48550/arXiv.2404.12404.
53. Moe, L., U.T. Nguyen, and B.T. Luu, *Mitigating Class Imbalance in Fact-Checking Datasets through LLM-Based Synthetic Data Generation*. 2025, ACM.
54. Gonzales, A., G. Guruswamy, and S.R. Smith, Synthetic data in health care: A narrative review. *PLoS Digital Health*, 2023. 2(1): p. e0000082.
55. Nadas, M., L. Diosan, and A. Tomescu, Synthetic data generation using large language models: Advances in text and code. *arXiv preprint*, 2025: p. arXiv:2503.14023. https://doi.org/10.48550/arXiv.2503.14023.
56. Xu, Y., et al., MedSyn: Text-guided anatomy-aware synthesis of high-fidelity 3-D CT images. *IEEE Transactions on Medical Imaging*, 2024. 43(10): p. 3648–3660.
57. Singhal, K., et al., Large language models encode clinical knowledge. *Nature*, 2023. 620(7972): p. 172–180.
58. Wornow, M., et al., Zero-shot clinical trial patient matching with LLMs. *NEJM AI*, 2025. 2(1): p. AIcs2400360.
59. Marks, M. and C.E. Haupt, AI chatbots, health privacy, and challenges to HIPAA compliance. *JAMA*, 2023. 330(4): p. 309–310.
60. Brown, T., et al., Language models are few-shot learners. *Advances in Neural Information Processing Systems*, 2020. 33: p. 1877–1901.
61. Brown, K.E., et al., Large language models are less effective at clinical prediction tasks than locally trained machine learning models. *Journal of the American Medical Informatics Association*, 2025. 32(5): p. 811–822.
62. Nori, H., et al., Capabilities of gpt-4 on medical challenge problems. *arXiv preprint*, 2023: p. arXiv:2303.13375.

63. Khattab, O., et al., DSPy: Compiling declarative language model calls into self-improving pipelines. *arXiv preprint*, 2023: p. arXiv:2310.03714. https://doi.org/10.48550/arXiv.2310.03714.
64. Wei, J., et al., Chain-of-thought prompting elicits reasoning in large language models. *Advances in Neural Information Processing Systems*, 2022. 35: p. 24824–24837.
65. Yao, S., et al., Tree of thoughts: Deliberate problem solving with large language models. *Advances in Neural Information Processing Systems*, 2023. 36: p. 11809–11822.
66. Besta, M., et al., Graph of thoughts: Solving elaborate problems with large language models, in *Proceedings of the AAAI Conference on Artificial Intelligence*. 2024.
67. Nachane, S.S., et al., Few shot chain-of-thought driven reasoning to prompt LLMs for open ended medical question answering. *arXiv preprint*, 2024: p. arXiv:2403.04890.
68. Mangrulkar, S., et al., *PEFT: State-of-the-art Parameter-Efficient Fine-Tuning Methods*. 2023, Hugging Face.
69. Hu, E.J., et al., Lora: Low-rank adaptation of large language models. *ICLR*, 2022. 1(2): p. 3.
70. Hanke, V., et al., Open LLMs are necessary for current private adaptations and outperform their closed alternatives. *Advances in Neural Information Processing Systems*, 2024. 37: p. 1220–1250.
71. Wolfe, R., et al., Laboratory-scale AI: Open-weight models are competitive with CHATGPT even in low-resource settings, in *Proceedings of the 2024 ACM Conference on Fairness, Accountability, and Transparency*. 2024.
72. Neha, F., D. Bhati, and D.K. Shukla, Retrieval-augmented generation (rag) in healthcare: A comprehensive review. *AI*, 2025. 6(9): p. 226.
73. Zakka, C., et al., Almanac—retrieval-augmented language models for clinical medicine. *NEJM AI*, 2024. 1(2): p. AIoa2300068.
74. Liu, S., A.B. McCoy, and A. Wright, Improving large language model applications in biomedicine with retrieval-augmented generation: A systematic review, meta-analysis, and clinical development guidelines. *Journal of the American Medical Informatics Association*, 2025. 32(4): p. 605–615.
75. Huang, K., et al., Biomni: A general-purpose biomedical AI agent. *biorxiv*, 2025.
76. Schmidgall, S., et al., AgentClinic: A multimodal agent benchmark to evaluate AI in simulated clinical environments. *arXiv preprint*, 2024: p. arXiv:2405.07960.
77. Gorenshtein, A., et al., AI agents in clinical medicine: A systematic review. *medRxiv*, 2025: p. 2025.08. 22.25334232.
78. LangChain, I., *LangGraph: Build Resilient Language Agents as Graphs*. 2024, LangChain, Inc.
79. Chase, H., *LangChain*. 2022, LangChain, Inc.
80. Wu, Q., et al., Autogen: Enabling next-gen LLM applications via multi-agent conversations, in *First Conference on Language Modeling*. 2024.
81. Lu, P., et al., Octotools: An agentic framework with extensible tools for complex reasoning. *arXiv preprint*, 2025: p. arXiv:2502.11271.
82. Goodfellow, I., Y. Bengio, and A. Courville, *Deep Learning*. 2016, MIT Press.
83. Sottana, A., et al., Evaluation metrics in the era of GPT-4: Reliably evaluating large language models on sequence to sequence tasks. *arXiv e-prints*, 2023: p. arXiv:2310.13800.

84. Li, B., I. Sigler, and Y. Xue, Evaluating large language models: Principles, approaches, and applications in NeurIPS, in *Tutorial Presented at the Thirty-Eighth Conference on Neural Information Processing Systems*. 2024.
85. Jeong, H., et al., The comparative trap: Pairwise comparisons amplifies biased preferences of LLM evaluators. *arXiv preprint*, 2024: p. arXiv:2406.12319.
86. Artstein, R. and M. Poesio, Survey article: Inter-coder agreement for computational linguistics. *Computational Linguistics*, 2008. 34(4): p. 555–596.
87. Lin, C.-Y., *ROUGE: A Package for Automatic Evaluation of Summaries*. 2004, Barcelona, Spain: Association for Computational Linguistics.
88. Papineni, K., et al., BLEU, in *Proceedings of the 40th Annual Meeting on Association for Computational Linguistics—ACL '02*. 2001, Association for Computational Linguistics. p. 311.
89. Banerjee, S. and A. Lavie, *METEOR: An Automatic Metric for MT Evaluation with Improved Correlation with Human Judgments*. 2005, Ann Arbor, Michigan: Association for Computational Linguistics.
90. Zhang, T., et al., BERTScore: Evaluating text generation with BERT. *arXiv preprint*, 2019: p. arXiv:1904.09675. https://doi.org/10.48550/arXiv.1904.09675.
91. Sellam, T., D. Das, and A.P. Parikh, BLEURT: Learning robust metrics for text generation. *arXiv e-prints*, 2020: p. arXiv:2004.04696.
92. Fraile Navarro, D., et al., Expert evaluation of large language models for clinical dialogue summarization. *Scientific Reports*, 2025. 15(1).
93. Kocaman, V., et al., Clinical large language model evaluation by expert review (CLEVER): Framework development and validation. *JMIR AI*, 2025. 4: p. e72153.
94. Williams, G., et al., Human evaluators vs. LLM-as-a-judge: Toward scalable, real-time evaluation of GenAI in global health. *medRxiv*, 2025: p. 2025.10.27.25338910.
95. Cheong, M., G. Bush, and M. Wildenauer, "Lost in the crowd": Ethical concerns in crowdsourced evaluations of LLMs. *AI and Ethics*, 2025. 5(4): p. 4407–4413.
96. Awasthi, R., et al., Human evaluation of large language models in healthcare: Gaps, challenges, and the need for standardization. *NPJ Health Systems*, 2025. 2(1).
97. Gu, J., et al., A survey on LLM-as-a-judge. *The Innovation*, 2024. 7(6): p. 1–30.
98. Chiang, C.-H. and H.-y. Lee, Can large language models be an alternative to human evaluations? *arXiv preprint*, 2023: p. arXiv:2305.01937. https://doi.org/10.48550/arXiv.2305.01937.
99. Shi, L., et al., Judging the judges: A systematic study of position bias in LLM-as-a-judge. *arXiv preprint*, 2024: p. arXiv:2406.07791. https://doi.org/10.48550/arXiv.2406.07791.
100. Chen, Z.-Y., et al., Beyond the surface: Measuring self-preference in LLM judgments. *arXiv preprint*, 2025: p. arXiv:2506.02592. https://doi.org/10.48550/arXiv.2506.02592.
101. Hua, A., et al., Flaw or artifact? Rethinking prompt sensitivity in evaluating LLMs, in *Proceedings of the 2025 Conference on Empirical Methods in Natural Language Processing*. 2025.
102. Verga, P., et al., Replacing judges with juries: Evaluating LLM generations with a panel of diverse models. *arXiv preprint*, 2024: p. arXiv:2404.18796. https://doi.org/10.48550/arXiv.2404.18796.
103. Macmillan, M.K., et al., Assessing post-encounter note documentation by examinees in a field test of a nationally administered standardized patient test. *Academic Medicine*, 2000. 75(10): p. S112–S114.

104. Harden, R.M., et al., Assessment of clinical competence using objective structured examination. *Br Med J*, 1975. 1(5955): p. 447–451.
105. Friedman, C., et al., Toward a science of learning systems: A research agenda for the high-functioning learning health system. *Journal of the American Medical Informatics Association*, 2014. 22(1): p. 43–50.
106. Greene, S.M., R.J. Reid, and E.B. Larson, Implementing the learning health system: From concept to action. *Annals of Internal Medicine*, 2012. 157(3): p. 207–210.
107. Enticott, J., A. Johnson, and H. Teede, Learning health systems using data to drive healthcare improvement and impact: A systematic review. *BMC Health Services Research*, 2021. 21(1).

11 AI at the Bedside

Courtney Reamer, Brian T. Garibaldi

11.1 CASE PRESENTATION

Mr. X is a 72-year-old male presenting with 3 months of increasing dyspnea on exertion and fatigue to an inpatient general medicine floor. How could artificial intelligence (AI) enhance Mr. X's overall clinical experience while supporting his physicians during the process of information gathering, diagnosis, and management reasoning?

11.2 INTRODUCTION

The encounter between a patient and physician remains the cornerstone of the practice of medicine. However, bedside clinical skills are in decline, in part due to a lack of time spent with patients, an overreliance on technology-based testing, and a lack of appreciation for the enduring value of bedside skills (1, 2). This decline in bedside clinical skills has led to an increase in diagnostic error, higher healthcare costs, and a lack of professional fulfilment, as providers care more for the digital representation of a patient than an actual person (3–5). While technology has contributed to the erosion of bedside skills, the road back to the bedside requires an appreciation of the power of emerging technology to supplement traditional bedside skills, to help clinicians calibrate those skills, and to develop new ways of teaching, learning, and practicing at the bedside (2). In fact, the whole idea of the "bedside" has been transformed in recent years. The explosion of telemedicine visits during the COVID-19 pandemic brought the bedside into patient homes on a scale previously unimaginable (6). The development of cheaper and more accurate remote monitoring has redefined the bedside to include wherever a patient is wearing a sensor (7). However, no other technological advance has the potential to change how we teach, learn, and interact with patients at the modern bedside than artificial intelligence (AI).

11.3 AI AT THE BEDSIDE IN CLINICAL PRACTICE

AI is ripe to transform how medicine is practiced. Not only is AI poised to help improve efficiency and workflows, but it also has the potential to transform the way we gather and synthesize information. Table 11.1 summarizes the ways in which AI can improve bedside clinical care and education.

11.3.1 Remote Patient Monitoring

One area in which AI can advance bedside medicine is remote patient monitoring (RPM). RPM involves the use of electronic tools to capture personal health data that can be shared remotely with care teams. RPM has shown promise in improving clinical care and enabling patient engagement outside of traditional care settings. RPM tools involve a wide range of technologies, including home monitors for heart rate or blood pressure as well as advanced sensors capable of detecting falls or interpreting electrocardiogram (ECG) recordings (8–11).

RPM, especially continuous RPM, generates an overwhelming volume of data. AI can help sift through this information faster than humans and can identify clinically meaningful trends while reducing noise (9–11). AI RPM tools can potentially help avoid hospitalizations, improve care, and lower costs (11). AI can detect early warning signs of clinical decompensation or identify patients at higher

DOI: 10.1201/9781003617167-11

Table 11.1 The Promise of AI at the Bedside

AI-Enabled Tool	Potential Benefits
Remote patient monitoring (RPM)	• AI can help find meaningful information from continuous remote patient monitoring data and help decrease noise. • AI can help obtain useful information from video monitoring; for example, AI analysis of gait videos can provide diagnostic and prognostic insights.
AI scribes	• AI scribes reduce documentation burden and allow clinicians to be more present with patients. • Encounter transcripts create new opportunities for education, feedback, and assessment. • Key risks include privacy concerns, changes in patient disclosure, consent transparency, and medico-legal uncertainty.
AI and visual processing	• AI can help with static image interpretation using convolutional neural networks and vision transformers, making it well suited for pattern recognition tasks across multiple specialties. • There are significant limitations to these models. For example, they are highly vulnerable to image artifacts and variability in image quality.
AI in dermatology	• AI algorithms have shown promise in analyzing dermatoscope images and classifying skin lesions as benign or malignant. • To help mitigate bias, it is important that AI algorithms are trained on diverse data sets.
AI in ophthalmology	• Currently several AI algorithms are FDA approved for the diagnosis of diabetic retinopathy from fundoscopic images. • AI-based retinal image analysis can also be used to help educate medical students and residents on how to interpret retinal images.
AI in gastroenterology	• Procedures such as upper endoscopy and colonoscopy rely heavily on visual interpretation, presenting an ideal setting for AI integration. • For example, colonoscopy assisted by AI can increase the detection of adenomas.
Point-of-care ultrasound (POCUS)	• POCUS is increasingly being incorporated into care and has been proven to help improve diagnostic accuracy. POCUS adoption is limited due to insufficient training opportunities. • AI can help improve POCUS interpretability, accuracy, and quality and help with image acquisition.
Digital stethoscopes	• Digital stethoscopes enable recording, playback, and data sharing of heart sounds and ECG tracings, which can enhance clinical documentation and medical education. • AI-enabled digital stethoscopes can help with rhythm interpretation and even screen for reduced ejection fraction.
AI and real-time clinical reasoning support	• AI can help synthesize information and generate a differential diagnosis and management plan. • It is critical that AI and clinicians work synergistically and that clinicians do not overly depend on AI models.
AI and bedside procedural education	• AI-based procedural training tools are a promising way to supplement traditional instruction, providing learners with individualized, data-driven feedback at the bedside or in simulation settings.
Case-based simulation and AI virtual patients	• Generative AI represents a way to develop a large number of cases and allows for students to practice their history taking, diagnostic skills, clinical reasoning, and clinical management in real time.

risk for poor outcomes (12–14). For example, Sundrani et al. developed VitalML to predict clinical decompensation of initially stable emergency room patients, using physiologic data from 15 minutes of monitoring. VitalML significantly outperformed conventional triage models (13). AI-enabled RPM can provide alerts about potential decompensation in heart failure patients (9, 10). RPM can also expand the capabilities of "hospital at home" programs. Currently, hospital at home is limited to the lowest acuity patients, and most programs do not allow for frequent vital sign checks. RPM can provide more frequent monitoring, further increasing the potentially eligible patient pool (8).

Invasive remote patient monitoring has also shown promise. The CHAMPION trial demonstrated that a pulmonary pressure monitoring system in heart failure patients led to reduced hospitalizations (15). Additionally, a study on patients with pulmonary arterial hypertension found that insertable cardiac monitors accurately identified changes in patients' physiology following an increase in therapy or prior to clinical worsening (16). These data can potentially be used to create AI algorithms to further predict decompensation and improve clinical management.

Video monitoring is another area of RPM that offers considerable promise. Machine learning analysis of gait recordings can help provide diagnostic and prognostic insights (17–21). Mizuguchi et al. developed a model that derives a clinical frailty score from gait videos of patients with heart failure; Zeng et al. created an algorithm that predicts cardiovascular disease status using similar video data (18, 19). Additionally, AI video monitoring can evaluate environments for fall risks and detect falls in real time (20, 21).

By enabling increased accessibility and interpretability of RPM data, AI can expand the "bedside" beyond traditional hospital wards and clinics, allowing clinicians to extend care to patients' daily lives and to gain deeper insight into their health.

11.3.2 AI Scribes

While RPM can extend care beyond the clinic visit, AI scribes and ambient listening can help improve care during the clinic visit. Historically, clinical encounters were centered around direct, uninterrupted interactions between the patient and physician. The introduction of computers and computerized notes into the clinical setting, however, created competing demands for clinicians' attention, often shifting focus away from the patient. Clinical encounters have also become increasingly fragmented by EHR chat message interruptions (22). The advent of AI-powered ambient scribe technology enables clinicians to refocus their attention on the patient while AI works in the background to generate the note for the encounter. Allowing physicians to be more "present" can help improve patient satisfaction and strengthen the doctor–patient relationship, all while decreasing physician documentation burden (23).

Additionally, AI scribes offer an opportunity to reduce the administrative "sludge" that has accumulated in clinical practice. Over time, continuity of care has been replaced by fragmented, disconnected encounters. This fragmentation has reduced diagnostic accuracy and decreased patient satisfaction. One tool in addressing this is removing the administrative tasks that unnecessarily consume a clinician's time—the "sludge"—and thereby create space for providers to build meaningful relationships with patients (24). AI scribes can support this effort by decreasing documentation burden and freeing up clinicians' time to focus more on their patients.

Beyond documentation, AI-generated transcripts have powerful implications for medical education. The transcripts of real clinical encounters can serve as rich, objective data sources for direct observation, feedback, and competency assessment (25). Educators can use these transcripts and note summaries to evaluate communication skills, diagnostic reasoning, and patient-centeredness. Furthermore, AI can analyze these recordings and provide direct, real-time feedback on patient interactions.

While there are many potential benefits to ambient listening, significant risks must also be considered. As with any AI technology, there are risks regarding data security and privacy. Beyond this, there are risks that it might alter the patient–physician interaction and alter trust in the healthcare system. For example, a recent study explored patient attitudes toward AI ambient documentation and found that patients were more likely to censor what they say when discussing sensitive topics such as mental health, sexual health, or illicit activities. Additionally, the study found that, when patients went through a more explicit informed consent process, including language that AI can make errors and that the technology is used in partnership with a for-profit company, fewer patients consented (26). This suggests there needs to be improved clarity and disclosure about ambient listening technologies. Providers also have understandable fears about the technology, including how the data is stored or used. Some providers are also concerned about malpractice risk. Ultimately, these findings highlight the need for heightened transparency around ambient listening.

11.3.3 AI Visual Processing

AI is adept at analyzing images (particularly static images), which has several applications at the bedside. These visual recognition AI models are built using convolutional neural networks or vision transformers that process images through mathematical filters that detect patterns, similar to how neurons in our brain function.

11.3.3.1 AI and Dermatology

AI capabilities in image analysis have been applied successfully to dermatology. For example, a convolutional neural network was able to identify upward of ten dermatologic diagnoses with an area under the curve of over 0.95 using photographs (27). Dermoscopy is a diagnostic procedure in which a practitioner uses a specialized magnifying glass (i.e., a dermatoscope) to evaluate skin lesions in detail. AI algorithms have shown promise in analyzing dermatoscope images and classifying skin lesions as benign or malignant (28). These algorithms can also be repurposed for bedside education purposes. For example, AI-assisted dermoscopy can provide immediate feedback on lesion characterization by learners. Reviewing AI classifications alongside expert annotations can help trainees develop important diagnostic skills.

While AI algorithms are skilled at classifying skin lesions, they are no substitute for the comprehensive clinical evaluation performed at the bedside. For example, when classifying a lesion as benign or malignant, AI algorithms analyzing skin lesions do not take into account other important clinical factors such as clinical history, degree of sun damage, and the rest of the skin examination (29). AI algorithms are trained to look at the image alone and classify it.

It is also imperative to discuss the risks of bias with AI. AI algorithms can only be as good as the data used during their training. If the data used to train the model do not represent the full diversity of patient characteristics, including skin tone, lesion types, or atypical presentations, then AI performance will suffer, potentially leading to misdiagnosis and inequitable care. Importantly, this lack of representation in training is not unique to AI; traditional medical education textbooks also underrepresent dermatologic conditions in patients with darker skin. In one study, both an AI algorithm and physicians performed worse on images of dark skin tones and uncommon diseases (30).

In short, AI-based lesion classification should be viewed as a decision-support tool. The clinician's role in incorporating all of the available data to determine an accurate diagnosis and management plan remains essential. Ultimately, the goal of AI in dermatology is to serve as an adjunctive tool that enhances clinical care.

11.3.3.2 AI in Ophthalmology

Since the invention of the ophthalmoscope in 1858 by Hermann von Helmholtz, ophthalmology has been at the forefront of visual analysis to aid in diagnosis (31). Unsurprisingly, ophthalmology was one of the first fields where AI was used for image interpretation. For example, retinal photos can be used to aid in the diagnosis of diabetic retinopathy, glaucoma, and macular degeneration. AI algorithms to analyze retinal images for diabetic retinopathy have achieved AUC values of 0.99 and sensitivity and specificities greater than 87% (32). Currently there are several AI algorithms that are FDA approved for the diagnosis of diabetic retinopathy (DR) from fundoscopic images (33). Beals et al. evaluated an AI program in primary care practice to expand screening for DR and increase access to ophthalmologic care. This program included clinician education, patient education, and screening for DR with an AI algorithm that evaluated fundoscopic photos to determine whether a patient should be referred to ophthalmology. The program led to a 23% increase in referrals to ophthalmology and a 27% increase in vascular endothelial growth factor treatment compared to controls (34).

Beyond diagnosis, AI-based retinal image analysis offers important opportunities for bedside medical education. Direct ophthalmoscopy by non-ophthalmologists is a dying art, with subsequent lost opportunities to make important diagnoses in real time at the bedside (35). Just as the Beals et al. program included clinician education, similar approaches could be extended to train medical students and residents to interpret and to act on retinal findings (34). For instance, AI can generate synthetic images on which students can practice interpretation (36). AI might even be able to help teach students to perform direct ophthalmoscopy and acquire adequate fundoscopic images for interpretation (37).

11.3.3.3 AI in Gastroenterology

Another promising use of AI and visual processing is endoscopy. Procedures such as upper endoscopy and colonoscopy rely heavily on visual interpretation, representing an ideal setting for AI integration. The COLO-DETECT study was an open-label randomized controlled trial that evaluated the use of GI Genius, an AI aid for polyp detection, compared with standard colonoscopy. It found that colonoscopy assisted by GI Genius led to increased detection of adenomas. (38)

Beyond clinical applications, AI also offers the potential for improved bedside training in GI. AI-assisted virtual reality simulators can help improve procedural skills by providing an immersive but low-risk setting for procedural practice. (39) AI-assisted endoscopy can also provide real-time feedback to trainees (39). Such computerized feedback has been shown to optimize practice and training patterns (40). However, as systems such as these are utilized more, thoughtful implementation is needed to ensure that providers obtain independent skills and don't become overly reliant on the technology.

AI can augment bedside visual diagnostic capabilities across specialties. AI algorithms, through the use of complex mathematical processes, are adept at analyzing visual images. However, these algorithms are still in their infancy, and it is critical to recognize their limitations. For example, they are highly vulnerable to image artifacts and variability in image quality. In the real-world retinal imaging AI implementation described by Beals et al., only 72% of captured retinal images were of sufficient quality for the AI system to render a diagnostic result (34). Additionally, unlike humans, AI does not use context and reasoning to further process information; it uses only the pixels from a given image.

These limitations highlight the continued need for clinician oversight when using AI in clinical practice. Additionally, although one of the goals of AI is to improve efficiency and reduce cost, evidence suggests that fully automated systems may not always be the most economical approach. Xie et al. compared the economic costs of a fully automated AI diabetic retinopathy (DR) detection program, a semiautomated program with a human in the loop, and a fully human assessment. They found that the semiautomated system was the most cost-effective (41). This underscores an important point: The combination of human expertise and AI's analytic capabilities has the greatest potential to enhance healthcare delivery.

11.3.4 POCUS

Point of care ultrasound (POCUS) is increasingly being implemented as part of bedside encounters. POCUS is already standard-of-care for most bedside procedures, including thoracentesis, paracentesis, and central line placement. POCUS is rapidly becoming an important part of bedside diagnosis (42). POCUS provides for a speedy, real-time evaluation of cardiovascular, respiratory, gynecologic, musculoskeletal, soft-tissue, and abdominal pathology. Unlike traditional imaging studies, POCUS allows the physician to obtain immediate answers at the bedside, enabling timely diagnostic reasoning. POCUS can help rapidly evaluate response to interventions and allows serial monitoring (43). Furthermore, POCUS devices are small and can be carried in the pocket, making it feasible for providers to easily incorporate them into their bedside encounters (43). Including POCUS as part of the encounter in hospitalized patients can lead to an earlier and more accurate diagnosis (44–46). POCUS can also increase patient satisfaction and engagement, as physicians can demonstrate pathophysiology in real time (47). POCUS in its current form can only be practiced at the bedside. As a result, excitement around POCUS brings physicians, learners, and patients together, which can further enhance patient satisfaction and physician professional fulfilment (2). Even though POCUS is an increasingly useful tool, adoption is limited due to insufficient training opportunities (48).

AI can be leveraged to augment POCUS capabilities and enhance image acquisition and training, thereby improving usage. AI can help improve POCUS interpretability, accuracy, and quality. POCUS AI tools can improve image quality, automatically calculate measurements, such as cardiac ejection fraction (EF), and detect abnormal pathologies (37, 49–52). By automatically calculating measurements on key ultrasound findings, AI algorithms can reduce inter-user variability (53). For example, one study found that an AI algorithm achieved an AUC of 0.93 on an external validation set for detecting B lines on lung ultrasound (48). The ability to detect abnormal pathologies using AI assistance may make POCUS more accessible by reducing the level of operator expertise required, thereby broadening its use in resource-limited settings and among clinicians less experienced with ultrasound (48, 52).

AI can also help address the POCUS training gap that limits its broader adoption. Currently, POCUS training is time and labor-intensive. POCUS training courses are usually expensive (54). Studies have compared conventional POCUS training to conventional training combined with AI guidance and found that the combined groups had more sustained skill retention (55) and were better able to acquire difficult-to-obtain cardiac views (54). Another study found that AI can help guide novices to obtain high-quality images by providing real-time feedback and adaptive guidance (37, 56). Further studies are needed to evaluate the effectiveness of AI-driven POCUS training as a stand-alone educational approach.

The integration of AI-enhanced POCUS into bedside medical education offers a novel tool to strengthen bedside teaching and diagnostic skill development. By providing real-time image interpretation, automated measurements, and guided instruction, AI allows trainees to practice diagnostic reasoning at the bedside while receiving immediate feedback. This not only strengthens POCUS education but also reinforces clinical reasoning, physical exam skills, and understanding of disease pathology. For example, learners can enhance their ability to detect a pleural effusion using traditional physical exam skills such as chest inspection, percussion, and auscultation by comparing their physical exam findings to POCUS images (42). In this way, AI-augmented POCUS can transform the bedside encounter into an interactive environment where learners can practice technical skills, visualize pathology, and enhance their overall diagnostic accuracy. Additionally, by expanding POCUS use and enhancing the explainability of ultrasound findings, AI has the potential to improve patient satisfaction, deepen patients' understanding of their disease, and strengthen the therapeutic relationship between patients and their providers (47, 57).

11.3.5 Digital Stethoscopes

The stethoscope is arguably one of the most important technological innovations in medicine over the last two centuries. Auscultation remains one of the cornerstones of diagnosis for many cardiac, pulmonary, vascular, and gastrointestinal issues (58). The stethoscope is also one of the most important symbols of the medical profession (59). Despite recent reports that the stethoscope is a dying relic, the analog stethoscope remains one of the most important diagnostic tools throughout most of the world. While the stethoscope is not going away any time soon (its market share increased dramatically during the COVID-19 pandemic), it has evolved in recent years to include digital models (60). The digital stethoscope can amplify heart sounds, allowing for the detection of faint murmurs and improving accessibility for clinicians with hearing impairments. Additionally, digital stethoscopes enable recording, playback, and data sharing, which enhance both clinical documentation and medical education. From a teaching perspective, the ability to store and to annotate heart or lung sounds allows learners to review findings repeatedly and compare their interpretations with expert analyses, supporting deliberate practice at the bedside.

One of the main challenges of traditional auscultation is its subjectivity. The diagnostic value of the stethoscope depends on the clinician's experience, training, and auditory perception. AI-enabled stethoscopes help address this limitation by providing standardized analysis of recorded sounds and visual representations of waveforms, thereby reducing interobserver variability. Additionally, digital stethoscopes can assist in reliably interpreting cardiac rhythms. For example, an AI algorithm was able to detect atrial fibrillation from cardiac sounds with a specificity of 0.90 and a sensitivity of 0.95 (61). Newer models also acquire an electrocardiogram (ECG), which further enhances diagnostic and teaching possibilities for cardiac abnormalities. For instance, Attia et al., found that an AI-algorithm was able to reliably detect patients with a low EF based on stethoscope and ECG recordings in standard auscultation positions (62). While further studies are needed, one could imagine how this capability could help triage patients with cardiopulmonary complaints or screen high-risk populations for cardiovascular disease.

AI algorithms have also been explored in relation to respiratory diseases. An AI analysis of recorded lung sounds yielded a sensitivity of 77% and specificity of 50% for diagnosing pulmonary tuberculosis (TB) (63). These findings highlight the potential of AI to support quicker, noninvasive screening across a range of cardiopulmonary diseases.

Additional studies are needed to determine the digital stethoscope's impact on clinical outcomes (58). At the same time, digital stethoscopes can be used to enhance bedside medical education by capturing, labeling, and sharing sounds at the bedside. One of the authors (BTG) routinely uses a digital stethoscope during bedside teaching sessions to show an ECG and a spectrophonograph while simultaneously transmitting heart sounds to the entire room through either a speaker or wireless headphones. When coupled with a hand-carried ultrasound, these bedside sessions enable real-time diagnosis at the bedside, while also calibrating traditional physical exam skills such as observation, palpation, percussion, and auscultation.

11.3.6 AI and Real-Time Clinical Reasoning Support

AI can provide useful, real-time clinical reasoning support. AI large language models (LLMs) can rapidly synthesize enormous amounts of data, generate a differential diagnosis, and propose follow-up questions and next-step tests—functions required for bedside clinical reasoning. For example in an emergency department study comparing ChatGPT (GPT-4) with resident physicians, GPT-4 demonstrated high diagnostic accuracy from real patient presentations, suggesting it could be used as an assistant to help with clinical reasoning (64). Another study evaluated clinicians' diagnostic accuracy from clinical vignettes and found that using AI models improved their accuracy compared to baseline (65). However, LLMs do not execute genuine logic and their use of nonlocal data may undermine clinical relevance. It is therefore imperative that AI and clinicians work in concert and that AI does not replace true human reasoning and judgment (66). To help decrease the risk of hallucinations or bias, AI outputs can be "grounded" in truth from clinical guidelines and other accurate and trusted sources (67). Additionally, when building AI into workflows to assist clinical reasoning, it will be imperative to ensure clinicians do not become overly reliant and accepting of the AI output. For example, the study evaluating physician's diagnostic accuracy from clinical vignettes also found that physician's accuracy decreased when using a biased AI model compared to their baseline reasoning without AI support, suggesting that physicians are at risk of accepting the computer output as true even when it is clearly not (65).

11.4 AI AND BEDSIDE MEDICAL EDUCATION

The amount of knowledge needed to master the medical field is continuously expanding. The extensive knowledge requirements for healthcare professionals requires new and innovative methods for teaching and learning. AI offers the ability to analyze data in real time, providing immediate feedback and personalized learning plans (68). In this section, we will specifically focus on how AI can improve bedside medicine education.

11.4.1 Bedside Procedural Education

Bedside procedural competence is a critical component of medical education. Bedside procedures, ranging from simple suturing to complex ultrasound-guided interventions, are traditionally taught through apprenticeship-style learning, where trainees observe experts, practice under supervision (often on a procedural simulator), and gradually gain independence. However, limited faculty time and training, variability in case exposure, and patient safety concerns can restrict opportunities for deliberate practice and feedback. AI-based procedural training tools can supplement traditional instruction, providing learners with individualized, data-driven feedback at the bedside or in simulations.

For example, a study using an AI-based video assessment of suturing and knot tying demonstrated a cross-validation accuracy of 0.83 for overall pass/fail classification (69). While refinement is needed, this form of bedside procedural education holds promise. It can allow for immediate, objective feedback without significant faculty time or resource requirements and enables learners to practice and to improve their skills in a low-pressure environment.

Ultrasound-guided procedures are another important part of medical care. Training in these procedures are limited by patient cases and patient safety. AI can help bridge this gap by providing realistic case simulation with real-time feedback. For example, one study created an agar model that mimicked human anatomy and built machine learning models to provide learners with real-time feedback on visualization of target structures. The model also assessed learners on their speed (defined as time to target tissue penetration) and accuracy (defined as penetration of the correct target tissue with the needle). The study evaluated the AI model's ability to correctly identify the needle, needle tip, and blood vessel and found it had an accuracy of 91.33%, positive predictive value of 89.94%, and a sensitivity of 99.31% (70).

Collectively, these innovations suggest that AI can transform bedside procedural education by enabling trainees to obtain realistic practice and more applicable, real-time feedback.

11.4.2 Case-Based Simulation and AI Virtual Patients

Experiential learning through case-based examples is a key component of medical education, particularly during the preclinical years. However, developing high-quality cases is time-consuming and resource intensive for faculty, which limits their availability. In addition, simulation-based learning requires significant infrastructure, including the need to obtain standardized patients, further increasing cost and limiting access for students. Generative AI can create a large number of cases and allow students to practice their history taking, diagnostic skills, clinical reasoning, and clinical management in real time. Working with an AI-based case simulation also allows students to obtain real-time feedback (71). These tools can serve as the gateway for bedside education during the preclinical years and also extend bedside education during the clinical years. For example, students can use AI-driven virtual patients to rehearse an approach to a symptom before encountering it in a real patient, or to debrief after patient encounters, comparing their diagnostic reasoning to that of the AI model. Integrating these tools allows for the promotion of adult learning principles such as just-in-time teaching, reinforcing previously acquired knowledge through contextual application and promoting experiential learning (72).

AI can also be integrated directly into the bedside encounter to improve clinical skills. For example, the authors created an AI application to help learners improve their physical exam skills. AI-PE uses available data about a patient to generate a limited differential diagnosis. The app then suggests high-yield physical exam maneuvers that will help sort through these diagnostic possibilities, alongside links to high-quality resources such as videos that demonstrate how to perform and interpret those maneuvers. AI-PE can help learners develop a repertoire of high-yield physical exam maneuvers they can use in their clinical practice, helping to reinvigorate the bedside clinical encounter. Tools like AI-PE speak to ways AI can be used in medical education more broadly. AI-augmented tools can help standardize teaching across different clinical environments and ensure trainees receive consistent, evidence-based instruction, even when faculty time for direct bedside teaching is limited. Additionally, such tools create opportunities for immediate, individualized feedback and allow learners to track their growth over time.

11.5 AI AT THE BEDSIDE—RISKS AND LIMITATIONS

While AI holds promise for clinical care and medical education, risks and challenges need to be addressed. Table 11.2 summarizes some of the most pressing issues surrounding the use of AI at the bedside.

Table 11.2 Risks and Limitations of AI at the Bedside

De-skilling	• Reliance on AI may weaken independent clinical skills and lead to performance declines when AI support is removed.
Never-skilling	• Overreliance on AI during training may prevent learners from developing independent clinical reasoning skills and increase susceptibility to automation bias, in which clinicians accept the computer output as true without questioning it. • To guard against never-skilling, it is paramount to ensure that learners develop the clinical competencies and critical thinking skills necessary for independent practice.
Equity and bias	• Many healthcare datasets lack diversity and representation (e.g., dermatology images skew toward lighter skin). • AI models inherit bias from biased training data. • If biased datasets are used, AI will underperform in certain populations and worsen existing health disparities. • These risks underscore the importance of transparent algorithm development, diverse and representative training data, and continuous model validation and evaluation across demographic groups and clinical contexts.
Data security and privacy	• AI at the bedside requires collection of sensitive clinical and educational data, raising concerns about HIPAA compliance, secure storage and use, transparency with trainees, access to learner analytics, and the costs of data storage and governance.
Regulatory oversight	• Currently, most AI and machine learning (ML)–based tools are regulated under the framework of Software as a Medical Device (SaMD), which encompasses software intended for medical purposes independent of hardware. However, the regulatory landscape is evolving rapidly.

11.5.1 De-Skilling

There is understandable concern that the use of AI may lead to de-skilling of clinicians. The evolution of technology has sometimes led to the loss of cognitive skills. For example, one study evaluated primary care physicians' experiences with electronic health records and quality improvement tools through interviews and found that their views and practices suggested de-skilling (73). The use of clinical guidelines and "boilerplate" templates made physicians feel they were thinking less about patients individually and were losing clinical knowledge (73). Similarly, as use of AI grows, there is a risk of that overreliance on AI could erode fundamental critical thinking skills (74).

However, evidence suggests that AI can enhance, rather than diminish, overall system performance and healthcare outcomes. In a study evaluating radiology residents' interpretation of chest radiographs, those who read chest radiographs with AI support made fewer diagnostic errors and demonstrated greater inter-reader agreement than those without AI support (74). Endoscopists' adenoma detection rates improved while using AI-assisted guidance during colonoscopy (38). However, de-skilling is a real phenomenon after exposure to AI-powered tools. Endoscopists' adenoma detection rate decreased to below pre-AI levels after returning to standard (non AI-guided) colonoscopy (38, 75). Reliance on a digital, AI-enhanced stethoscope may diminish provider's ability to recognize subtle findings. However, this concern echoes earlier transitions in medicine. For example, before the invention of the stethoscope, physicians placed an ear directly on the patient's chest (so-called direct auscultation), a practice now lost with the use of the stethoscope. While this shift transformed the way clinicians gathered information, it ultimately improved diagnostic accuracy. In the same way, digital and AI-assisted stethoscopes can serve to improve diagnostic accuracy through amplifying subtle sounds, visualizing waveforms, and offering immediate AI-supported interpretation (76). Rather than replacing bedside skills, they can promote a deeper understanding of physiology and make bedside medicine more accessible and clinically useful.

11.5.2 Never-Skilling

Overdependence on AI also introduces the risk of never-skilling—a phenomenon in which learners never acquire the foundational competencies in the first place because AI is performing the tasks for them. If students and trainees routinely rely on AI to guide clinical reasoning, they have less opportunity to develop this skill independently (77). Clinicians serve a critical role in maintaining independent judgment and critically evaluating AI outputs. If future clinicians are not trained to think independently, overreliance on automated recommendations may exacerbate automation bias, defined as the tendency to automatically accept algorithmic outputs (65, 78). Emerging evidence supports this fear: one study found a negative correlation between frequent use of AI tools and critical thinking skills (77, 79). Another study evaluated clinicians' diagnostic reasoning using clinical vignettes with and without AI support and found evidence of automation bias. When clinicians were provided recommendations from a deliberately biased AI model that generated questionable outputs, their diagnostic accuracy declined compared with their baseline, non-AI-supported performance. These findings suggest that clinicians were more likely to defer to the AI's recommendations rather than rely on their own independent judgment (65). To guard against never-skilling, it will be paramount to ensure that learners develop the clinical competencies and critical thinking skills necessary for independent practice. This will require coordinated efforts from multidisciplinary groups to design curricula, oversight structures, and learning environments that balance AI assistance with deliberate skill building.

Technological advances have always reshaped clinical skills. While it is essential to remain aware of potential skill erosion, it is also important to recognize that the nature of essential clinical skills evolves over time as tools advance. Ultimately, maintaining a balance between preserving core reasoning abilities and skills and embracing technological augmentation is key to optimizing both clinician competence and patient care.

11.5.3 Equity and Bias

One major limitation and ethical concern with the use of AI at the bedside is the potential for biased algorithms, which can lead to increased inequity and reinforce or worsen existing health disparities. It is therefore imperative that rigorous evaluation of AI algorithms occur prior to implementation in the clinical setting.

AI algorithms will have bias if they are trained using biased data. For example, an AI algorithm used to detect skin cancer was more likely to classify lesions as malignant if they contained a ruler, as examples of melanomas in the training data were more likely to contain a ruler (29). Much of the historical healthcare data used to train AI is known to contain biases. For example, dermatology training datasets tend to mainly consist of Caucasian patients, thus leading to algorithms that are less accurate in patients with darker skin tones (80). Even the previously discussed AI-assisted assessment of suturing could be biased as the algorithm had less training with left-hand dominant videos (69). One could imagine left-handed individuals being more likely to fail the AI assessment!

These biases can manifest in consequential ways if implemented at the bedside or in medical education. AI tools used for real-time diagnosis, physiologic monitoring, or image interpretation may underperform in patients with underrepresented skin tones, body types, or disease presentations, potentially reinforcing existing health disparities in a systemic manner. For example, pulse oximetry is more likely to underestimate hypoxemia in individuals with darker skin. During COVID-19, missed hypoxemia was associated with a higher risk of readmission and was more likely to occur in Black patients (81–83).

Likewise, if AI-driven educational tools provide feedback based on biased data, trainees from diverse backgrounds or with differing physical approaches (perhaps due to a physical disability) might receive unfair assessments, impacting both learning and confidence. These risks underscore the importance of transparent algorithm development, diverse and representative training data, and continuous model validation and evaluation across demographic groups and clinical contexts.

11.5.4 Data Security and Privacy

AI at the bedside and in bedside education relies on the collection of a large volume of data, including protected health information (PHI), and audio and video recordings of patient encounters. This raises significant privacy and data security concerns. Systems relying on PHI must adhere to the Health Insurance Portability and Accountability Act (HIPAA) and ensure data is securely stored, encrypted, and only used for authorized purposes (84). Additional issues arise when using data to generate insights about learners. The use of AI should be disclosed to trainees, and clear guidelines established about who will have access to the insights generated from such data. For example, should prospective employees or even patients be able to see information about the clinical skills of their providers? The costs of data collection and storage also need to be factored into decisions about whether to use AI tools to aid in learner evaluation and assessment (85).

11.5.5 Regulatory Oversight

The regulatory landscape for artificial intelligence (AI) in healthcare is rapidly evolving. Currently, most AI and machine learning (ML)–based tools are regulated under the framework of Software as a Medical Device (SaMD), which encompasses software intended for medical purposes independent of hardware. In 2025, the FDA issued draft guidance on AI-enabled device software functions, providing recommendations for marketing submissions and emphasizing bias mitigation, validation, and continuous oversight (86). Despite these efforts, regulatory challenges remain, particularly regarding adaptive models that evolve post-deployment, the transparency of "black box" systems, and ensuring that training data represent diverse patient populations (87).

11.6 AN AI-AUGMENTED CLINIC VISIT OF THE FUTURE—A CASE EXAMPLE

Overall, AI has the ability to augment bedside medicine through many avenues. The best way to illustrate its impact might be through returning to the patient from the beginning of the chapter.

In an AI-enabled bedside visit, ambient listening technology could record the encounter and automatically generate documentation, allowing the medical team to remain fully engaged with Mr. X. The audio recording could be used to analyze speech patterns and to screen for neurodegenerative disease (88). Furthermore, the data from the AI scribe could be used to provide immediate feedback to the medical student who admitted Mr. X. Video-based gait analysis could determine frailty or fall risk during Mr. X's hospitalization, identifying extra resources to help him if needed (18). An ECG-enabled digital stethoscope could help determine if Mr. X had a valvular disorder, decreased ejection fraction, or atrial fibrillation as the cause of his shortness of breath (61, 62, 89–91). Additionally, POCUS could be used to estimate his EF and to look for structural heart disease (37, 50, 51, 92). Within a single bedside visit, these integrated AI-driven tools could generate actionable insights into Mr. X's frailty, fall risk, cardiovascular disease, and neurodegenerative disease transforming the routine bedside encounter into a more comprehensive, data-enhanced evaluation.

An AI analysis of the ECG-enabled digital stethoscope recording from Mr. X shows a high likelihood of paroxysmal atrial fibrillation and a reduced EF, prompting confirmation with POCUS, a formal echocardiogram, and a cardiology consultation. The medical student uses AI-PE and identifies an elevated JVP and a mitral regurgitation murmur, findings which inform subsequent testing and questions for the cardiology consultant. AI-powered analysis of Mr. X's speech suggests mild cognitive impairment. Upon further discussion, the care team uncovers some memory concerns. He is then referred to neurology and connected to appropriate resources at discharge, once his cardiovascular evaluation has been completed.

RPM enables providers to further extend their care beyond discharge. Mr. X is enrolled in an RPM program that tracks his vital signs and ECG in real time. The AI system continuously analyzes these data and provides alerts for early signs of clinical deterioration so that his care team can intervene before he calls the office with worsening shortness of breath again (9, 10, 93).

11.7 CONCLUSION

AI has the potential to transform the modern bedside encounter and bedside education by helping clinicians gather, synthesize, and act on clinical information more effectively. AI-enhanced tools such as RPM, POCUS, digital stethoscopes, and ambient listening can improve care efficiency and quality. Additionally, AI can improve medical education by providing real-time decision support, coaching, and feedback. AI can also enhance simulation experiences by creating virtual patient encounters and providing feedback on communication and procedural skills. However, for AI to be beneficial, it needs to be implemented and used in a thoughtful manner. AI must remain an assistive tool rather than a substitute for clinical judgment. Safeguards must be in place to prevent never-skilling, de-skilling, and automation bias and to reduce overall biases. Protecting privacy, ensuring transparency, and meeting evolving regulatory and security requirements are essential to safe and proper use.

REFERENCES

1. Garibaldi BT, Elder A. Seven reasons why the physical examination remains important. *J R Coll Physicians Edinb.* 2021;51(3):211–4.
2. Garibaldi BT, Russell SW. Strategies to reinvigorate the bedside clinical encounter. *The New England Journal of Medicine.* 2025;393(21):2142–50.
3. Newman-Toker DE, McDonald KM, Meltzer DO. How much diagnostic safety can we afford, and how should we decide? A health economics perspective. *BMJ Quality & Safety.* 2013;22(Suppl 2):ii11–ii20.
4. Neumann M, Edelhauser F, Tauschel D, Fischer MR, Wirtz M, Woopen C, *et al.* Empathy decline and its reasons: A systematic review of studies with medical students and residents. *Acad Med.* 2011;86(8):996–1009.
5. Costanzo C, Verghese A. The physical examination as ritual: Social sciences and embodiment in the context of the physical examination. *Med Clin North Am.* 2018;102(3):425–31.
6. Demeke HB, Merali S, Marks S, Pao LZ, Romero L, Sandhu P, *et al.* Trends in use of telehealth among health centers during the COVID-19 pandemic—United States, June 26-November 6, 2020. *MMWR Morb Mortal Wkly Rep.* 2021;70(7):240–4.

7. Cherian J, Mascia G, Kairamkonda D, Fisher A, McGinnis RS, Ray TR. Wearable sensing for clinical physiology monitoring: Emerging paradigms. *Physiology (Bethesda)*. 2025;41(4):310–324.
8. Whitehead D, Conley J. The next frontier of remote patient monitoring: Hospital at home. *J Med Internet Res*. 2023;25:e42335.
9. Chi WN, Reamer C, Gordon R, Sarswat N, Gupta C, White VanGompel E, *et al*. Continuous remote patient monitoring: Evaluation of the heart failure cascade soft launch. *Appl Clin Inform*. 2021;12(5):1161–73.
10. Reamer C, Chi WN, Gordon R, Sarswat N, Gupta C, Gaznabi S, *et al*. Continuous remote patient monitoring in patients with heart failure (cascade study): Protocol for a mixed methods feasibility study. *JMIR Res Protoc*. 2022;11(8):e36741.
11. Dubey A, Tiwari A. Artificial intelligence and remote patient monitoring in US healthcare market: A literature review. *J Mark Access Health Policy*. 2023;11(1):2205618.
12. Huete-Garcia A, Rodriguez-Lopez S. Development and implementation of an artificial intelligence-enhanced care model to improve patient safety in hospital wards in Spain. *Acute Crit Care*. 2024;39(4):488–98.
13. Sundrani S, Chen J, Jin BT, Abad ZSH, Rajpurkar P, Kim D. Predicting patient decompensation from continuous physiologic monitoring in the emergency department. *NPJ Digit Med*. 2023;6(1):60.
14. Khan MM, Shah N. AI-driven wearable sensors for postoperative monitoring in surgical patients: A systematic review. *Comput Biol Med*. 2025;196(Pt B):110783.
15. Abraham WT, Adamson PB, Bourge RC, Aaron MF, Costanzo MR, Stevenson LW, *et al*. Wireless pulmonary artery haemodynamic monitoring in chronic heart failure: A randomised controlled trial. *Lancet (London, England)*. 2011;377(9766):658–66.
16. Middleton JT, Binmahfooz S, Zafar H, Patel J, Ashraf C, Jake, *et al*. Remote monitored physiological response to therapeutic escalation and clinical worsening in patients with pulmonary arterial hypertension. *medRxiv*. 2024:2023.04.27.23289153.
17. Ozates ME, Yaman A, Salami F, Campos S, Wolf SI, Schneider U. Identification and interpretation of gait analysis features and foot conditions by explainable AI. *Sci Rep*. 2024;14(1):5998.
18. Mizuguchi Y, Nakao M, Nagai T, Takahashi Y, Abe T, Kakinoki S, *et al*. Machine learning-based gait analysis to predict clinical frailty scale in elderly patients with heart failure. *Eur Heart J Digit Health*. 2024;5(2):152–62.
19. Zeng J, Lin S, Li Z, Sun R, Yu X, Lian X, *et al*. Association between gait video information and general cardiovascular diseases: A prospective cross-sectional study. *Eur Heart J Digit Health*. 2024;5(4):469–80.
20. Núñez-Marcos A, Arganda-Carreras I. Transformer-based fall detection in videos. *Engineering Applications of Artificial Intelligence*. 2024;132:107937.
21. Moore J, Celik Y, Stuart S, McMeekin P, Walker R, Hetherington V, *et al*. Using video technology and AI within Parkinson's disease free-living fall risk assessment. *Sensors (Basel)*. 2024;24(15).
22. Baratta LR, Harford D, Sinsky CA, Kannampallil T, Lou SS. Characterizing the patterns of electronic health record-integrated secure messaging use: Cross-sectional study. *J Med Internet Res*. 2023;25:e48583.
23. Zulman DM, Haverfield MC, Shaw JG, Brown-Johnson CG, Schwartz R, Tierney AA, *et al*. Practices to foster physician presence and connection with patients in the clinical encounter. *JAMA*. 2020;323(1):70–81.
24. Sinsky CA, Shanafelt TD, Ristow AM. Radical reorientation of the US health care system around relationships: Rebalancing the transactional model. *Mayo Clin Proc*. 2022;97(12):2194–205.

25. Gordon M, Daniel M, Ajiboye A, Uraiby H, Xu NY, Bartlett R, *et al.* A scoping review of artificial intelligence in medical education: BEME Guide No. 84. *Med Teach.* 2024;46(4):446–70.
26. Lawrence K, Kuram VS, Levine DL, Sharif S, Polet C, Malhotra K, *et al.* Informed consent for ambient documentation using generative AI in ambulatory care. *JAMA Netw Open.* 2025;8(7):e2522400.
27. Mathur J, Chouhan V, Pangti R, Kumar S, Gupta S. A convolutional neural network architecture for the recognition of cutaneous manifestations of COVID–19. *Dermatol Ther.* 2021;34(2):e14902.
28. Haggenmuller S, Maron RC, Hekler A, Utikal JS, Barata C, Barnhill RL, *et al.* Skin cancer classification via convolutional neural networks: Systematic review of studies involving human experts. *Eur J Cancer.* 2021;156:202–16.
29. Liopyris K, Gregoriou S, Dias J, Stratigos AJ. Artificial intelligence in dermatology: Challenges and perspectives. *Dermatol Ther (Heidelb).* 2022;12(12):2637–51.
30. Daneshjou R, Vodrahalli K, Novoa RA, Jenkins M, Liang W, Rotemberg V, *et al.* Disparities in dermatology AI performance on a diverse, curated clinical image set. *Sci Adv.* 2022;8(32):eabq6147.
31. Walker HK. The origins of the history and physical examination. In: Walker HK, Hall WD, Hurst JW, editors. *Clinical Methods: The History, Physical, and Laboratory Examinations.* Butterworth-Heinemann, 3rd ed. Boston, 1990.
32. Gulshan V, Peng L, Coram M, Stumpe MC, Wu D, Narayanaswamy A, *et al.* Development and validation of a deep learning algorithm for detection of diabetic retinopathy in retinal fundus photographs. *JAMA.* 2016;316(22):2402–10.
33. Huang X, Wang H, She C, Feng J, Liu X, Hu X, *et al.* Artificial intelligence promotes the diagnosis and screening of diabetic retinopathy. *Front Endocrinol (Lausanne).* 2022;13:946915.
34. Beals D, Simon L, Rogers F, Pogroszewski S. Revolutionizing diabetic retinopathy screening: Integrating AI-based retinal imaging in primary care. *J CME.* 2025;14(1):2437294.
35. Mackay DD, Garza PS, Bruce BB, Newman NJ, Biousse V. The demise of direct ophthalmoscopy: A modern clinical challenge. *Neurol Clin Pract.* 2015;5(2):150–7.
36. Tabuchi H, Engelmann J, Maeda F, Nishikawa R, Nagasawa T, Yamauchi T, *et al.* Using artificial intelligence to improve human performance: Efficient retinal disease detection training with synthetic images. *Br J Ophthalmol.* 2024;108(10):1430–5.
37. Cheema BS, Walter J, Narang A, Thomas JD. Artificial intelligence-enabled POCUS in the COVID-19 ICU: A new spin on cardiac ultrasound. *JACC Case Rep.* 2021;3(2):258–63.
38. Seager A, Sharp L, Neilson LJ, Brand A, Hampton JS, Lee TJW, *et al.* Polyp detection with colonoscopy assisted by the GI Genius artificial intelligence endoscopy module compared with standard colonoscopy in routine colonoscopy practice (COLO-DETECT): A multicentre, open-label, parallel-arm, pragmatic randomised controlled trial. *Lancet Gastroenterol Hepatol.* 2024;9(10):911–23.
39. Farooq F, Warraich MUT, Ud Din MM, Saleem N, Asif MS, Khan H. Role of artificial intelligence in gastroenterology training (2005–2025): Trends, tools, and challenges. *Cureus.* 2025;17(8):e90085.
40. Vilmann AS, Norsk D, Svendsen MBS, Reinhold R, Svendsen LB, Park YS, *et al.* Computerized feedback during colonoscopy training leads to improved performance: A randomized trial. *Gastrointest Endosc.* 2018;88(5):869–76.

41. Xie Y, Nguyen QD, Hamzah H, Lim G, Bellemo V, Gunasekeran DV, *et al.* Artificial intelligence for teleophthalmology-based diabetic retinopathy screening in a national programme: An economic analysis modelling study. *Lancet Digit Health.* 2020;2(5):e240–e9.
42. Kumar A, Liu G, Chi J, Kugler J. The role of technology in the bedside encounter. *Med Clin North Am.* 2018;102(3):443–51.
43. Rice JA, Brewer J, Speaks T, Choi C, Lahsaei P, Romito BT. The POCUS consult: How point of care ultrasound helps guide medical decision making. *Int J Gen Med.* 2021;14:9789–806.
44. Laursen CB, Sloth E, Lassen AT, Christensen R, Lambrechtsen J, Madsen PH, *et al.* Point-of-care ultrasonography in patients admitted with respiratory symptoms: A single-blind, randomised controlled trial. *Lancet Respir Med.* 2014;2(8):638–46.
45. Chavez MA, Shams N, Ellington LE, Naithani N, Gilman RH, Steinhoff MC, *et al.* Lung ultrasound for the diagnosis of pneumonia in adults: A systematic review and meta-analysis. *Respir Res.* 2014;15(1):50.
46. Andersen CA, Holden S, Vela J, Rathleff MS, Jensen MB. Point-of-care ultrasound in general practice: A systematic review. *Ann Fam Med.* 2019;17(1):61–9.
47. Balmuth EA, Luan D, Jannat-Khah D, Evans A, Wong T, Scales DA. Point-of-care ultrasound (POCUS): Assessing patient satisfaction and socioemotional benefits in the hospital setting. *PLoS One.* 2024;19(2):e0298665.
48. Arntfield R, Wu D, Tschirhart J, VanBerlo B, Ford A, Ho J, *et al.* Automation of lung ultrasound interpretation via deep learning for the classification of normal versus abnormal lung parenchyma: A multicenter study. *Diagnostics (Basel).* 2021;11(11).
49. Wong A, Roslan NL, McDonald R, Noor J, Hutchings S, D'Costa P, *et al.* Clinical obstacles to machine-learning POCUS adoption and system-wide AI implementation (The COMPASS-AI survey). *Ultrasound J.* 2025;17(1):32.
50. Lin X, Yang F, Chen Y, Chen X, Wang W, Li W, *et al.* Echocardiography-based AI for detection and quantification of atrial septal defect. *Front Cardiovasc Med.* 2023;10:985657.
51. Darwich F, Devaraj S, Liebe JD. AI-supported echocardiography for the detection of heart diseases—a scoping review. *Stud Health Technol Inform.* 2024;317:219–27.
52. Zgool T, Antico M, Edwards C, Fontanarosa D. Point-of-care ultrasound imaging for automated detection of abdominal haemorrhage: A systematic review. *Ultrasound Med Biol.* 2025;51(11):1888–900.
53. Michard F, Mulder MP, Gonzalez F, Sanfilippo F. AI for the hemodynamic assessment of critically ill and surgical patients: Focus on clinical applications. *Ann Intensive Care.* 2025;15(1):26.
54. Karni O, Shitrit IB, Perlin A, Jedwab R, Wacht O, Fuchs L. AI-enhanced guidance demonstrated improvement in novices' Apical-4-chamber and Apical-5-chamber views. *BMC Med Educ.* 2025;25(1):558.
55. Johnson S, Feldman S, Gessouroun R, Fuller M, Stafford-Smith M, Bronshteyn YS, *et al.* AI-augmented vs. conventional cardiac POCUS training: A pilot study among obstetric anesthesiologists. *Int J Obstet Anesth.* 2024;60:104238.
56. Kumar A, Baum E, Parmer-Chow C, Kugler J. Limited echocardiogram acquisition by novice clinicians aided with deep learning: A randomized controlled trial. *Biol Methods Protoc.* 2025;10(1):bpaf083.
57. Andersen CA, Brodersen J, Rudbaek TR, Jensen MB. Patients' experiences of the use of point-of-care ultrasound in general practice—a cross-sectional study. *BMC Fam Pract.* 2021;22(1):116.

58. van der Harst P, Nathoe H. Transforming cardiology with AI: The Eko CORE 500 digital stethoscope. *Neth Heart J*. 2025;33(4):141–2.
59. Mangione S. The stethoscope as metaphor. *Cleve Clin J Med*. 2012;79(8):545–6.
60. *Stethoscope Market Size to Hit US$ 950 Million by 2030: BioSpace*; 2022. Available from: https://www.biospace.com/stethoscope-market-size-to-hit-us-950-million-by-2030.
61. Guo Y, Lin H, Chen H, Wu X, Luo Y. Detection of atrial fibrillation via artificial intelligence-assisted auscultation. *BMC Cardiovasc Disord*. 2025;25(1):795.
62. Attia ZI, Dugan J, Rideout A, Maidens JN, Venkatraman S, Guo L, *et al*. Automated detection of low ejection fraction from a one-lead electrocardiogram: Application of an AI algorithm to an electrocardiogram-enabled Digital Stethoscope(). *Eur Heart J Digit Health*. 2022;3(3):373–9.
63. Cox H, Rani Y, Nakiyingi L, Francia KA, Xie Y, Hoang C, *et al*. Diagnostic accuracy of a commercial AI digital stethoscope for diagnosis of TB. *IJTLD Open*. 2025;2(10):610–5.
64. Hoppe JM, Auer MK, Struven A, Massberg S, Stremmel C. ChatGPT with GPT-4 outperforms emergency department physicians in diagnostic accuracy: Retrospective analysis. *J Med Internet Res*. 2024;26:e56110.
65. Jabbour S, Fouhey D, Shepard S, Valley TS, Kazerooni EA, Banovic N, *et al*. Measuring the impact of AI in the diagnosis of hospitalized patients: A randomized clinical vignette survey study. *JAMA*. 2023;330(23):2275–84.
66. Xu H, Wang Y, Xun Y, Shao R, Jiao Y. Artificial intelligence for clinical reasoning: The reliability challenge and path to evidence-based practice. *QJM*. 2025;118(11):802–4.
67. Oniani D, Wu X, Visweswaran S, Kapoor S, Kooragayalu S, Polanska K, *et al*. Enhancing large language models for clinical decision support by incorporating clinical practice guidelines. *Proc (IEEE Int Conf Healthc Inform)*. 2024;2024:694–702.
68. Tozsin A, Ucmak H, Soyturk S, Aydin A, Gozen AS, Fahim MA, *et al*. The role of artificial intelligence in medical education: A systematic review. *Surg Innov*. 2024;31(4):415–23.
69. Nagaraj MB, Namazi B, Sankaranarayanan G, Scott DJ. Developing artificial intelligence models for medical student suturing and knot-tying video-based assessment and coaching. *Surg Endosc*. 2023;37(1):402–11.
70. Xu FWX, Choo AMH, Ting PLM, Ong SJ, Khoo D. Leveraging AI in postgraduate medical education for rapid skill acquisition in ultrasound-guided procedural techniques. *J Imaging*. 2023;9(10).
71. Scherr R, Halaseh FF, Spina A, Andalib S, Rivera R. ChatGPT interactive medical simulations for early clinical education: Case study. *JMIR Med Educ*. 2023;9:e49877.
72. Yilmaz Y, Papanagnou D, Fornari A, Chan TM. The learning loop: Conceptualizing just-in-time faculty development. *AEM Educ Train*. 2022;6(1):e10722.
73. Hoff T. deskilling and adaptation among primary care physicians using two work innovations. *Health Care Manage Rev*. 2011;36(4):338–48.
74. Savardi M, Signoroni A, Benini S, Vaccher F, Alberti M, Ciolli P, *et al*. Upskilling or deskilling? Measurable role of an AI-supported training for radiology residents: A lesson from the pandemic. *Insights Imaging*. 2025;16(1):23.
75. Budzyn K, Romanczyk M, Kitala D, Kolodziej P, Bugajski M, Adami HO, *et al*. Endoscopist deskilling risk after exposure to artificial intelligence in colonoscopy: A multicentre, observational study. *Lancet Gastroenterol Hepatol*. 2025;10(10):896–903.

76. Umans V. Transforming cardiology with AI: The eko CORE 500 digital stethoscope. *Neth Heart J.* 2025;33(9):286.
77. Abdulnour RE, Gin B, Boscardin CK. Educational strategies for clinical supervision of artificial intelligence use. *The New England Journal of Medicine.* 2025;393(8):786–97.
78. Goddard K, Roudsari A, Wyatt JC. Automation bias: A systematic review of frequency, effect mediators, and mitigators. *J Am Med Inform Assoc.* 2012;19(1):121–7.
79. Gerlich M. AI tools in society: Impacts on cognitive offloading and the future of critical thinking. *Societies.* 2025;15(1):6.
80. Adamson AS, Smith A. Machine learning and health care disparities in dermatology. *JAMA Dermatol.* 2018;154(11):1247–8.
81. Fawzy A, Ali H, Dziedzic PH, Potu N, Calvillo E, Golden SH, *et al.* Skin pigmentation and pulse oximeter accuracy in the intensive care unit: A pilot prospective study. *Am J Respir Crit Care Med.* 2024;210(3):355–8.
82. Fawzy A, Wu TD, Wang K, Robinson ML, Farha J, Bradke A, *et al.* Racial and ethnic discrepancy in pulse oximetry and delayed identification of treatment eligibility among patients with COVID–19. *JAMA Intern Med.* 2022;182(7):730–8.
83. Fawzy A, Wu TD, Wang K, Sands KE, Fisher AM, Arnold Egloff SA, *et al.* Clinical outcomes associated with overestimation of oxygen saturation by pulse oximetry in patients hospitalized with COVID–19. *JAMA Netw Open.* 2023;6(8):e2330856.
84. Health Insurance Portability and Accountability Act of 1996 (HIPAA), Pub. L. No. Pub. L. 104–191(1996).
85. Garibaldi BT, Hollon M, Knopp MI, Winkel AF, Burk-Rafel J, Caretta-Weyer HA. How data analytics can be leveraged to enhance graduate clinical skills education. *J Grad Med Educ.* 2025;17(2 Suppl):37–41.
86. Administration USFaD. *Artificial Intelligence-Enabled Device Software Functions: Lifecycle Management and Marketing Submission Recommendations.* Silver Spring, MD: U.S. Department of Health and Human Services, Food and Drug Administration, 2025.
87. Abulibdeh R, Celi LA, Sejdic E. The illusion of safety: A report to the FDA on AI healthcare product approvals. *PLoS Digit Health.* 2025;4(6):e0000866.
88. Martinez-Nicolas I, Llorente TE, Martinez-Sanchez F, Meilan JJG. Ten years of research on automatic voice and speech analysis of people with Alzheimer's disease and mild cognitive impairment: A systematic review article. *Front Psychol.* 2021;12:620251.
89. Lin C, Kuo FC, Chau T, Shih JH, Lin CS, Chen CC, *et al.* Artificial intelligence-enabled electrocardiography contributes to hyperthyroidism detection and outcome prediction. *Commun Med (Lond).* 2024;4(1):42.
90. Attia ZI, Noseworthy PA, Lopez-Jimenez F, Asirvatham SJ, Deshmukh AJ, Gersh BJ, *et al.* An artificial intelligence-enabled ECG algorithm for the identification of patients with atrial fibrillation during sinus rhythm: A retrospective analysis of outcome prediction. *Lancet (London, England).* 2019;394(10201):861–7.
91. Roquemen-Echeverri V, Jacobs PG, Shalen EF, Schulman PM, Heitner SB, Denfeld Q, *et al.* External evaluation of a commercial artificial intelligence-augmented digital auscultation platform in valvular heart disease detection using echocardiography as reference standard. *Int J Cardiol.* 2025;419:132653.
92. Blaivas M, Blaivas L. Machine learning algorithm using publicly available echo database for simplified "visual estimation" of left ventricular ejection fraction. *World J Exp Med.* 2022;12(2):16–25.
93. Oikonomou EK, Khera R. Artificial intelligence-enhanced patient evaluation: Bridging art and science. *Eur Heart J.* 2024;45(35):3204–18.

12 AI and Clinical Reasoning

Peter G. Brodeur, Adam Rodman

12.1 INTRODUCTION

Artificial intelligence (AI) includes large language models such as ChatGPT, which have the capability of producing text seemingly generated by humans. Large language models (LLMs) have achieved feats previously thought to be unique to humans such as passing the United States Medical Licensing Exam[1,2] or outperforming human physicians on diagnostic reasoning in real emergency department cases.[3] As such, there has been a surge in the ad hoc use of LLMs by not only medical students[4] but also practicing physicians.[5] This rapid adoption pushes the inevitable responsibility of oversight and implementation of AI into training onto medical educators. Specifically in fields with a heavy cognitive load, such as internal medicine, educators must harness the use of AI in medical education to ensure the adequate development of clinical reasoning skills.[6] In this chapter, we hope to serve medical educators by providing a broad overview of clinical reasoning as a construct and review the role of AI in the teaching and assessment of clinical reasoning. We will begin by outlining our current understanding of clinical reasoning and the subsequent assessments currently in practice. Building on this foundation, we will explore the history of clinical decision support tools up to modern-day LLMs and their impact on the reasoning processes of a physician.

12.2 HISTORY OF CLINICAL REASONING

Most would agree that developing clinical reasoning skills is a core component of medical education. However, there has been significant disagreement on the best way to train doctors to approach diagnostic challenges and subsequent management decisions. Unlike teaching pathophysiology or physical exam skills, clinical reasoning is a psychological construct that lacks clear definitions; even reasoning researchers rely on consensus working definitions of clinical reasoning as "the integration of knowledge and contextual information" or "interplay between individual healthcare provider, patient, and environmental components."[7]

Rudimentary forms of clinical reasoning can be traced back to the Hippocratics, when "rules of thumbs" or heuristics were taught primarily as mechanisms for diagnosis. In contrast to other ancient teachings, these heuristics were largely based on the experience of the clinician rather than inductive or formal logical mechanisms.[8] In the 19th century, clinical reasoning evolved from an elicitation of symptoms (often called semiotics) to the gathering and analysis of clinical data with the advent of new techniques and technologies such as auscultation and thermometry. Increase in structured data collection led to the concepts of the differential diagnosis—a combination of intuition supported by scientific aid such as patient data and underlying knowledge of pathophysiological processes.[9] For the most part, the study—and teaching—of the process to move from symptom to diagnosis remained obscure, largely taught by example.

One of the first comprehensive frameworks for clinical reasoning was the hypothetico-deductive approach, initially proposed by Elstein et al. In this model, the clinician generates a set of hypotheses to guide information gathering that they then use to rule in or out these hypotheses in an iterative process. It was quickly noted that this universal approach to clinical reasoning did not fully explain

DOI: 10.1201/9781003617167-12

clinical reasoning. For example, experienced physicians generated both fewer and better hypotheses than medical students, resulting in more accurate conclusions.[10, 11] Furthermore, Elstein then coined the term "content specificity" when it was found that success on one problem was poorly correlated with success on a second problem using this framework, reflecting that specific content knowledge such as biomedical processes was essential to the clinical reasoning process. In other words, "critical thinking" mattered far less to diagnostic success than knowledge. This foundational work showed that clinical reasoning could not be captured by a one-size-fits-all general reasoning process but was dependent on other factors such as content knowledge, experience, and intuition. Early work also focused on memory recall, derived from emerging literature on chess masters.[12] However, experimental data showed that recall of content knowledge indicative of expertise was not necessarily in the form of specific clinical data pertaining to a certain case and that intentional memory was not an adequate measure of clinical expertise.[13,14]

Further inquiry investigated not just volume of knowledge but *kinds of knowledge* and *how it is structured*. This led to a seminal framework proposed by Schmidt: *illness scripts*.[15] Illness scripts function much like other psychological scripts: a sequence of events in a stereotyped order.[16] Illness scripts are emergent as a part of a larger process of development throughout medical training and are proposed to follow four steps.[15]

- Trainees start by developing cognitive scaffolds that represent how objects, events, or concepts are interrelated. These information nodes are then automatically accessed and applied to rationale when thinking through a case.
- Second, these elaborated informational networks learned largely in medical school are refined and bridged through exposure to patient care. Through this process, learners develop heuristics or shortcuts as they encounter the same case again and no longer need to activate large quantities of knowledge. For example, novice students are much more verbose, regurgitating clinical signs and symptoms of sepsis, whereas the experienced student is brief in recognizing a presentation as sepsis and simply stating this.[13]
- The third stage is the emergence of illness scripts, which unfolds as students transition to clinical practice. Through seeing many varieties of patient presentations, physicians start to understand how diseases unfold, in which contexts, and how this varies with different factors. As doctors practice, their scripts become even more divorced from the pathophysiology taught in medical school.[17,18] Illness scripts add nuance to the idea of "content specificity" since two physicians may develop entirely different illness scripts for specific diseases but can arrive at the same conclusion. This also explains how even expert clinicians may struggle on certain disease presentations if their illness script is insufficiently developed.
- In the fourth and final stage, clinicians will develop exemplars—they will engage memories of previous patients and find similarities among these previous patient encounters when approaching a new case.

When the four stages are complete, "the recollections of prior patients, indexed by the relevant illness scripts, are stored in episodic memory, which makes them very easily accessible."[15]

Illness scripts focus on knowledge structure and activation, but, of course, there are also cases that seem to require much more deliberate critical thinking. It is posited that illness scripts still allow for previously dense networks of knowledge developed in medical school to remain accessible when physicians encounter a case for which we have no illness script. Embedded into the use of illness scripts is the concept of the interplay between nonanalytic (system 1) and analytic (system 2) reasoning.[19–21] Nonanalytical reasoning is often referred to as *pattern recognition,* and it is commonly both unconscious and automatic. For example, clinicians may have seen the presentation of pulmonary embolism countless times and can readily match it among the available illness scripts or exemplars. As experts often rely on nonanalytic reasoning, it requires adequate experience to make this approach feasible. Unsurprisingly nonanalytical thinking may be fraught with cognitive biases and is a known source of diagnostic error.[22] Nonanalytical reasoning can also be influenced by contextual factors, such as the clinical setting and surrounding environment. Despite a popular imagination of the distinctiveness of nonanalytical and analytical thinking, current models stress that these two processes are not discrete.[23] In fact, there is a combined approach where both nonanalytic and analytic interact with the mental representation of the case presented,[19] in which a clinician forms a problem representation upon hearing the patient's presentation, generates hypotheses that inform which illness scripts and exemplars to search for, which creates a feedback loop whereby the identification of an illness script drives further pointed data acquisition. The analytical thinking is triggered when a case is sufficiently complex.[24]

While illness scripts remain the dominant explanatory model of clinical reasoning, other schemas have been proposed, such as probability-based Bayesian analysis, which we will revisit later in the evaluation process of reasoning such as with script concordance testing.[22,25–27] This schema implies that physicians develop an a priori probability of each diagnosis and update those probabilities as more information becomes available. Decision trees beginning with clinical presentation and ending with diagnoses have also been proposed.[28,29] Finally, there are semantic aspects of reasoning, known as semantic qualifiers—adjectives or adverbs describing symptoms that give the clinician a hint on the clinical meaning to apply. Often these are paired, for example, joint pain is either polyarticular or monoarticular. This in turn gives the clinician the ability to compare and contrast diagnostic possibilities.[30]

To recap, the definition of clinical reasoning is variable among physicians. In addition, the theorized clinical reasoning processes have iteratively been defined from heuristics based on experience to a *one-size-fits-all* hypothetico-deductive reasoning process to a flexible, personalized, fine-tuned network of illness scripts based on clinical experience that interplays with fast and slow critical thinking processes after developing a sufficient problem representation and hypotheses.

12.3 ASSESSMENT OF CLINICAL REASONING

As the construct of clinical reasoning has gained complexity, so too has the task of clinical educators. Given such a flexible framework of clinical reasoning, how can medical education craft—and assess—expert clinical reasoners?

Scientific medicine, most famously advocated by Abraham Flexner in the early 20th century, centered around a connection between clinical teaching and laboratory medicine. Flexner applied the scientific process to student learning, believing that a "more or less bungled" experiment by the student in the clinical setting was an invaluable learning experience.[8,31,32] While this may have been the goal, critical observers throughout the 20th century noted that this type of learning was haphazard and most teaching by instructors was centered around their previous clinical experience.[8,33] The major challenge to "eminence-based medicine" came from Elstein in the 1970s, whose findings, as just detailed, also had the important implication of pointing out that, just as reasoning processes were often invisible to clinicians, so too were the strategies to teach it.[34] This insight led to a science of teaching clinical reasoning. What should a curriculum to teach expert reasoners look like? A psychological focus has sometimes been used to argue against the emphasis of basic science education. If physicians don't often access that information when solving cases, what is the value? Schmidt argues that, even if we do not access this information routinely, it remains encapsulated for later access should we choose to call on it in complex cases.[13,19,35] Thus it remains an essential contribution to content specificity.

In parallel with the accumulation of basic science and clinical knowledge, educational strategies should also encourage structuring of knowledge. Medical educators should be aware of both nonanalytic and analytic reasoning[19] and teach students the value of both processes. Despite the increasing popularity of script theory with early learners, educators need to imbue a healthy amount of caution regarding nonanalytic reasoning as novice learners often lack robust clinical experiences that allow experts to refine their scripts. Instead, medical education should center around examples of clinical cases, preferably actual patients, in addition to variable contexts to build robust scripts that do not fall victim to distractors in different contexts. This is especially important when teaching takes the form of organ systems whereby the nature of hypothesis generation is blunted by the learner knowing a case is being presented during a cardiovascular disease session. The development of accurate illness scripts should be pressure tested by the educators, ideally through prompting. For example, asking for a problem representation can ensure the learner creates a fruitful foundation for further hypothesis generation. Additionally, prompting learners to uncover otherwise invisible reasoning process may be a useful tactic to exercise their reasoning skills. Having learners justify their responses helps create the necessary linkages early on in the development of networks of knowledge.[24,36]

The flexibility of the clinical reasoning process necessitates a reciprocal flexibility of medical educators in handling learners of all stages and also warrants a multifaceted approach so that all aspects of illness scripts are covered. This "multiple-biopsy" approach of using multiple-choice questions, oral examinations, time on the clinical wards, etc. ensures that all aspects of knowledge may be integrated into reasoning processes and the development of well-rounded illness scripts.[19]

Modern medical educators have a variety of reasoning assessments used at all stages of training. In a review of clinical reasoning assessments, Daniel et al. outline three main categories for which assessment of clinical reasoning is carried out—non-workplace assessments, assessments in simulated clinical environments, and workplace-based assessments.[37]

- Non-workplace assessments consist of methods such as multiple-choice questions, short/long answer essays, oral examinations, or script concordance testing, which in essence tests Bayesian reasoning by presenting learners with new information about a case and asking how it changes their answers. Non-workplace assessments contribute to the development of content specificity in a consistent way across all learners and are thus most often used for high stakes assessments. However, these assessments most often fall under the criticism of measuring fewer components of the reasoning process.

- Assessments in simulated clinical environments often take the form of objective structured clinical examinations (OSCE) or clinical scenarios with virtual patients or patient dummies. These assessments have the similar advantage of non-workplace assessments in that there is strong content validity and standardization. They improve the reasoning assessment process by forcing the medical student to create problem representations and subsequent hypotheses.

However, despite these improvements, they are resource intensive and may drown out contextual factors in real life that serve as distractors.

- Lastly, workplace assessments take the form of direct observation of clinical skills in real clinical settings or assessment of clinical notes that have been evaluated using validated psychometric scores such as the revised-IDEA.[38] Workplace assessments have the advantage of allowing global assessments of the reasoning process and the inclusion of the most diverse set of reasoning processes in real contexts. Drawbacks include the possibility of biased assessments by preceptors, limited validity evidence, and the possibility of lacking a diverse amount of clinical cases.[37]

We will see later in this chapter how clinical decision support tools and modern-day AI have a recurring role in the non-workplace assessments and assessments in simulated clinical environments.

12.4 HISTORY OF AI AND CLINICAL REASONING

In the previous section, we outlined the development of a psychological model of clinical reasoning. Despite this rigorous knowledge of the reasoning process, diagnostic error still remains common, and reasoning is subject to cognitive errors such as anchoring, framing effects, overconfidence, and omission bias, among others, thus making clinical decision support tools an attractive adjunct to physician cognition.[22] Attempts to symbolically model clinician reasoning via AI both predate and were influential in the development of our modern psychological theories. The linkage between clinical reasoning and AI is best thought of as an ouroboros, where innovations in one field directly influence the other. After all, the output product of medical diagnostic abilities has been shown to yield far from perfect results. It has been reported that diagnostic error may lead to approximately one million Americans becoming permanently disabled or experience death annually.[39,40] This also appears to affect women and those from minority racial and ethnic groups as opposed to white men, shedding light on potential cognitive biases in the diagnostic process.[41] Furthermore, among malpractice claims, misdiagnosis is the most common, most costly, and most dangerous, as nearly double the number of claims are in the setting of significant injury as opposed to other allegation groups.[40] As the clinical reasoning process is often hidden, this makes addressing diagnostic error challenging. Several approaches have been taken such as increasing simulation experience,[42] debiasing,[43–45] conscious reflection,[46,47] clinical algorithms,[22] second opinions,[48,49] and clinical decision support tools.[50,51]

Concerns about poor reasoning leading to diagnostic errors is not a new concept. In recognition of this, in 1918 Bernard Shaw first imagined the possible impact of electronic decision support on error reduction, citing:

> the observation of the symptoms is extremely fallible, depending not only on the personal condition of the doctor (who has possibly been dragged to the case by his nightbell after an exhausting day), but upon the replies of the patient to questions which are not always properly understood, and for lack of the necessary verbal skills could not be properly answered if they were understood. From such sources of error machinery is free.[52]

In the 1950s, also alluding to diagnostic error reduction, Ledley and Lusted began advocating for a reasoning process based on Bayesian probability theory that could be harnessed by computers to aid in the diagnostic process.[50,51] Wardle similarly argued the value proposition for computer assistance in medicine to not only improve diagnostic accuracy but also diagnostic reliability, speed of diagnosis, cost reduction, improving training in diagnostic techniques, and research.[53]

In light of this optimism, the development of computer diagnostic tools took off in the 1960s. Citing Ledley and Lusted, Warner et al. employed a Bayesian approach to diagnosing congenital heart disease, assigning conditional probabilities to symptoms, arguing that "the differential diagnosis resulting from the solution of the equation is frequently more complete and, in retrospect, often appears more logical to the clinicians than the differential diagnosis listed by each of them prior to seeing the equation's prediction." This same system was also used to teach medical students a logical approach to diagnostics.[54] Similar early models trended toward one chief complaint, such as abdominal pain; in 1974, computer-aided diagnosis was shown to increase the diagnostic performance of clinicians[55] or antibiotic selection as exhibited by the expert system MYCIN—a computer-based consultation device providing physicians with antimicrobial therapy advice.[56] Not only did MYCIN provide this advice, it also allowed the physician to query the model for rationale by simple prompts such as asking "why?" after which the model would express its logic, providing a sense of education on its reasoning process. This insight into the backend underlying logic is something that we will see remains in a theme in modern-day AI systems.[56]

Shortly thereafter came the task of creating models capable of generating differential diagnoses across a variety of disease types. Tackling diagnostics in pediatrics, in the 1970s MEDITEL considered the correct diagnosis in 83% of cases in which the final correct diagnosis had not been considered on initial presentation.[57] In complex cases, the computer system considered the correct diagnosis at the same rate as physicians and considered the correct diagnosis more often than physicians when the diagnosis was not made within 48 hours of presentation.[58] Expert systems began to explicitly model psychological clinical reasoning processes, most notably INTERNIST-1 in the early 1980s, a differential diagnosis generator for general internal medicine. Early analysis of INTERNIST-1 showed similar performance on the *New England Journal of Medicine* clinicopathological conference cases (CPCs) compared to hospital clinicians but worse performance compared to the specialist case discussants.[59] Early limitations noted for INTERNIST-1 included lack of ability on complicated multisystem problems with an "inability to look at several problems areas simultaneously," lack of temporal or anatomical reasoning, and no ability for the clinician to see the rationale behind the output. As the model matured (and was renamed the Quick Medical Reference [QMR]),[60] the focus shifted from purely differential diagnosis generators to useful diagnostic aids in the reasoning process. This prompted the physician to consider diagnoses along with access to additional information about the knowledge bank from which the output differentials were derived. QMR also contained a case simulator for educational purposes, which residents found useful.[61] Studies of QMR demonstrated that students could generate the correct diagnosis on CPCs nearly half the time,[62] improved the performance of medical interns on diagnostically challenging cases,[63] and were even applicable to emergency department presentations.[64] Other studies revealed limited effectiveness of QMR as a diagnostic tool, only reaching ~40% diagnostic accuracy within the first five diagnoses on undifferentiated medicine patients at the time of referral,[65] whereas on CPCs, entering all information into QMR allowed the system to reach 93% diagnostic accuracy within the first five diagnoses.[66] Accuracy was also noted to be dependent on the quality of information provided by QMR.[67]

Other diagnostic computer systems surrounding this era included ILIAD and DxPlain. ILIAD had the ability to provide a differential diagnosis, suggest next steps in working up a patient, and a simulation mode in which the user can work up a simulated patient to receive feedback. When used as part of a medical curriculum, ILIAD boosted the performance of medical students in diagnosing uncommon diseases,[68] and improved the diagnostic reasoning process of nurse practitioner students.[69] DxPlain was designed to be particularly user friendly and was based off a curated database of medical information from the American Medical Association's Current Medical Information and Terminology, which contained summaries of nearly 3000 diseases.[70] With the many systems available, head-to-head studies commenced. Berner et al. compared the diagnostic ability ILIAD, Dxplain, Meditel, and QMR and found that the programs performed equally with the proportion of correct diagnoses included in the output ranging from 0.52 to 0.71, which suggested modest sensitivity. Berner also astutely pointed out that, while these systems provide the correct diagnoses, in the hands of the inexperienced clinician, the long list of output contains several distractors that could lead to unnecessary testing.[71] While the systems apparently had human-like performance in many settings, did they truly improve the performance of the physician?

Early studies were equivocal. Elstein et al. showed that, in difficult cases with incomplete information, in over 70% of cases, ILIAD did not change the position of the correct diagnosis.[72] Friedman et al., using a similar methodology, found that diagnostic quality scores did differ modestly after consultation with the decision support system among attendings, residents, and medical students. Additionally, the likelihood that the correct diagnosis appeared in the differential increased by roughly 6%. They particularly highlighted the improved performance of medical students citing a potential educational role for these systems.[73]

With the explosion of work in the 1980s, the promise of computers led the field to embrace a mindset that these systems were "oracles" and that physicians were largely passive recipients of the expert output.[72,74] However, toward the late 1980s and into the 1990s, it was clear that computer-aided diagnosis had significant limitations. Literature that was highly critical of these systems began to be published in the early 1990s, particularly an editorial in the *New England Journal of Medicine* titled "A Report Card on Computer-Assisted Diagnosis—the Grade: C." Critiques of these systems raised several concerns. Evidence that they improved patient outcomes was limited, and consultations often took too long for busy physicians. The systems also required clinicians to enter information using restrictive language, a process many users found cumbersome. Studies showed that these models performed well only when supplied with data curated by expert users. More fundamentally, they were built on the assumption that diagnostic errors stemmed from a single point of failure in a physician's reasoning process, rather than from the complex, multifactorial nature of clinical decision-making. Like much early AI, these systems depended on large, hand-crafted knowledge bases that required continual updating as new medical evidence emerged—a costly and time-consuming undertaking. [72,74,75] As enthusiasm waned, the term "clinical oracle" gradually gave way to the more modest label "clinical decision support" (CDS).

These limitations in medicine coincided with a broader period of disillusionment and disinvestment in AI, sometimes called an AI winter. Just as in the broader field, innovations in CDS similarly declined. The notable exception was ISABEL, starting in the early 2000s. ISABEL, initially developed for pediatrics but extended to adult medicine, was available on the internet and a tool that allowed free text—even copy and paste—for the user.[76] It was the first commercial model to make use of natural language processing and search algorithms to develop its output. Due to the ability to accept free text, ISABEL reduced time of use and improved the sensitivity of its diagnoses. A study on CPCs from the *New England Journal of Medicine* found that ISABEL included the correct diagnosis in its output up to 96% of the time with the missed diagnoses only being due to not having that particular diagnosis in its knowledge base.[76] In a landmark study by Bond et al. in 2011 evaluating ISABEL, DiagnosisPro, Dxplain, and PEPID, researchers found questions on Medical Knowledge Self-Assessment Program (MKSAP) and CPCs from the *New England Journal of Medicine*; Dxplain and ISABEL were equivalent but superior to other CDS tools.[77] As a follow-up to the aforementioned study by Friedman et al.,[73] ISABEL's impact on the differential length and inclusion of the correct diagnosis was evaluated as to whether CDS was used early or late in the patient encounter. In both cases, there was an improvement of 7–8% in the likelihood that the correct diagnosis emerged in the differential with effects most notable for medical students and residents.[78] Lastly, a 2022 study by Fritz et al. of Memem7 and ISABEL showed 56% and 68% of the time the systems could include the correct diagnosis in the output on complex cases from the *New England Journal of Medicine*.[79] Together, these studies established newer CDS tools as a pivotal bridge between the stagnation of CDS and the modern resurgence of AI in clinical reasoning.

12.5 AI AND CLINICAL REASONING EDUCATION

Previous generations of CDS displayed promise and in experimental settings showed human-equivalent performance; however, they often failed at more general real-world implementations, and their aforementioned limitations prevented the widespread adoption of their use in clinical practice. While disease-specific machine learning (ML) algorithms showed promise in specific domains such as the detection of diabetic retinopathy,[80] it was the development of LLMs (i.e., transformer-based text encoding and decoding algorithms) that drove new breakthroughs in clinical reasoning. By 2022, LLMs had encoded enough broad medical knowledge to pass the United States Medical Licensing Exam, a generalizable feat previously only accomplishable by humans that created shock waves through the medical education community.[1,2] LLMs are uniquely well suited to multiple-choice questions (MCQs) and "gold standard" answers. However, as previously noted, MCQs do not encompass the full range of skills considered to be clinical reasoning, serving as only one piece of the "multiple biopsy" approach to assessing clinical reasoning.

More robust analyses drawn from previous generations of CDS systems followed. An early study of Google Bard versus physicians showed similar performance with a slight edge in favor of physicians.[81] Compared to medical students, Open AI's GPT-4 outperformed historical data from first- and second-year medical students on clinical reasoning examinations.[82] In a study by Kanjee et al., it was shown that GPT-4 could include the correct diagnosis 64% of the time on *New England Journal of Medicine* CPCs; 39% of the time, the top diagnosis was the final diagnosis, in line with previous studies using ISABEL and Memem7.[79,83] Despite being language prediction engines, LLMs also had significant abilities in probabilistic reasoning. GPT-4 was superior to humans in a simple pretest and posttest probability exercise after a negative test result. However, GPT-4 did not perform as well following positive test results.[84]

Continuing the multiple biopsy approach, LLMs could also textually display their reasoning. Cabral *et al.* evaluated GPT-4 clinical reasoning abilities versus attending physicians and residents. GPT-4 and attendings/residents were provided with twenty cases at four time points: triage presentation, review of systems, physical exam, and results of diagnostic testing. A validated score for assessing clinical reasoning in documentation—the revised-IDEA (R-IDEA) score—was used to grade clinical reasoning. GPT-4 outperformed attendings and residents in clinical reasoning documentation while performing similarly on "cannot miss" diagnoses at triage and diagnostic accuracy.[85] Similar to the early days of CDS systems, once diagnostic capabilities were established, there was a need to move away from the "oracle" model of the relationship between physicians and AI. Does modern-day AI augment physician reasoning abilities? Goh et al. showed that physicians with GPT-4 outperformed physicians with conventional resources (Google, UpToDate, etc.) in management reasoning tasks,[86,87] while the two groups performed similarly on diagnostic reasoning tasks.[88]

AI models are continuously being trained, and, subsequently, new versions are being released. Particularly relevant was the advent of reasoning models. It was noted that chain-of-thought (CoT) prompting, whereby a model is prompted to perform a step-by-step approach to problem-solving, could result in improved model output, which resulted in model creators baking in a CoT process at run time. In September 2024, OpenAI released o1-preview—a model that seemingly thinks before responding and runs through a step-by-step "thinking out loud" reasoning process akin to prompting a medical student to think aloud.[89] Similar to the dual process approach to clinical reasoning (system 1 and system 2 thinking), this approach by the models is similar to system 2 thinking required of physicians when facing a diagnostic challenge that cannot be resolved via more simplistic thought processes. The authors of this chapter have since evaluated this new reasoning o1-preview model, applying several of the methods in previous studies of earlier models of GPT. On CPCs from the *New England Journal of Medicine*, the o1-preview included the final diagnosis in 78% of its differentials and the first diagnosis was correct 52% of the time. The model was also shown to outperform GPT-4, attending, and resident physicians in clinical reasoning documentation, as well as improve management reasoning processes of physicians. Additionally, o1-preview was shown to outperform internal medicine physicians diagnostically on real cases coming through an emergency department.[3] Yet, even with the emergency department case analysis, a fair criticism remains that the AI was spoon-fed history and physical information that was collected by a human. However, patient-facing LLMs have also shown great promise in history taking from standardized patients.[90]

As seen previously, throughout the past 70 years, CDS systems have had the primary aim of improving the diagnostic process but also have demonstrated the secondary benefit of improving medical student clinical reasoning abilities. LLMs have similarly shown to improve medical student performance on several aspects of clinical reasoning, such as history taking.[91,92] Within non-workplace assessments, LLMs can develop MCQs that are indistinguishable from human-generated questions in a time-efficient manner.[93–95] Furthermore, LLMs may be able to improve student performance on MCQs.[96,97] LLMs may also be used to generate simulated clinical environments[98] and thus may be able to alleviate the resource-intensive nature. For example, grading of OSCEs may be able to be shifted toward AI. A zero-shot LLM architecture with minimal prompt engineering was able to successfully grade OSCEs and significantly reduce the turnaround time for feedback.[99] Additionally, routine feedback has been posited as a core component of developing reasoning skills.[22] Students who prepare for OSCEs using text AI simulated training outperformed students without access to this training.[100] Fields such as urology have also seen improvements in evaluation exercises when using LLMs for training.[101] While evaluations of AI tools on the development of reasoning skills are in its infancy, there is a clear call for integration of AI into physician training.[6]

12.6 CONCLUSIONS

AI has its limitations. First, there remains the issue of hallucinations whereby the models confidently generate incorrect material.[102] Second, there are patient information privacy concerns—we do not endorse the input of protected health information into publicly available models. Third, these models have been shown to be subject to cognitive biases that often plague physicians, such as racial and gender biases.[103,104] Given these limitations, we believe that, in the near term, AI clinical reasoning is more likely to be deployed with a human in the loop and thus more likely to be used to augment a physician's reasoning abilities rather than automate.

It is not hard to fathom that these models will inevitably be formally deployed in the clinical setting. In fact, resources such as OpenEvidence[105] and GPT models are already frequently used by physicians.[4,5] What will be the subsequent impact on clinical reasoning skills? Many medical students already prefer ChatGPT to conventional teaching methods, such as professors and textbooks.[106] In order to teach clinical reasoning, the educator must be familiar not only with the facility of reasoning but also with the tools at the disposal of the learner. Medical students will undoubtedly begin to develop early illness scripts from LLMs and adapt them to clinical practice. It is imperative that educators recognize this and be in favor of LLMs as a future core competency. Furthermore, medical educators should take advantage of the use cases for AI in medical education such as the generation of teaching cases,[107] providing feedback on clinical documentation[82] and perhaps even help lead educational sessions such as morning reports.[2,83] It is crucial with the rapid development and improvement of AI systems that leaders in medical education embrace the integration of AI into the reasoning process across all levels of training.

REFERENCES

1. Kung, T. H. et al. Performance of ChatGPT on USMLE: Potential for AI-assisted medical education using large language models. *PLoS Digit. Health* 2, e0000198 (2023).
2. Singhal, K. et al. Large language models encode clinical knowledge. *Nature* 620, 172–180 (2023).
3. Brodeur, P. G. et al. Superhuman performance of a large language model on the reasoning tasks of a physician. *arXiv preprint* arXiv:2412.10849 (2024). https://doi.org/10.48550/ARXIV.2412.10849.
4. Zhang, J. S., Yoon, C., Williams, D. K. A. & Pinkas, A. Exploring the usage of ChatGPT among medical students in the United States. *J. Med. Educ. Curric. Dev.* 11, 23821205241264695 (2024).
5. Fried, A. J. et al. Large language models in internal medicine residency: Current use and attitudes among internal medicine residents. *Discov. Artif. Intell.* 4, 70 (2024).
6. Cooper, A. & Rodman, A. AI and medical education—a 21st-century Pandora's box. *N. Engl. J. Med.* 389, 385–387 (2023).
7. Young, M. et al. Drawing boundaries: The difficulty in defining clinical reasoning. *Acad. Med. J. Assoc. Am. Med. Coll.* 93, 990–995 (2018).
8. Custers, E. J. F. M. Training clinical reasoning: Historical and theoretical background. In *Principles and Practice of Case-Based Clinical Reasoning Education: A Method for Preclinical Students* (eds ten Cate, O., Custers, E. J. F. M. & Durning, S. J.) (Springer, Cham (CH), 2018).
9. Maude, J. Differential diagnosis: The key to reducing diagnosis error, measuring diagnosis and a mechanism to reduce healthcare costs. *Diagnosis* 1, 107–109 (2014).

10. Elstein, Arthur S., Lee S. Sh*ulman, and Sarah A. Sprafka, et al. Medical Problem Solving: An Analysis of Clinical Reasoning.* Cambridge, Massachusetts: Harvard University Press, 1978. *Newsl. Sci. Technol. Hum. Values* 3, 50–51 (1978).
11. Barrows, H. S., Norman, G. R., Neufeld, V. R. & Feightner, J. W. The clinical reasoning of randomly selected physicians in general medical practice. *Clin. Investig. Med. Med. Clin. Exp.* 5, 49–55 (1982).
12. Robbins, T. W. et al. Working memory in chess. *Mem. Cognit.* 24, 83–93 (1996).
13. Schmidt, H. G., Boshuizen, H. P. A. & Hobus, P. P. M. Transitory stages in the development of medical expertise the 'intermediate effect' in clinical case representation studies. *Proc. Annu. Meet. Cogn. Sci. Soc.* 10 (1988).
14. Norman, G. R., Brooks, L. R. & Allen, S. W. Recall by expert medical practitioners and novices as a record of processing attention. *J. Exp. Psychol. Learn. Mem. Cogn.* 15, 1166–1174 (1989).
15. Schmidt, H. G., Norman, G. R. & Boshuizen, H. P. A cognitive perspective on medical expertise: Theory and implication. *Acad. Med. J. Assoc. Am. Med. Coll.* 65, 611–621 (1990).
16. Barrows, H. S. & Feltovich, P. J. The clinical reasoning process. *Med. Educ.* 21, 86–91 (1987).
17. Patel, V. L., Evans, D. A. & Groen, G. J. Biomedical knowledge and clinical reasoning. In: *Cognitive Science in Medicine: Biomedical Modeling* (eds Evans, D. A., Patel, V. L.) (MIT Press, Cambridge (MA), 1989). 53–112.
18. Boshuizen, H. P. A., Schmidt, H. G. & Coughlin, L. D. On the application of medical basic-science knowledge in clinical reasoning: Implications for structural knowledge differences between experts and novices. *Proc. Annu. Meet. Cogn. Sci. Soc.* 10 (1988).
19. Eva, K. W. What every teacher needs to know about clinical reasoning. *Med. Educ.* 39, 98–106 (2005).
20. Pelaccia, T., Tardif, J., Triby, E. & Charlin, B. An analysis of clinical reasoning through a recent and comprehensive approach: The dual-process theory. *Med. Educ. Online* 16, 10.3402/meo.v16i0.5890 (2011).
21. Norman, G., Pelaccia, T., Wyer, P. & Sherbino, J. Dual process models of clinical reasoning: The central role of knowledge in diagnostic expertise. *J. Eval. Clin. Pract.* 30, 788–796 (2024).
22. Elstein, A. S. Thinking about diagnostic thinking: A 30-year perspective. *Adv. Health Sci. Educ. Theory Pract.* 14(Suppl. 1), 7–18 (2009).
23. Croskerry, P. A universal model of diagnostic reasoning. *Acad. Med. J. Assoc. Am. Med. Coll.* 84, 1022–1028 (2009).
24. Bowen, J. L. Educational strategies to promote clinical diagnostic reasoning. *N. Engl. J. Med.* 355, 2217–2225 (2006).
25. Weinstein, M. C. & Fineberg, H. V. *Clinical Decision Analysis.* W.B. Saunders, 1980.
26. Wigton, R. S. Use of linear models to analyze physicians' decisions. *Med. Decis. Mak. Int. J. Soc. Med. Decis. Mak.* 8, 241–252 (1988).
27. Lubarsky, S., Dory, V., Duggan, P., Gagnon, R. & Charlin, B. Script concordance testing: From theory to practice: AMEE guide no. 75. *Med. Teach.* 35, 184–193 (2013).
28. Mandin, H., Jones, A., Woloschuk, W. & Harasym, P. Helping students learn to think like experts when solving clinical problems. *Acad. Med. J. Assoc. Am. Med. Coll.* 72, 173–179 (1997).
29. Coderre, S., Mandin, H., Harasym, P. H. & Fick, G. H. Diagnostic reasoning strategies and diagnostic success. *Med. Educ.* 37, 695–703 (2003).

30. Bordage, G. & Lemieux, M. Semantic structures and diagnostic thinking of experts and novices. *Acad. Med. J. Assoc. Am. Med. Coll.* 66, S70–72 (1991).
31. Turner, A. L. *Medical Education: A Comparative Study*. By Abraham Flexner. New York: The MacMillan Company, 1925. *J. Laryngol. Otol.* 40, 486–488 (1925).
32. Flexner, A. *Medical Education in Europe: A Report to the Carnegie Foundation for the Advancement of Teaching*. D.B. Updike, 1912.
33. Becker, H. S., Geer, B., Hughes, E. C. & Strauss, A. L. *Boys in White: Student Culture in Medical School*. Lemur Press, 2021.
34. Elstein, A. S., Kagan, N., Shulman, L. S., Jason, H. & Loupe, M. J. Methods and theory in the study of medical inquiry. *J. Med. Educ.* 47, 85–92 (1972).
35. Norman, G. R., Trott, A. D., Brooks, L. R. & Smith, E. K. M. Cognitive differences in clinical reasoning related to postgraduate training. *Teach. Learn. Med.* 6, 114–120 (1994).
36. Connell, K. J., Bordage, G., Chang, R. W., Howard, B. A. & Sinacore, J. Measuring the promotion of thinking during precepting encounters in outpatient settings. *Acad. Med. J. Assoc. Am. Med. Coll.* 74, S10–12 (1999).
37. Daniel, M. et al. Clinical reasoning assessment methods: A scoping review and practical guidance. *Acad. Med. J. Assoc. Am. Med. Coll.* 94, 902–912 (2019).
38. Schaye, V. *et al.* Development of a clinical reasoning documentation assessment tool for resident and fellow admission notes: A shared mental model for feedback. *J. Gen. Intern. Med.* 37, 507–512 (2022).
39. Newman-Toker, D. E. et al. Burden of serious harms from diagnostic error in the USA. *BMJ Qual. Saf.* 33, 109–120 (2024).
40. Saber Tehrani, A. S. et al. 25-Year summary of US malpractice claims for diagnostic errors 1986–2010: An analysis from the National Practitioner Data Bank. *BMJ Qual. Saf.* 22, 672–680 (2013).
41. Newman-Toker, D. E. et al. *Diagnostic Errors in the Emergency Department: A Systematic Review*. Rockville, MD: Agency for Healthcare Research and Quality (US), 2022.
42. Bond, W. et al. The use of simulation in the development of individual cognitive expertise in emergency medicine. *Acad. Emerg. Med. Off. J. Soc. Acad. Emerg. Med.* 15, 1037–1045 (2008).
43. *Cognitive Interventions to Reduce Diagnostic Error: A Narrative Review*. BMJ Quality & Safety. https://qualitysafety.bmj.com/content/21/7/535#ref-163.
44. Sherbino, J., Yip, S., Dore, K. L., Siu, E. & Norman, G. R. The effectiveness of cognitive forcing strategies to decrease diagnostic error: An exploratory study. *Teach. Learn. Med.* 23, 78–84 (2011).
45. Tversky, A. & Kahneman, D. Judgment under uncertainty: Heuristics and biases. *Sci. New Ser.* 185, 1124–1131 (1974). http://www.jstor.org.
46. Coderre, S., Wright, B. & McLaughlin, K. To think is good: Querying an initial hypothesis reduces diagnostic error in medical students. *Acad. Med.* 85, 1125–1129 (2010).
47. Mamede, S. et al. Effect of availability bias and reflective reasoning on diagnostic accuracy among internal medicine residents. *JAMA* 304, 1198–1203 (2010).
48. Duijm, L. E. M., Groenewoud, J. H., Fracheboud, J. & de Koning, H. J. Additional double reading of screening mammograms by radiologic technologists: Impact on screening performance parameters. *J. Natl. Cancer Inst.* 99, 1162–1170 (2007).
49. Kwek, B. H., Lau, T. N., Ng, F. C. & Gao, F. Non-consensual double reading in the Singapore Breast Screening Project: Benefits and limitations. *Ann. Acad. Med. Singapore* 32, 438–441 (2003).
50. Lusted, L. B. Medical electronics. *N. Engl. J. Med.* 252, 580–585 (1955).

51. Ledley, R. S. & Lusted, L. B. Reasoning foundations of medical diagnosis; symbolic logic, probability, and value theory aid our understanding of how physicians reason. *Science* 130, 9–21 (1959).
52. Shaw, B. *Doctors' Delusions: Crude Criminology and Sham Education*. Constable, 1932.
53. Wardle, A. & Wardle, L. Computer aided diagnosis—a review of research. *Methods Inf. Med.* 17, 15–28 (1978).
54. Warner, H. R., Toronto, A. F., Veasey, L. G. & Stephenson, R. A Mathematical approach to medical diagnosis: Application to congenital heart disease. *JAMA* 177, 177–183 (1961).
55. De Dombal, F. T., Leaper, D. J., Horrocks, J. C., Staniland, J. R. & McCann, A. P. Human and computer-aided diagnosis of abdominal pain: Further report with emphasis on performance of clinicians. *Br. Med. J.* 1, 376–380 (1974).
56. Shortliffe, E. H. et al. Computer-based consultations in clinical therapeutics: Explanation and rule acquisition capabilities of the MYCIN system. *Comput. Biomed. Res. Int. J.* 8, 303–320 (1975).
57. Swender, P. T., Tunnessen, W. W., Jr. & Oski, F. A. Computer-assisted diagnosis. *Am. J. Dis. Child.* 127, 859–861 (1974).
58. Wexler, J. R., Swender, P. T., Tunnessen, W. W. & Oski, F. A. Impact of a system of computer-assisted diagnosis. Initial evaluation of the hospitalized patient. *Am. J. Dis. Child. 1960* 129, 203–205 (1975).
59. Miller, R. A., Pople, H. E. & Myers, J. D. Internist-1, an experimental computer-based diagnostic consultant for general internal medicine. *N. Engl. J. Med.* 307, 468–476 (1982).
60. Miller, R. A., McNeil, M. A., Challinor, S. M., Masarie, F. E. & Myers, J. D. The INTERNIST-1/QUICK MEDICAL REFERENCE project—status report. *West. J. Med.* 145, 816–822 (1986).
61. Arene, I., Ahmed, W., Fox, M., Barr, C. E. & Fisher, K. Evaluation of quick medical reference (QMR) as a teaching tool. *MD Comput. Comput. Med. Pract.* 15, 323–326 (1998).
62. Gozum, M. E. Emulating cognitive diagnostic skills without clinical experience: A report of medical students using Quick Medical Reference and Iliad in the diagnosis of difficult clinical cases. *Proc. Symp. Comput. Appl. Med. Care* 991 (1994).
63. Bacchus, C. M., Quinton, C., O'Rourke, K. & Detsky, A. S. A randomized crossover trial of Quick Medical Reference (QMR) as a teaching tool for medical interns. *J. Gen. Intern. Med.* 9, 616–621 (1994).
64. Graber, M. A. & VanScoy, D. How well does decision support software perform in the emergency department? *Emerg. Med. J. EMJ* 20, 426–428 (2003).
65. Lemaire, J. B. et al. Effectiveness of the Quick Medical Reference as a diagnostic tool. *CMAJ Can. Med. Assoc. J. J. Assoc. Medicale Can.* 161, 725–728 (1999).
66. Caratozzolo, V. Use of expert systems in internal medicine. Analysis of performance and reliability of the Quick Medical Reference. *Recenti Prog. Med.* 86, 492–495 (1995).
67. Berner, E. S., Maisiak, R. S., Cobbs, C. G. & Taunton, O. D. Effects of a decision support system on physicians' diagnostic performance. *J. Am. Med. Inform. Assoc. JAMIA* 6, 420–427 (1999).
68. Lincoln, M. J. et al. Iliad training enhances medical students' diagnostic skills. *J. Med. Syst.* 15, 93–110 (1991).
69. Lange, L. L. et al. Use of Iliad to improve diagnostic performance of nurse practitioner students. *J. Nurs. Educ.* 36, 36–45 (1997).
70. Barnett, G. O., Cimino, J. J., Hupp, J. A. & Hoffer, E. P. DXplain. An evolving diagnostic decision-support system. *JAMA* 258, 67–74 (1987).

71. Berner, E. S. et al. Performance of four computer-based diagnostic systems. *N. Engl. J. Med.* 330, 1792–1796 (1994).
72. Elstein, A. S. et al. Effects of a decision support system on the diagnostic accuracy of users: A preliminary report. *J. Am. Med. Inform. Assoc. JAMIA* 3, 422–428 (1996).
73. Friedman, C. P. et al. Enhancement of clinicians' diagnostic reasoning by computer-based consultation: A multisite study of 2 systems. *JAMA* 282, 1851–1856 (1999).
74. Miller, R. A. & Masarie, F. E. The demise of the 'Greek Oracle' model for medical diagnostic systems. *Methods Inf. Med.* 29, 1–2 (1990).
75. Kassirer, J. P. A report card on computer-assisted diagnosis—the grade: C. *N. Engl. J. Med.* 330, 1824–1825 (1994).
76. Graber, M. L. & Mathew, A. Performance of a web-based clinical diagnosis support system for internists. *J. Gen. Intern. Med.* 23, 37–40 (2008).
77. Bond, W. F. et al. Differential diagnosis generators: An evaluation of currently available computer programs. *J. Gen. Intern. Med.* 27, 213–219 (2012).
78. Sibbald, M. et al. Should electronic differential diagnosis support be used early or late in the diagnostic process? A multicentre experimental study of Isabel. *BMJ Qual. Saf.* 31, 426–433 (2022).
79. Fritz, P. et al. Evaluation of medical decision support systems (DDX generators) using real medical cases of varying complexity and origin. *BMC Med. Inform. Decis. Mak.* 22, 254 (2022).
80. Gulshan, V. et al. Development and validation of a deep learning algorithm for detection of diabetic retinopathy in retinal fundus photographs. *JAMA* 316, 2402–2410 (2016).
81. Hirosawa, T., Mizuta, K., Harada, Y. & Shimizu, T. Comparative evaluation of diagnostic accuracy between google bard and physicians. *Am. J. Med.* 136, 1119–1123.e18 (2023).
82. Strong, E. et al. Chatbot vs medical student performance on free-response clinical reasoning examinations. *JAMA Intern. Med.* 183, 1028–1030 (2023).
83. Kanjee, Z., Crowe, B. & Rodman, A. Accuracy of a generative artificial intelligence model in a complex diagnostic challenge. *JAMA* 330, 78–80 (2023).
84. Rodman, A., Buckley, T. A., Manrai, A. K. & Morgan, D. J. Artificial intelligence vs clinician performance in estimating probabilities of diagnoses before and after testing. *JAMA Netw. Open* 6, e2347075 (2023).
85. Cabral, S. et al. Clinical reasoning of a generative artificial intelligence model compared with physicians. *JAMA Intern. Med.* 184, 581–583 (2024).
86. Goh, E. et al. Large language model influence on management reasoning: A randomized controlled trial. *medRxiv Prepr. Serv. Health Sci.* 2024.08.05.24311485 (2024) https://doi.org/10.1101/2024.08.05.24311485.
87. Goh, E. et al. GPT-4 assistance for improvement of physician performance on patient care tasks: A randomized controlled trial. *Nat. Med.* 31, 1233–1238 (2025).
88. Goh, E. et al. Large language model influence on diagnostic reasoning. *JAMA Netw. Open* 7, e2440969 (2024).
89. *Introducing OpenAI o1.* OpenAI. https://openai.com/index/introducing-openai-o1-preview/.
90. Tu, T. et al. Towards conversational diagnostic artificial intelligence. *Nature* 642, 442–450 (2025).
91. Brügge, E. et al. Large language models improve clinical decision making of medical students through patient simulation and structured feedback: A randomized controlled trial. *BMC Med. Educ.* 24, 1391 (2024).

92. Yamamoto, A. et al. Enhancing medical interview skills through AI-simulated patient interactions: Nonrandomized controlled trial. *JMIR Med. Educ.* 10, e58753 (2024).
93. Camarata, T. et al. LLM-Generated multiple choice practice quizzes for preclinical medical students. *Adv. Physiol. Educ.* 49, 758–763 (2025).
94. Cheung, B. H. H. et al. ChatGPT versus human in generating medical graduate exam multiple choice questions-A multinational prospective study (Hong Kong S.A.R., Singapore, Ireland, and the United Kingdom). *PLoS One* 18, e0290691 (2023).
95. Jackson, F. I. et al. Large language model clinical vignettes and multiple-choice questions for postgraduate medical education. *Acad. Med.* 10.1097/ACM.0000000000006137 (2025) https://doi.org/10.1097/ACM.0000000000006137.
96. Kalam, K. A. *et al.* ChatGPT as a learning tool for medical students: Results from a randomized controlled trial. *Cureus* 17, e85767 (2025).
97. Li, J., Yin, K., Wang, Y., Jiang, X. & Chen, D. Effectiveness of generative artificial intelligence-based teaching versus traditional teaching methods in medical education: A meta-analysis of randomized controlled trials. *BMC Med. Educ.* 25, 1175 (2025).
98. Scherr, R., Halaseh, F. F., Spina, A., Andalib, S. & Rivera, R. ChatGPT interactive medical simulations for early clinical education: Case study. *JMIR Med. Educ.* 9, e49877 (2023).
99. Jamieson, A. R. et al. Rubrics to prompts: Assessing medical student post-encounter notes with AI. *NEJM AI* 1, AIcs2400631 (2024).
100. Lavigne, E. et al. AI-standardized clinical examination training on OSCE performance. *NEJM AI* 2, AIoa2500066 (2025).
101. Hui, Z., Zewu, Z., Jiao, H. & Yu, C. Application of ChatGPT-assisted problem-based learning teaching method in clinical medical education. *BMC Med. Educ.* 25, 1–7 (2025).
102. Mello, M. M. & Guha, N. ChatGPT and physicians' malpractice risk. *JAMA Health Forum* 4, e231938 (2023).
103. Wang, J. & Redelmeier, D. A. Cognitive biases and artificial intelligence. *NEJM AI* 1, AIcs2400639 (2024).
104. Zack, T. et al. Assessing the potential of GPT-4 to perpetuate racial and gender biases in healthcare: A model evaluation study. *Lancet Digit. Health* 6, e12–e22 (2024).
105. *About.* OpenEvidence. https://www.openevidence.com.
106. Zhang, J. S., Yoon, C., Williams, D. K. A. & Pinkas, A. Exploring the usage of ChatGPT among medical students in the United States. *J. Med. Educ. Curric. Dev.* 11, 23821205241264695 (2024).
107. Coşkun, Ö., Kıyak, Y. S. & Budakoğlu, I. İ. ChatGPT to generate clinical vignettes for teaching and multiple-choice questions for assessment: A randomized controlled experiment. *Med. Teach.* 47, 268–274 (2025).

Index

Note: Page numbers in *italics* indicate a figure and page numbers in **bold** indicate a table on the corresponding page. Page numbers followed by "n" with numbers refer to notes.

D

E

F

I

J

K

L

M

N

O

For Product Safety Concerns and Information please contact our EU
representative GPSR@taylorandfrancis.com
Taylor & Francis Verlag GmbH, Kaufingerstraße 24, 80331 München, Germany

www.ingramcontent.com/pod-product-compliance
Lightning Source LLC
LaVergne TN
LVHW021127031026
849361LV00019B/230
9781041033042